MEDICAL
INTELLIGENCE
UNIT 4

Ribozymes in the Gene Therapy of Cancer

Kevin J. Scanlon, Ph.D.
Berlex Biosciences
Cancer Research Department
Richmond, California, U.S.A.

Mohammed Kashani-Sabet, M.D.
U.C.S.F. Cancer Center
University of California San Francisco
San Francisco, California, U.S.A.

R.G. LANDES
COMPANY
AUSTIN, TEXAS
U.S.A.

MEDICAL INTELLIGENCE UNIT

Ribozymes in the Gene Therapy of Cancer

R.G. LANDES COMPANY
Austin, Texas, U.S.A.

Copyright © 1998 R.G. Landes Company

All rights reserved.
No part of this book may be reproduced or transmitted in any form or by any means, electronic or mechanical, including photocopy, recording, or any information storage and retrieval system, without permission in writing from the publisher.
Printed in the U.S.A.

Please address all inquiries to the Publishers:
R.G. Landes Company, 810 South Church Street, Georgetown, Texas, U.S.A. 78626
Phone: 512/ 863 7762; FAX: 512/ 863 0081

ISBN: 1-57059-552-6

While the authors, editors and publisher believe that drug selection and dosage and the specifications and usage of equipment and devices, as set forth in this book, are in accord with current recommendations and practice at the time of publication, they make no warranty, expressed or implied, with respect to material described in this book. In view of the ongoing research, equipment development, changes in governmental regulations and the rapid accumulation of information relating to the biomedical sciences, the reader is urged to carefully review and evaluate the information provided herein.

Library of Congress Cataloging-in-Publication Data

Ribozymes in gene therapy of cancer / [edited by] Kevin J. Scanlon, Mohammed Kashani-Sabet.
      p. cm.--(Biotechnology intelligence unit)
  Includes bibliographical references and index.
  ISBN 1-57059-552-6
  1. Cancer--Gene therapy. 2. Catalytic RNA--Therapeutic use. I. Scanlon, Kevin J., 1947- . II. Kashani-Sabet, Mohammed. III. Series.
  [DNLM: 1. Neoplasms--therapy. 2 RNA, Catalytic--therapeutic use. 3. Gene Therapy--methods. QZ 266 R486 1998]
  RC271.G45R53 1998
  616.99'4042--dc21
  DNLM/DLC   98-28767
  for Library of Congress   CIP

Publisher's Note

Landes Bioscience produces books in six Intelligence Unit series: *Medical, Molecular Biology, Neuroscience, Tissue Engineering, Biotechnology* and *Environmental*. The authors of our books are acknowledged leaders in their fields. Topics are unique; almost without exception, no similar books exist on these topics.

Our goal is to publish books in important and rapidly changing areas of bioscience for sophisticated researchers and clinicians. To achieve this goal, we have accelerated our publishing program to conform to the fast pace at which information grows in bioscience. Most of our books are published within 90 to 120 days of receipt of the manuscript. We would like to thank our readers for their continuing interest and welcome any comments or suggestions they may have for future books.

Judith Kemper
Production Manager
R.G. Landes Company

CONTENTS

Section I: Biochemistry of Ribozymes

1. **The Biochemistry of the Hammerhead Ribozyme** 3
   Philip C. Turner
   - The Hammerhead Motif 3
   - Mutagenesis and Sequence Requirements 4
   - Hammerhead Ribozyme Structure 5
   - Reaction Mechanism and Kinetics 5
   - Specificity 7
   - Modified Hammerhead Ribozymes 8
   - Pharmacokinetic and Cellular Uptake Studies 9
   - Making Hammerhead Ribozymes Work In Vivo 9
   - Target Site Selection 10
   - Hammerhead Ribozyme Design for In Vivo Expression 10
   - Conclusion 11

2. **Biochemistry of the Hairpin Ribozyme** 15
   Andrew Siwkowski and Arnold Hampel
   - Introduction 15
   - Biochemistry and Mechanism of the Reaction 15
   - Conclusions 21

3. **Biochemistry of Hepatitis Delta Virus Catalytic RNAs** 23
   N. Kyle Tanner
   - Introduction 23
   - Properties of HDV 23
   - Properties of the Catalytic Domains 24
   - Strain Comparisons 27
   - Data Summary 28
   - Self-Cleavage Reaction 30
   - Biological Relevance 30
   - Trans-Cleaving Activity 32
   - Applications 34
   - Concluding Remarks 34

Section II: Expression and Delivery of Ribozymes 39

4. **Exogenous Delivery of Ribozymes** 41
   Mark A. Reynolds
   - Introduction 41
   - Tissue Culture Studies 41
   - Localized Delivery In Vivo 45
   - Systemic Delivery 50
   - Future Applications 54

5. **Novel RNA Motif (Dimeric Minizyme) Capable of Cleaving L6 BCR-ABL Fusion (b2a2) mRNA with High Specificity** 61
   Tomoko Kuwabara, Masaki Warashina and Kazunari Taira
   Introduction 61
   Current Research 62
   Future Prospects 74

6. **Using Ribozymes to Attenuate Gene Expression in Transgenic Mice** 79
   Shimon Efrat
   Introduction 79
   Examples of Ribozyme Applications in Transgenic Mice 79
   Future Directions 85

7. **Retroviral Delivery of Ribozymes** 87
   Lun-Quan Sun and Geoff Symonds
   Retroviral Properties and Life Cycle 87
   Retroviral Vectors and Their Design 87
   Cell Type Specific Promoters 90
   Packaging Cell Lines 90
   Targeting of Retroviruses 90
   Ribozyme Action 91
   Murine Model Systems for Retroviral-Ribozyme Delivery
   and Inhibition of Gene Expression 92
   Anti-HIV Retroviral Ribozyme Constructs 93
   General Aspects of Retroviral and Other Delivery Systems ... 95
   Clinical Application of Retroviral Delivery of Ribozymes 96
   Concluding Remarks 97

8. **Adeno-Associated Virus (AAV) Mediated Ribozyme Expression in Mammalian Cells** 101
   Piruz Nahreini and Beth Roberts
   Introduction 101
   Generation of Recombinant AAV 104
   rAAV Infection and Transgene Expression 109
   Concluding Remarks 116

Section III: Ribozyme Targets for Gene Therapy 123

9. **Applications of Anti-Oncogene Ribozymes for the Treatment of Bladder Cancer** 125
   Akira Irie and Eric J. Small
   Overview of Bladder Cancer 125
   Molecular Genetics of Bladder Cancer 126
   H-*ras* Oncogene in Bladder Cancer 127

	Anti-Oncogene Ribozymes Against Bladder Cancer 128
	Delivery of Ribozymes to Bladder Tumors 130
	Conclusions 131

10. **Gene Therapy of Breast Cancer** 135
    T. Suzuki and B. Anderegg
    Introduction 135
    Anti-c-*erb*B-2 Ribozyme Strategy 135
    Anti-c-*erb*B-2 Ribozyme Expression 136
    Future Prospects 138
    Conclusions 139

11. **Therapeutic Application of an Anti-*ras* Ribozyme in Human Pancreatic Cancer** 143
    Hiroshi Kijima and Kevin J. Scanlon
    Abstract 143
    Introduction 143
    Results 144
    Discussion 146
    Conclusion 147

12. **The Use of Ribozymes for Gene Therapy of Lung Cancer** 151
    Alex W. Tong, Yu-An Zhang, David Y. Bouffard, John Nemunaitis
    Summary 151
    Introduction 152
    Growth Inhibition by Antisense Oligonucleotides (AS-ODN) 152
    Growth Inhibition by Ribozyme 153
    Future Considerations 158

13. **Ribozymes in Gene Therapy of Prostate Cancer** 165
    Dale J. Voeks, Gary A. Clawson, and James S. Norris
    Introduction 165
    Ribozymes in Prostate Cancer 166
    Conclusions 170

14. **Ribozymes in Targeting Tumor Suppressor Genes** 175
    Tapas Mukhopadhyay and Jack A. Roth
    Introduction 175
    General Considerations for Ribozyme Function 176
    Targets for Ribozymes in Cancer 176
    Cellular Genes Targeted by Ribozyme Molecules 177
    Conclusion 180

15. **Inhibition of the Multidrug Resistance Phenotype by Different Delivery Systems of an Anti-mdr Ribozyme** 183
    Per Sonne Holm, David T. Curiel and Manfred Dietel
    Introduction 183
    Catalytic Activity of the mdr Ribozyme 184
    Delivery Systems of the Anti-*mdr* Ribozyme 186
    Conclusion 191

16. **Anti-BCR-ABL Ribozymes** 195
    Lance H. Leopold, Scott K. Shore and E. Premkumar Reddy
    Introduction 195
    Current Research 196
    Future Directions 206

17. **Potential Design and Facilitation of Hammerhead Ribozyme Turnover by Cellular Proteins** 213
    Mouldy Sioud
    Introduction 213
    General Aspects for Ribozyme Design 214
    Effect of Proteins on Ribozyme Cleavage 215
    Ribozymes as Gene Therapy in Cancer Treatment 216

18. **Human Papillomaviruses** 223
    E.J. Shillitoe
    Introduction 223
    Papillomaviruses 223
    The Viral Genome 224
    Mechanism of Oncogenesis 224
    Anti-Papillomavirus Gene Therapy 226
    Antisense Inhibition of Expression of HPV-Genes 226
    Inhibition of HPV by Ribozymes 227
    Delivery Methods for Anti-HPV Ribozymes 228
    Future Directions for Research 229

Index 235

EDITORS

Kevin J. Scanlon, Ph.D.
Cancer Research Department
Berlex Biosciences
Richmond, California, U.S.A.
Chapter 11

Mohammed Kashani-Sabet, M.D.
U.C.S.F. Cancer Center
University of California San Francisco
San Francisco, California, U.S.A.

CONTRIBUTORS

B. Anderegg, Ph.D.
Department of Cancer Research
Berlex Biosciences
Richmond, Califonia, U.S.A.
Chapter 10

David Y. Bouffard, Ph.D.
Berlex Biosciences
Richmond, California, U.S.A.
Chapter 12

Gary A. Clawson
Penn State University
Hershey, Pennsylvania, U.S.A.
Chapter 13

David T. Curiel, M.D.
Gene Therapy Program
The University of Alabama at
 Birmingham
Birmingham, Alabama, USA
Chapter 15

Manfred Dietel, Prof., M.D.
Universitätsklinikum Charité
Institute of Pathology
Berlin, Germany
Chapter 15

Shimon Efrat
Department of Molecular
 Pharmacology
Albert Einstein College of Medicine
Bronx, New York, U.S.A.
Chapter 6

Arnold Hampel, Ph.D.
Department of Biological Sciences
Northern Illinois University
DeKalb, Illinois, U.S.A.
Chapter 2

Per Sonne Holm, Ph.D.
Universitätsklinikum Charité
Institute of Pathology
Berlin, Germany
Chapter 15

Akira Irie, M.D.
Department of Cancer Research
Berlex Biosciences
Richmond, California, U.S.A.
Chapter 9

Hiroshi Kijima, M.D.
Department of Pathology
Tokai University School of Medicine
Bohseidai, Isehara, Kanagawa, Japan
Chapter 11

Tomoko Kuwabara, Ph.D.
National Institute for Advanced
   Interdisciplinary Research
National Institute of Bioscience and
   Human Technology; and
Institute of Applied Biochemistry
University of Tsukuba
Tsukuba Science City, Japan
Chapter 5

Lance H. Leopold, M.D.
The Fels Institute for Cancer Research
   and Molecular Biology
Temple University School of Medicine
Philadelphia, Pennsylvania, U.S.A.
Chapter 16

Tapas Mukhopadhyay, Ph.D.
Section of Thoracic Molecular
   OncologyDepartment of Thoracic
   and Cardiovascular Surgery
The University of Texas M.D. Anderson
   Cancer Center
Houston, Texas, U.S.A.
Chapter 14

Piruz Nahreini, Ph.D.
Ribozyme Pharmaceuticals Inc.
Boulder, Colorado, U.S.A.
Chapter 8

John Nemunaitis, M.D.
Mary Crowley Cancer Research Program
Baylor Research Institute
Baylor University Medical Center
Dallas, Texas, U.S.A.
Chapter 12

James S. Norris, Ph.D.
Medical University of South Carolina
Charleston, South Carolina, U.S.A.
Chapter 13

E. Premkumar Reddy, Ph.D.
Department of Biochemistry
Temple University
Philadelphia, Pennsylvania, U.S.A.
Chapter 16

Mark A. Reynolds, Ph.D.
Ribozyme Pharmaceuticals, Inc.
Boulder, Colorado, U.S.A.
Chapter 4

Beth Roberts, M.S.
Ribozyme Pharmaceuticals Inc.
Boulder, Colorado, U.S.A.
Chapter 8

Jack A. Roth, M.D.
Section of Thoracic Molecular Oncology
Department of Thoracic and
   Cardiovascular Surgery *and*
Department of Tumor Biology
The University of Texas M.D. Anderson
   Cancer Center
Houston, Texas, U.S.A.
Chapter 14

E.J. Shillitoe
Department of Microbiology and
   Immunology
SUNY College of Medicine
Syracuse, New York, U.S.A.
Chapter 18

Scott K. Shore
The Fels Institute for Cancer Research
   and Molecular Biology
Temple University School of Medicine
Philadelphia, Pennsylvania, U.S.A.
Chapter 16

Mouldy Sioud
Department of Immunology
Institute for Cancer Research
The Norwegian Radium Hospital
Montebello, Oslo, Norway
Chapter 17

Andrew Siwkowski, M.S.
Department of Biological Sciences
Northern Illinois University
DeKalb, Illinois, U.S.A.
Chapter 2

Eric J. Small
Department of Medicine and Urology
University of California at San Francisco
San Francisco, California, U.S.A.
Chapter 9

Lun-Quan Sun, Ph.D.
Johnson & Johnson Research
    Laboratories
Sydney, Australia
Chapter 7

T. Suzuki, M.D.
Department of Cancer Research
Berlex Biosciences
Richmond, California, U.S.A.
Chapter 10

Geoff Symonds, Ph.D.
Johnson & Johnson Research
    Laboratories
Sydney, Australia
Chapter 7

Kazunari Taira, Prof. Ph.D.
National Institute for Advanced
    Interdisciplinary Research
National Institute of Bioscience and
    Human Technology; and
Institute of Applied Biochemistry
University of Tsukuba
Tsukuba Science City, Japan
Chapter 5

N. Kyle Tanner, Ph.D.
Département de Biochimie Médicale
Centre Médical Univeritaire
Genéve, Switzerland
Chapter 3

Alex W. Tong, Ph.D.
Cancer Immunology Research
    Laboratory
Baylor-Sammons Cancer Center
Baylor University Medical Center
Dallas, Texas, U.S.A.
Chapter 12

Philip C. Turner, Ph.D.
School of Biological Sciences
University of Liverpool
Liverpool, U.K.
Chapter 1

Dale J. Voeks
Medical University of South Carolina
Charleston, South Carolina, U.S.A.
Chapter 13

Masaki Warashina, Ph.D.
National Institute for Advanced
    Interdisciplinary Research
National Institute of Bioscience and
    Human Technology; and
Institute of Applied Biochemistry
University of Tsukuba
Tsukuba Science City, Japan
Chapter 5

Yu-An Zhang
Cancer Immunology Research
    Laboratory
Baylor-Sammons Cancer Center
Baylor University Medical Center
Dallas, Texas, U.S.A.
Chapter 12

FOREWORD

The field of ribozymes has come a long way since the initial observations of cis-acting self-cleaving molecules in *Tetrahymena* and RNase P. Along with the discovery of different types of catalytic RNAs in diverse biological systems has come the demonstration of the biological utility of ribozyme-mediated genetic manipulation. Ribozymes have clearly found a place alongside antibodies and antisense oligonucleotides in the armamentarium used to disrupt target-specific gene expression. Beyond target validation, ribozymes are being increasingly investigated for their therapeutic potential.

The time is therefore ripe to review some of the recent developments in the field of ribozyme biochemistry and to examine their use in biological systems related to cancer. Advances in gene therapy offer the promise of a significant impact on the management of intractable diseases. Cancer represents one of the most important targets of gene therapy studies and, not surprisingly, much of the biological investigations using ribozymes have occurred in the realm of cancer.

In order to conduct a comprehensive review of the relevant aspects of ribozyme technology, this Medical Intelligence Unit volume is composed of three sections. The first section serves as an overview of the biochemistry of hammerhead, hairpin and hepatitis delta ribozymes. This is followed by five chapters discussing the ways in which optimal delivery and expression of ribozymes may be achieved. The issue of adenoviral delivery of ribozymes has been left to the individual chapters in which this modality has been utilized. The final section contains manuscripts discussing the multiple targets of ribozyme action with relevance to cancer research. We hope that the reader will enjoy these up-to-date discussions on the latest developments in ribozyme technology which will pave its path to the clinical arena.

Mohammed Kashani-Sabet, M.D.
Kevin J. Scanlon, Ph.D.

Section I
Biochemistry of Ribozymes

CHAPTER 1

The Biochemistry of the Hammerhead Ribozyme

Philip C. Turner

Experiments in the early nineteen eighties led to the discovery of catalytic RNAs (ribozymes), including self-cleaving introns[1,2] and the RNA component of the tRNA processing enzyme RNase P.[3,4] Later, examples of the class of ribozymes known as hammerhead ribozymes were discovered during studies of the replication of plant viruses and virusoids.[5-7] These small, pathogenic plant RNAs undergo a self-catalyzed cleavage reaction to generate monomeric genomes, and this reaction can be replicated in vitro at neutral pH in the presence of Mg^{2+}.[8,9] Other types of ribozymes have been discovered, including the hairpin ribozyme[10,11] and the hepatitis delta virus ribozyme[12] which are discussed in chapters 2 and 3.

The Hammerhead Motif

By comparing sequences of the hammerhead catalytic motif from a variety of sources, and combining it with information from mutagenesis studies, the conserved and important features of the motif have been elucidated; they are shown in Figure 1.1. For a recent detailed review, see ref. 13. It was found to consist of 3 base paired helices, or stems, (I-III), with helices I and III flanking the cleavage site which is on the 3' side of an unpaired, or bulged, nucleotide. Helix II is connected to the other helices by two single-stranded regions that contain most of the conserved nucleotides in the hammerhead motif. The numbering system of Hertel et al[14] is useful for descriptive and comparative purposes and is used in Figure 1.1. As shown, of the nucleotides in the single stranded regions which presumably form the hammerhead's catalytic core, only the U7 position shows variations in nature.[15] The sequences of helices I-III show little conservation except at the ends of helix II, where a purine, R10.1, pairs with a pyrimidine Y11.1, and helix III where A15.1 base pairs with U16.1.

Hammerhead ribozymes, as they exist in nature, self-cleave and hence work in cis. This is achieved by the RNA folding to form loops at the ends of two of the helices. In vitro, however, it is possible to assemble the catalytically active motif shown in Figure 1.1 in a variety of ways, using either 1, 2 or 3 RNA molecules.[16-20] If only one RNA molecule is involved, then two of the helices are joined by loops and cleavage is in cis (self-cleavage). If two RNA molecules are used, then only one loop is required between a pair of helices and cleavage occurs in trans.[20] Finally, using 3 RNA molecules there are no loops connecting the ends of the helices and cleavage is also in trans. In the case of two RNA molecules, there are three ways of dividing the hammerhead motif, which have been called I/II, II/III and I/III

Ribozymes in the Gene Therapy of Cancer, edited by Kevin J. Scanlon and Mohammed Kashani-Sabet.
©1998 R.G. Landes Company.

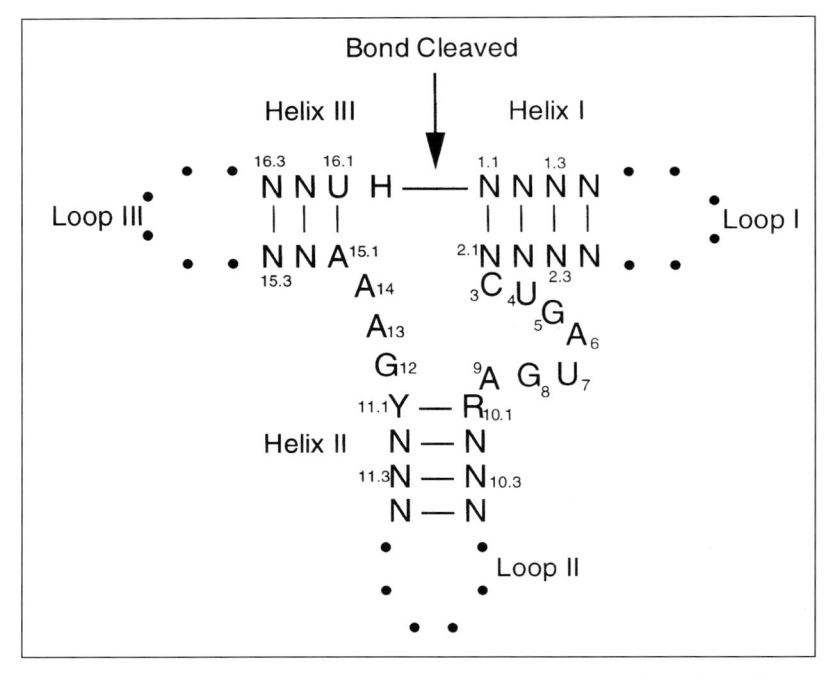

Fig. 1.1. Diagram of the hammerhead ribozyme. The bond cleaved is indicated by an arrow. N stands for any nucleotide, H is A, C or U, but not G. Y (pyrimidine) is C or U and R (purine) is A or G. Numbering is according to ref. 14. In nature one of the helices is not terminated by a loop. Conserved nucleotides are all those other than N, with the exception of U7. Domain I of the catalytic core is nucleotides C3-A6 and domain II is U7-A9 and G12-A14.

depending on which helices are used to bind to the substrate, or cleaved, strand. The design called I/III, in which the remaining loop terminates helix II, contains almost all the conserved residues in the enzyme strand.[17] Hence, the substrate strand has only a minimal sequence requirement (5'-U-H-3'). This design has been widely utilized because it is not only ideal for use in attempts to downregulate gene expression, but also permits relatively easy chemical synthesis of the short enzyme strand of RNA. In this design the substrate strand is commonly referred to as the target RNA which is to be cleaved, and the enzyme strand is generally called the ribozyme.

Mutagenesis and Sequence Requirements

In the single stranded regions of the hammerhead ribozyme's catalytic core, nucleotide substitutions at all positions except U7 destroy catalytic activity and this fact can be utilized to create non-cleaving ribozymes as negative controls, for example, to determine antisense effects. Ruffner et al[15] have shown that catalytic rates in vitro are best with U at position 7, but G>A>C, which is only 20% as active.

Conserved nucleotides are not present in helix I, but helix II contains two immediately adjacent to the catalytic core. These are most commonly a G-C base pair at R10.1 - Y11.1, and this combination is the most active in vitro. Although only one nucleotide pair is conserved in helix II, its absolute length has an effect on ribozyme activity in vitro.[7,15,21,22] If helix II is shorter than 2 bp, activity is severely reduced. The loop terminating helix II, which is usually 4 nucleotides long, has little apparent influence on activity in vitro and can even be replaced by non-nucleoside linkers[23-25] or deoxynucleotides[26] without total loss of activity.

Helix III contains the conserved A15.1 - U16.1 base pair and the U16.1 is found as part of the cleaved triplet, which is most often 5'-GUC-3', although the triplets 5'-GUA-3' and 5'-AUA-3' are seen as cleavage sites in nature, though rarely.[27,28] In vitro analysis of systematic mutations in the GUC sequence in the target have shown that cleavage can occur after any NUH triplet[15,29-31] (H means any nucleotide but G), though efficiency is usually much reduced compared to GUC. Shimayama et al[30] showed that, in vitro, the efficiency of cleavage at the various triplet combinations depended on the relative concentrations of the ribozyme and substrate. If either were saturating, cleavage depended on k_{cat} and GUC, AUC>GUA, AUA, CUC were much more efficient than other versions of NUH. If ribozyme or substrate was limiting, then GUC>CUC and all other combinations were much less efficient. The extent to which these observations can be applied to cleavage in vivo, particularly of long target RNAs by either chemically modified, exogenously applied ribozymes or ribozymes transcribed in vivo which contain additional sequences, is not clear and at least one report suggests they are not applicable.[32]

Hammerhead Ribozyme Structure

The structure of the hammerhead ribozyme has been studied both in solution[32-35] and in crystalline form.[36,37] Two X-ray diffraction crystal structures show that the hammerhead ribozyme has a y-shape in which helices II and III stack colinearly with helix I adjacent to helix II (Fig. 1.2). General features of the crystal structures agree with the proposed solution structures. In the colinear stacking of helices II and III, nucleotides in part of the catalytic core, called domain II (consisting of G12, A13, A14 and U7, G8, A9) form non-Watson-Crick base pairs and result in a pseudocontinuous helix. Domain I of the catalytic core (C3, U4, G5, A6) forms a uridine turn motif, allowing the sugar phosphate backbone of helix II (at U7) to turn and form the bottom of helix I (after C3).

In trying to account for the hammerhead ribozyme's catalytic requirement for Mg^{2+}, at least two Mg^{2+} binding sites have been proposed.[37] One of these is thought to be mainly structural and involves a pentahydrated Mg^{2+}, binding mainly to the 5' phosphate of A9 with additional contacts to G8, G10.1 and G12. Another site, in which $Mg(H_2O)_6^{2+}$ may bind to C3 and C17 as well as other groups in the vicinity of the catalytic pocket, is closer to the cleavage site (3' to C17) and is thought to be involved in the catalytic mechanism by facilitating deprotonation of the 2'-hydroxyl of C17.[37,38] Electrophoretic mobility studies[39] indicate that there is a Mg^{2+} threshold above which helix I is adjacent to helix II (as in the crystal and catalytically active form) and below which helix I is adjacent to helix III.

Reaction Mechanism and Kinetics

Magnesium ions, or certain other divalent metal ions, are essential for hammerhead ribozyme catalysis. As suggested by the structural studies, the divalent metal ions are required firstly to promote correct folding of the catalytic core, and secondly as a reaction cofactor.[40] Zn^{2+} and Cd^{2+} can only perform this second, cofactor function and therefore require spermine to help fold the RNA. By studying variation in reaction rates with pH and with pK_a values of hydrated metal ions, it was concluded that the metal ion acts as a base in the reaction mechanism and that only one deprotonation event was involved.[41] Although some details of the reaction mechanism are still unclear (such as a second metal ion requirement), the overall cleavage reaction is outlined in Figure 1.3. A hydrated Mg^{2+} acts as a base to attack the essential 2'-OH group of C17, which then acts as a nucleophile attacking the scissile phosphate. After cleavage, C17 has a 2',3' cyclic phosphate and N1.1 has a 5'-OH.

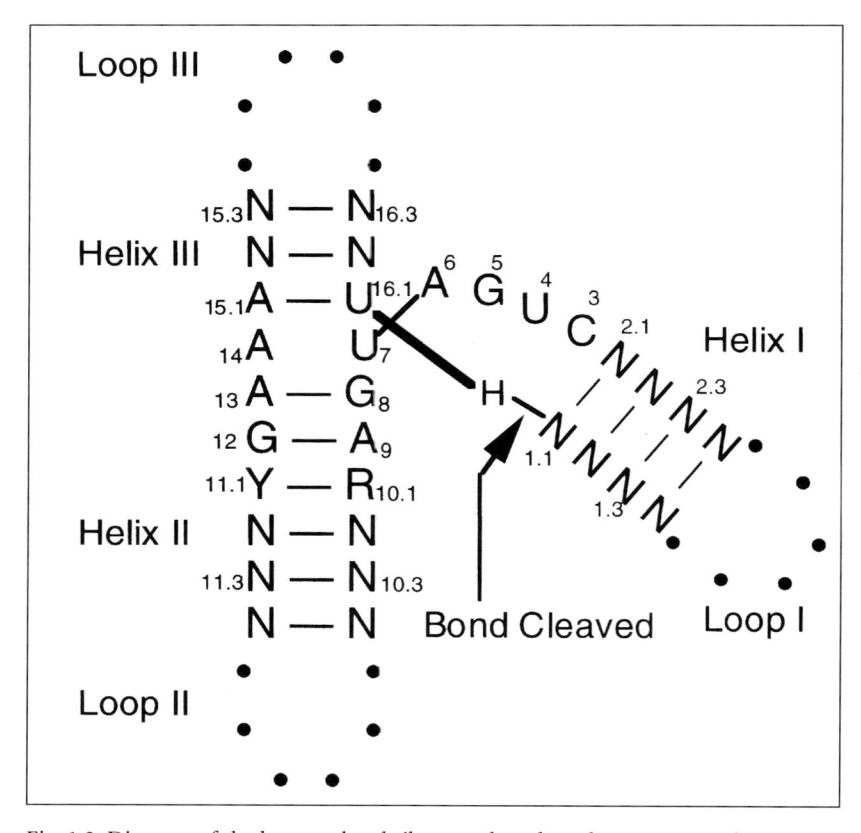

Fig. 1.2. Diagram of the hammerhead ribozyme based on the X-ray crystal structure. For explanation of symbols see Fig. 1.1. Note how helix III stacks colinearly with helix II. Reversed-Hoogsteen base pairs form between A9 and G12 and between G8 and A13 and non-Watson Crick base pairs are also present between U7 and A14 as well as between A15.1 and U16.1.

The hammerhead ribozyme catalytic reaction can be fitted to the Michalis-Menten equation as long as:
1. the ribozyme concentration is much less than the substrate concentration;
2. the step R + S ⇌ R.S is rapid and reversible; and
3. the rate determining step is R.S ⇌ R.P (where R = ribozyme, S = substrate and P = products).[42-45]

Under these multiple turnover conditions, the values derived from the Michalis-Menten equation for K_m (which is a measure of the ribozyme's affinity for substrate) are usually around 50-500 nM and for k_{cat} (which is the rate of product production) are about 1 min^{-1}, which is much lower than for protein enzymes (≈500 min^{-1}). These conditions are usually only met in vitro, and for short ribozyme and target molecules, where alternative (probably inactive) conformations for ribozyme and substrate are few or nonexistent.[46,47] When these conditions are not met, K_m and k_{cat} can often be determined under single turnover conditions where the ribozyme concentration is made to exceed the substrate concentration.[48]

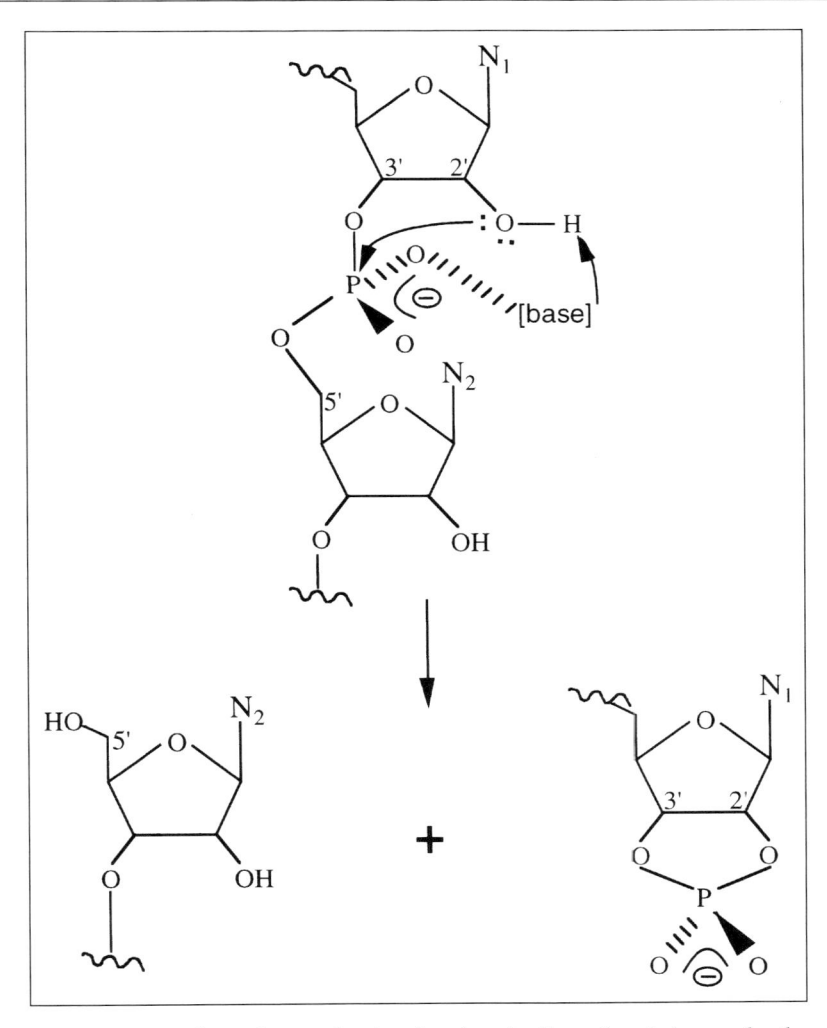

Fig. 1.3. Proposed reaction mechanism for phosphodiester bond cleavage by the hammerhead ribozyme. A hydrated Mg^{2+} ion deprotonates the 2' OH of N_1 and the 2' oxygen acts as a nucleophile to attack the scissile phosphate. A 2',3' cyclic phosphate is formed on N_1.

Specificity

Ribozymes bind to target RNAs according to the rules of RNA duplex formation, at a rate of around 5×10^8 M, the association being largely independent of length and sequence.[49] The specificity of a ribozyme is its ability to cleave at one particular site and is usually a very important consideration when one intends to cleave only one target RNA species in a complex mixture, in which some RNAs could be similar to the target. Most studies on the specificity of hammerhead ribozymes have been performed in vitro with simple ribozyme and substrate molecules and in these conditions specificity is determined by the rate of cleavage compared to substrate dissociation.[50] Higher specificity will be achieved with a slower cleavage step or an increased rate of substrate dissociation.

Hertel et al examined the effects of shortening helices I and III, combined with introducing single mismatches in helix III, and concluded that the total target recognition length (of helices I and III) could be 12 nucleotides without a reduction in specificity.[51] These experimental conditions differ from those expected in vivo, and hence it is likely that high specificity can be retained in vivo with duplex regions longer than 12 bp, especially if the number of G-C base pairs is not excessive. Mismatches close to the cleavage site can also be used to give high specificity such as when targeting a mutant oncogene transcript which may differ by only one nucleotide from the wild type mRNA.[52]

Modified Hammerhead Ribozymes

A considerable variety of modifications to the basic, all-RNA type I/III hammerhead ribozyme have been carried out, mostly with the intention of improving the efficiency of target cleavage by the ribozyme as a way of developing these molecules as therapeutic compounds for exogenous delivery. Some modifications, such as the asymmetric hammerhead ribozyme design, can also be applied when ribozymes are to be transcribed within cells from gene constructs.

Chemical modifications of the hammerhead ribozyme that have been tried include replacement of some of the 2'-OH moieties with allyl, amino, deoxy, fluoro or O-methyl groups.[53-55] In addition, the modification of parts of the backbone of the ribozyme from phosphates to phosphorothioates has the dramatic effect of increasing the resistance of the ribozyme to the action of cellular and serum nucleases.[56] The key nucleases are pyrimidine-specific endonucleases, which will attack C3, U4 and U7 of the unmodified core, as well as 3'-exonucleases. Most of these chemical modifications do not significantly increase the catalytic activity; in fact reductions are more common. However, significant increases in stability and/or useful pharmacological properties outweigh these drawbacks and make modified hammerhead ribozymes an exciting class of potential therapeutic reagents. The positions U4 and U7 have been modified and stabilized to pyrimidine-specific endonucleases by both 2'-C-allyl and 2'-amino nucleotides without loss of catalytic activity,[54,56] and there is one report of improved catalytic activity by replacing U7 with pyrimidine-4-one.[57] Some very encouraging results have been obtained by direct injection of such chemically protected ribozymes into mouse jaws[58] and rabbit knee joints[59] in which specific target mRNA levels were transiently reduced or eliminated. Both chemically modified and unmodified ribozymes have also been delivered to cells encapsulated in cationic liposomes[60-62] and have resulted in the desired phenotypic changes, such as restoration of drug sensitivity,[63] cell proliferation[60] and secretion of TNFα.[64] Liposomes do have some drawbacks and other delivery systems are being evaluated.[65]

Modifications to reduce helix II and its connecting loop have established a minimum version of the hammerhead ribozyme called a minizyme which has no base pairs in helix II, such that A9 is connected to G12 only by a loop that can be DNA or RNA.[26,66] When helix II still retains 1 bp the ribozyme is called a miniribozyme. These kinds of modifications can reduce the costs of chemical synthesis, but generally yield ribozymes with decreased chemical cleavage rates as measured using short targets in vitro. However, against long target RNAs in vivo, this may not be a problem, as cleavage is not likely to be rate limiting in this situation.[66,67] The introduction of DNA, or DNA combined with some of the other modifications listed above, into helices I and III, but not helix II, can not only make the ribozyme more nuclease resistant, but may also stimulate the overall reaction several fold. This may work by enhancing either the cleavage rate or the turnover rate.[26]

Asymmetric hammerhead ribozymes are a modification of the basic hammerhead ribozyme in which either helix I or helix III is significantly longer. Where the long helix is greater than about 30 residues, these molecules are best produced by transcription. Shorter types can be made by either chemical synthesis or transcription. In vitro experiments with relatively short substrates have shown that asymmetric hammerhead ribozymes can cleave their target when helix I is as short as 2 or 3 bp.[51] Interestingly, by varying helix I and III lengths, it has also been observed that, in vitro, longer helix III ribozyme constructs could cleave one to two orders of magnitude more rapidly than longer helix I constructs with the same total base pairing capacity.[48] This would be an important design feature if generally true and applicable in vivo.

An additional form of modification of the hammerhead ribozyme that may be generally beneficial in vivo has been reported by Sioud and Jespersen.[68] A region of a TNFα ribozyme that is bound by the enzyme GAPDH in cells can be linked to other ribozymes and causes their catalytic activity to be increased in vitro and in vivo.

Pharmacokinetic and Cellular Uptake Studies

For chemically modified hammerhead ribozymes to be used as therapeutic compounds, it is important to study their pharmacokinetic properties and the first comprehensive study has recently appeared.[69] A symmetric 38-mer ribozyme against a cytochrome P450 containing 2'-O-allyl ribonucleotides at all positions outside the catalytic core and at positions C3, U4 and U7 was administered as a single intravenous injection of 0.25 mg into adult male rats. This ribozyme binds to serum albumin at binding site I, as do linear phosphorothioate oligonucleotides. The plasma elimination half life, at 6.5 hours, was shorter than that of these more stable phosphorothioates, but intact ribozyme was still detectable after 48 hours. Metabolism is via endonuclease attack on the internal residues that are not 2'-O-allyl protected, and a 27-mer metabolite was found to accumulate in brain tissue, which does not happen with phosphorothioates. The main organs of accumulation were kidney and liver. Renal excretion of the ribozyme was minor compared to phosphorothioates, perhaps due to high reabsorption in the proximal tubule. As no tissue toxicity was observed, the 2'-O-allyl modified ribozyme seemed promising as a therapeutic.

The cellular uptake properties of a 2'-O-methyl modified hammerhead ribozyme containing 2'-amino groups on residues U4 and U7 have recently been examined.[70] This symmetric ribozyme against EGFR had 7 bp arms and was taken up by glioma cells in a temperature, energy and pH dependent fashion which could be competed with a variety of other oligonucleotides and polyanions. The ribozyme had a punctate, extranuclear localization. Overall, ribozyme uptake seemed to be via a similar endocytic mechanism to that for other oligodeoxynucleotides and also showed some cell-type specific differences.[70,71]

Making Hammerhead Ribozymes Work In Vivo

There are two distinct parts to this problem. The first involves selection of a suitable and efficient site for cleavage in the target molecule, which is usually an mRNA molecule of several hundred nucleotides in length. The second problem involves the optimal design of the ribozyme. A significant part of this second problem concerns how the ribozyme will be administered, i.e., will it be transcribed from a gene that is introduced into cells (endogenous expression), or will the ribozyme be synthesized and administered as a drug (exogenously delivered)? The engineering of hammerhead ribozymes for exogenous delivery has recently been reviewed[55] and the mechanics of delivery are considered in chapter 4 of this text and hence will not be further discussed. As chapters 5-8 cover various aspects of expressing ribozymes endogenously, only general points regarding hammerhead ribozyme design for endogenous expression will be made here.

Target Site Selection

Naturally occurring RNA molecules that may be chosen for cleavage by hammerhead ribozymes are sufficiently long that they can fold into complex secondary and tertiary structures. This means that not all of the 5'-UH-3' sequences along the target RNA will be equally accessible to ribozyme attack. Initial attempts to predict accessible 5'-UH-3' sites using computer programs[72-74] did demonstrate some successes, but this method does not guarantee that any particular 5'-UH-3' sequence would be efficiently cleavable in vitro, let alone in vivo. A more empirical method of selecting accessible target sites is to determine experimentally which parts of a target RNA molecule are able to bind short antisense oligodeoxynucleotides and thus be sites of nuclease (RNase H) sensitivity.[60,75,76] Usually these sites at which oligodeoxynucleotides can anneal are also accessible to ribozymes, at least in vitro. Sites chosen in this way might well be cleavable in vivo, but may not be the best possible sites for in vivo cleavage.

A method which permits selection of efficient ribozyme cleavage sites from a large number of possibilities in an in vivo system would clearly be superior. Lieber and Strauss[77] have developed one such system in which a library of ribozymes, containing a constant ribozyme core sequence but random hybridizing arm sequences, is mixed with target RNA in cellular extracts. The various ribozymes will cleave the target RNA in different positions and to different degrees, but the most efficient will produce cleavage products that are the most abundant. The cleavage products are cloned by making cDNA and using PCR, and the sequences of the cleavage sites determined by sequencing the clones. With this knowledge of the cleavage site, efficient ribozymes can be designed that work well in vivo.[78]

Some other in vivo methods of selecting efficient ribozyme target sites are being developed, but as yet do not permit exhaustive screening of all possible sites. Luciferase has been used as a reporter in which target sequences have been linked upstream of the luciferase gene. Ribozymes introduced, or co-expressed, in cells expressing the construct should cause a reduction in luciferase activity if they are active.[32,79] An *E. coli* based system utilizing positive selection with trimethoprim for hammerhead ribozymes cleaving in cis[80] and a yeast system that requires cell cycle arrest[81] may also be worth considering if they are further developed.

Hammerhead Ribozyme Design for In Vivo Expression

For hammerhead ribozymes expressed in vivo, there seems little point in changing the length of helix II and its terminating loop as, in vivo, extensions to helix II seem to inhibit activity.[82] Maintaining the standard catalytic core, except when creating an inactive ribozyme control, is also prudent. Altering the length of the arms that anneal to the target RNA is an important factor, but it is not yet clear what the best design is for in vivo activity. Conflicting reports exist in the literature, some suggesting that short arms of 6-8 nucleotides are more efficient[77,82,83] and others that hybridizing arms need to be in excess of 25 nt.[84,85] These differences in efficiency are most likely due to differences in the accessibility of the various target sites used, but differences in the sequences adjacent to the ribozyme, as well as the cell system and cellular compartment in which cleavage was being tested, will also play a part. A recent study looking at both subcellular localization and the length of helix III of asymmetric hammerhead ribozymes concluded that shorter ribozymes were superior when injected into the cytoplasm, whereas the helix III region needed to be greater than 51 nt to be effective when injected into the nucleus.[86] Clearly, efforts should be made to express ribozymes in a way that will ensure an appropriate subcellular localization for the target in question.

Conclusion

Since their discovery less than 15 years ago, hammerhead ribozymes have become the most studied type of catalytic RNA. Armed with this accruing knowledge, which includes the recent crystal structure and the wealth of information on mutagenesis and chemical modification, researchers in the field of medicine have engineered hammerhead ribozymes which are now poised to become essential therapeutic agents.[87] They hold promise for exogenous administration in a variety of disorders, and will be invaluable tools for gene therapists in their efforts to combat genetic disease and cancer, as is described in Section III.

References

1. Kruger K, Grabowski PJ, Zuang AJ et al. Self-splicing RNA: Autoexcision and autocyclization of the ribosomal RNA intervening sequence of *Tetrahymena*. Cell 1982; 31:147-157.
2. Cech TR. Self-splicing of group I introns. Annu Rev Biochem 1990; 59:543-568.
3. Guerrier-Takada C, Gardiner K, Marsh T et al. The RNA moiety of ribonuclease P is the catalytic subunit of the enzyme. Cell 1983; 35:849-857.
4. Altman S. Ribonuclease P. J Biol Chem 1990; 265:20053-20056.
5. Buzayan JM, Gerlach WL, Bruening G. Non-enzymic cleavage and ligation of RNAs complementary to a plant virus satellite RNA. Nature 1986; 323:349-353.
6. Forster AC, Symons RH. Self-cleavage of plus and minus RNAs of a virusoid and a structural model for the active sites. Cell 1987; 49:211-220.
7. Symons RH. Small catalytic RNAs. Annu Rev Biochem 1992; 61:641-671.
8. Hutchins CJ, Rathjen PD, Forster AC et al. Self-cleavage of plus and minus RNA transcripts of avocado sunblotch viroid. Nucleic Acids Res 1986; 14:3627-3640.
9. Prody GA, Bakos JT, Buzayan JM et al. Autolytic processing of dimeric plant virus satellite RNA. Science 1986; 231:1577-1580.
10. Haseloff J, Gerlach WL. Sequences required for self-catalyzed cleavage of the satellite RNA of tobacco ringspot virus. Gene 1989; 82:43-52.
11. Hampel A, Tritz R. RNA catalytic properties of the minimum (-)sTRSV sequence. Biochemistry 1989; 28:4929-4933.
12. Wu H-N, Lin Y-J, Lin F-P et al. Human hepatitis delta virus RNA subfragments contain an autocleavage activity. Proc Natl Acad Sci USA 1989; 86:1831-1835.
13. Birikh KR, Heaton PA, Eckstein F. The structure, function and application of the hammerhead ribozyme. Eur J Biochem 1997; 245:1-16.
14. Hertel KJ, Pardi A, Uhlenbeck OC et al. Numbering system for the hammerhead ribozyme. Nucleic Acids Res 1992; 20:3252.
15. Ruffner DE, Stormo GD, Uhlenbeck OC. Sequence requirements of the hammerhead RNA self-cleavage reaction. Biochemistry 1990; 29:10695-10702.
16. Uhlenbeck OC. A small catalytic oligoribonucleotide. Nature 1987; 328:596-600.
17. Haseloff J, Gerlach WL. Simple RNA enzymes with new and highly specific endoribonuclease activity. Nature 1988; 334:585-591.
18. Jeffries AC, Symons RH. A catalytic 13-mer ribozyme. Nucleic Acids Res 1989; 17:1371-1377.
19. Odai O, Hiroaki H, Tanaka T et al. Properties of a hammerhead-type RNA enzyme system that consists of 3 RNA oligomer strands. Nucleosides and Nucleotides 1994; 13:1569-1579.
20. Clouet-D'Orval B, Uhlenbeck OC. Kinetic characterisation of I/II format hammerhead ribozymes. RNA 1996; 2:483-491.
21. Tuschl T, Eckstein F. Hammerhead ribozymes: Importance of stem-loop II for activity. Proc Natl Acad Sci USA 1993; 90: 6991-6994.
22. Nakamaye KL, Eckstein F. AUA-Cleaving hammerhead ribozymes: Attempted selection for improved cleavage. Biochemistry 1994; 33:1271-1277.
23. Benseler F, Fu D-J, Ludwig J et al. Hammerhead-like molecules containing non-nucleoside linkers are active RNA catalyzts. J Am Chem Soc 1993; 115:8483-8484.
24. Thomson JB, Tuschl T, Eckstein F. Activity of hammerhead ribozyme containing non-nucleotidic linkers. Nucleic Acids Res 1993; 21:5600-5603.

25. Fu D-J, Benseler F, McLaughlin LW. Hammerhead ribozymes containing non-nucleoside linkers are active RNA catalysts. J Am Chem Soc 1994; 116:4591-4598.
26. Hendry P, McCall MJ, Santiago FS et al. In vitro activity of minimised hammerhead ribozymes. Nucleic Acids Res 1995; 23:3922-3927.
27. Keese P, Bruening G, Symons RH. Comparative sequence and structure of circular RNAs from two isolates of lucerne transient streak virus. FEBS Lett 1983; 159:185-190.
28. Miller WA, Hercus T, Waterhouse PM et al. A satellite RNA of barley yellow dwarf virus contains a novel hammerhead structure in the self-cleaving domain. Virology 1991; 183:711-720.
29. Perriman R, Delves A, Gerlach WL. Extended target-site specificity for a hammerhead ribozyme. Gene 1992; 113:157-163.
30. Shimayama T, Nishikawa S, Taira K. Generality of the NUX rule—kinetic analysis of the results of systematic mutations in the trinucleotide at the cleavage site of hammerhead ribozymes. Biochemistry 1995; 34:3649-3654.
31. Zoumadakis M, Tabler M. Comparative analysis of cleavage rates after systematic permutation of the NUX' consensus target motif for hammerhead ribozymes. Nucleic Acids Res 1995; 23:1192-1196.
32. Kawasaki H, Ohkawa J, Tanishige N et al. Selection of the best target site for ribozyme-mediated cleavage within a fusion gene for adenovirus E1A-associated 300 kDA protein (p300) and luciferase. Nucleic Acids Res 1996; 24:3010-3016.
33. Amiri KMA, Hagerman PJ. Global conformation of a self-cleaving hammerhead RNA. Biochemistry 1994; 33:13172-13177.
34. Tuschl T, Gohlke C, Jovin TM et al. A three-dimensional model for the hammerhead ribozyme based on fluorescence measurements. Science 1994; 266:785-789.
35. Bassi GS, Mollegaard NE, Murchie AIH et al. Ionic interactions and the global conformations of the hammerhead ribozyme. Nat Struct Biol 1995; 2:45-55.
36. Pley HW, Flaherty KM, McKay DB. Three-dimensional structure of a hammerhead ribozyme. Nature 1994; 372:68-74.
37. Scott WG, Finch JT, Klug A. The crystal structure of an all-RNA hammerhead ribozyme—a proposed mechanism for RNA catalytic cleavage. Cell 1995; 81:991-1002.
38. Murray JB, Adams CJ, Arnold JRP et al. The roles of the conserved pyrimidine bases in hammerhead ribozyme catalysis—evidence for a magnesium ion binding site. Biochem J 1995; 311:487-494.
39. Bassi GS, Murchie AIH, Lilley DMJ. The ion-induced folding of the hammerhead ribozyme: Core sequence changes that perturb folding into the inactive conformation. RNA 1996; 2:756-768.
40. Dahm SC, Uhlenbeck OC. Role of divalent metal ions in the hammerhead ribozyme cleavage reaction. Biochemistry 1991; 30:9464-9469.
41. Dahm SC, Derrick WB, Uhlenbeck OC. Evidence for the role of solvated metal hydroxide in the hammerhead cleavage mechanism. Biochemistry 1993; 32:13040-13045.
42. McConnell T. Theoretical considerations in measuring reaction parameters. In: Turner PC, ed. Ribozyme Protocols. Totowa: Humana Press Inc., 1997:187-198.
43. McConnell T. Experimental approaches for measuring reaction parameters. In: Turner PC, ed. Ribozyme Protocols. Totowa: Humana Press Inc., 1997:199-208.
44. DeYoung MB, Siwkowski A, Hampel A. Determination of catalytic parameters for hairpin ribozymes. In: Turner PC, ed. Ribozyme Protocols. Totowa: Humana Press Inc., 1997:209-220.
45. Hendry P, McCall MJ, Lockett TJ. Characterising ribozyme cleavage reactions. In: Turner PC, ed. Ribozyme Protocols. Totowa: Humana Press Inc., 1997:221-229.
46. Fedor MJ, Uhlenbeck OC. Kinetics of intermolecular cleavage by hammerhead ribozymes. Biochemistry 1992; 31:12042-12054.
47. Hertel KJ, Herschlag D, Uhlenbeck OC. A kinetic and thermodynamic framework for the hammerhead ribozyme reaction. Biochemistry 1994; 33:3374-3385.
48. Hendry P, McCall MJ. Unexpected anisotropy in substrate cleavage rates by asymmetric hammerhead ribozymes. Nucleic Acids Res 1996; 24:2679-2684.

49. Nelson JW, Tinoco I Jr. Comparison of the kinetics of ribo-oligonucleotide, deoxyribo-oligonucleotide and hybrid oligonucleotide double-strand formation by temperature-jump kinetics. Biochemistry 1982; 21:5289-5295.
50. Herschlag D. Implications of ribozyme kinetics for targeting the cleavage of specific RNA molecules in vivo: More isn't always better. Proc Natl Acad Sci USA 1991; 88:6921-6925.
51. Hertel KJ, Herschlag D, Uhlenbeck OC. Specificity of hammerhead ribozyme cleavage. EMBO J 1996; 15:3751-3757.
52. Funato T, Shitara T, Tone T et al. Suppression of H-*ras*-mediated transformation in NIH3T3 cells by a *ras* ribozyme. Biochem Pharmacol 1994; 48:1471-1475.
53. Pieken WA, Olsen DB, Benseler F et al. Kinetic characterisation of ribonuclease-resistant 2'-modified hammerhead ribozymes. Science 1991; 253:314-317.
54. Heidenreich O, Benseler F, Fahrenholz A et al. High activity and stability of hammerhead ribozymes containing 2'-modified pyrimidine nucleosides and phosphorothioates. J Biol Chem 1994; 269:2131-2138.
55. Usman N, Beigelman L, McSwiggen JA. Hammerhead ribozyme engineering. Curr Opin Struct Biol 1996; 1:527-533.
56. Beigelman L, McSwiggen JA, Draper KG et al. Chemical modification of hammerhead ribozymes: Catalytic activity and nuclease resistance. J Biol Chem 1995; 270:25702-25708.
57. Burgin AB, Gonzalez C, Matulic-Adamic J et al. Chemically modified hammerhead ribozymes with improved catalytic rates. Biochemistry 1996; 35:14090-14097.
58. Lyngstdaas SP, Risnes S, Sproat BS et al. A synthetic, chemically modified ribozyme eliminates amelogenin, the major translation product in developing mouse enamel in vivo. EMBO J 1995; 14:5224-5229.
59. Flory CM, Pavco PA, Jarvis TC et al. Nuclease-resistant ribozymes decrease stromelysin mRNA levels in rabbit synovium following exogenous delivery to the knee joint. Proc Natl Acad Sci USA 1996; 93:754-758.
60. Jarvis TC, Alby JA, Beaudry AA et al. Inhibition of vascular smooth muscle cell proliferation by ribozymes that cleave c-myb mRNA. RNA 1996; 2:419-428.
61. Castanotto D, Bertrand E, Rossi JJ. Exogenous cellular delivery of ribozymes and ribozyme encoding DNAs. In: Turner PC, ed. Ribozyme Protocols. Totowa: Humana Press Inc., 1997:429-439.
62. Brown SA, Jarvis TC. Optimization of lipid-mediated ribozyme delivery to cells in culture. In: Turner PC, ed. Ribozyme Protocols. Totowa: Humana Press Inc., 1997:441-449.
63. Kiehntopf M, Brach MA, Licht T et al. Ribozyme-mediated cleavage of the MDR-1 transcript restores chemosensitivity in previously resistant cancer cells. EMBO J 1994; 13:4645-4652.
64. Kisich KO, Stecha PF, Harter HA et al. Inhibition of TNF-alpha secretion by murine macrophages following in vivo and in vitro ribozyme treatment. J Cell Biochem 1995; 19A:221.
65. Leopold HL, Shore SK, Newkirk TA et al. Multiunit ribozyme-mediated cleavage of bcr-abl mRNA in myeloid leukemias. Blood 1995; 85:2162-2170.
66. McCall MJ, Hendry P, Lockett TJ. Minimized hammerhead ribozymes. In: Turner PC, ed. Ribozyme Protocols. Totowa: Humana Press Inc., 1997:151-159.
67. Sioud M. Effects of variations in length of hammerhead ribozyme antisense arms upon the cleavage of longer RNA substrates. Nucleic Acids Res 1997; 25:333-338.
68. Sioud M, Jespersen L. Enhancement of hammerhead ribozyme catalysis by glyceraldehyde-3-phosphate dehydrogenase. J Mol Biol 1996; 257:775-789.
69. Desjardins JP, Sproat BS, Beijer B et al. Pharmacokinetics of a synthetic, chemically-modified hammerhead ribozyme against the rat cytochrome-P-450 3A2 messenger-RNA after single intravenous injections. J Pharmacol Exp Ther 1996; 278:1419-1427.
70. Fell PL, Hudson AJ, Reynolds MA. Cellular uptake properties of a 2'-amino/2'-O-methyl-modified chimeric hammerhead ribozyme targeted to the epidermal growth factor receptor mRNA. Antisense and Nucleic Acid Drug Development 1997; 7:319-326.
71. Hawley P, Gibson I. Interaction of oligodeoxynucleotides with mammalian cells. Antisense and Nucleic Acid Drug Development 1996; 6:185-195.

72. Christoffersen RE, McSwiggen J, Konings D. Application of computational technologies to ribozyme biotechnology products. J Mol Struct 1994; 311:273-284.
73. Sczakiel G, Tabler M. Computer-aided calculation of the local folding potential of target RNA and its use for ribozyme design. In: Turner PC, ed. Ribozyme Protocols. Totowa: Humana Press Inc., 1997:11-15.
74. James W, Cowe E. Computational approaches to the identification of ribozyme target sites. In: Turner PC, ed. Ribozyme Protocols. Totowa: Humana Press Inc., 1997:17-26.
75. Frank BL, Goodchild J. Selection of accessible sites for ribozymes on large RNA transcripts. In: Turner PC, ed. Ribozyme Protocols. Totowa: Humana Press Inc., 1997:37-43.
76. Birikh KR, Berlin YA, Soreq H et al. Probing accessible sites for ribozymes on human acetylcholinesterase RNA. 1997; 3:429-437.
77. Lieber A, Strauss M. Selection of efficient cleavage sites in target RNAs by using a ribozyme expression library. Mol Cell Biol 1995; 15:540-551.
78. Lieber A, Kay MA. Adenovirus mediated expression of ribozymes in mice. J Virol 1996; 70:3153-3158.
79. Scherr M, Grez R, Ganser A. Specific hammerhead ribozyme-mediated cleavage of mutant N-*ras* mRNA in vitro and ex vivo—oligoribonucleotides as therapeutic agents. J Biol Chem 1997; 272:14304-14313.
80. Fujita S, Koguma T, Ohkawa J. Discrimination of a single base change in a ribozyme using the gene for dihydrofolate reductase as a selective marker in *Escherichia coli*. Proc Natl Acad Sci USA 1997; 94:391-396.
81. Ferbeyre G, Bratty J, Chen H et al. Cell-cycle arrest promotes trans-hammerhead ribozyme action in yeast. J Biol Chem 1996; 271:19318-19323.
82. Homann M, Tabler M, Tzortzakaki S et al. Extension of helix II of an HIV-1-directed hammerhead ribozyme with long antisense flanks does not alter kinetic parameters in vitro but causes loss of inhibitory potential in living cells. Nucleic Acids Res 1994; 22:3951-3957.
83. Bertrand EL, Rossi JJ. Facilitation of hammerhead ribozyme catalysis by the nucleocapsid protein of HIV-1 and the heterogeneous nuclear ribonucleoprotein A1. EMBO J 1994: 13:2904-2912.
84. Crissell P, Thompson S, James W. Inhibition of HIV-1 replication by ribozymes that show poor catalytic activity in vitro. Nucleic Acids Res 1993; 21:5251-5255.
85. Beck J, Nassal M. Efficient hammerhead ribozyme-mediated cleavage of the structured hepatitis B virus encapsidation signal in vitro and in cell extracts, but not in intact cells. Nucleic Acids Res 1995; 23:4954-4962.
86. Hormes R, Homann M, Oelze I et al. The subcellular localization and length of hammerhead ribozymes determine efficacy in human cells. Nucleic Acids Res 1997; 25:769-775.
87. James HA, Gibson I. The therapeutic potential of ribozymes. Blood 1998; 91:371-382.

CHAPTER 2

Biochemistry of the Hairpin Ribozyme

Andrew Siwkowski and Arnold Hampel

Introduction

The observation that the 359 nt negative strand of the satellite RNA of tobacco ringspot virus [(-)sTRSV] was autocatalytic[1] led to identification of the minimal catalytic center consisting of a 50 nt enzyme-like RNA and a 14 nt substrate.[2] This structure was named the hairpin ribozyme.[3] The ribozyme/substrate consisted of 4 helices, helices 1, 2, 3, 4, and five loops, loops 1, 2, 3, 4, and 5 (Fig. 2.1). Helix 1, between the ribozyme and substrate, can vary in length and have a variable sequence as long as base pairing is maintained. Helix 2, also between the ribozyme and substrate is fixed at 4 bp; however it also can vary in sequence as long as base pairing is maintained. Helix 3 is a 4 bp helix found in the ribozyme separated from helix 2 by a single unpaired A15, which serves as a hinge.[4-6] Helix 4, in the native sequence, contains three Watson-Crick base pairs and one non-canonical A:G base pair.[7] Thus a total of 18 bp exist in the two-dimensional structure of the hairpin ribozyme.

The helices are separated by five single stranded loop regions. Loop 5 is dispensable and can be replaced by other structures as long as a strong helix 4 is maintained. Loops 1, 2, 4, and 5, however, contain required bases. Thus the hairpin ribozyme consists of essentially two domains—domain I (helices 1 and 2; loops 1 and 5) and domain II (helices 3 and 4 and loops 2 and 4).[8]

Cleavage takes place in the substrate at loop 5 by breakage of the phosphodiester bond at ApG to produce a 5' cleavage fragment with a 2',3'-cyclic phosphate terminus and 3' cleavage fragment with a 5'-OH terminus. The hairpin ribozyme can also produce a ligated product.[9] The ligation reaction uses the same termini as produced with cleavage, and thus appears to be a simple reversal of the forward (cleavage) reaction.[10]

Biochemistry and Mechanism of the Reaction

The (-)sTRSV ribozyme supports multiple cleavage events, has a temperature optimum of 37°C, and an energy of activation of 19 kcal/mol.[2] Recent reports of kinetic parameters for the cleavage event, determined by several groups,[11-14] fall within a range of 19-96 nM for K_m and 0.12-0.36/min for k_{cat}. Substrate dissociation rates are so much slower than cleavage rates that virtually every substrate that binds is cleaved, and the rate of ligation was found to be 10X faster than cleavage—indicating that the hairpin ribozyme is truly a unique catalytic system among known catalytic RNAs.[12]

The hairpin ribozyme catalyzes cleavage of substrate containing an R_p phosphorothioate substitution at ApG of the cleavage site.[15] The cleavage reaction proceeds with inversion of configuration of the phosphorus in the product with respect to that of the substrate, suggesting an in-line attack mechanism.[16] A low sulfur effect was associated with catalysis at an

---

Ribozymes in the Gene Therapy of Cancer, edited by Kevin J. Scanlon and Mohammed Kashani-Sabet. ©1998 R.G. Landes Company.

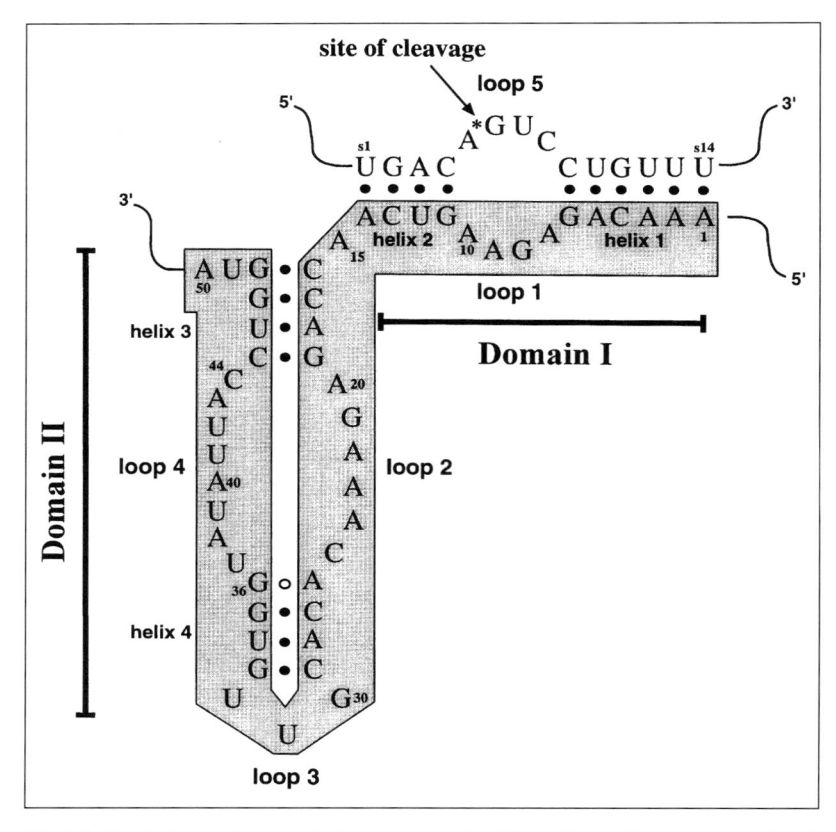

Fig. 2.1. The hairpin ribozyme/substrate complex. The hairpin ribozyme complexed with its substrate forms a structure with four helical regions interspersed by five loop regions. These exist as two domains, domain I and domain II.

R_p phosphorothioate substitution at the cleavage site.[17,18] Efficient cleavage of the S_p phosphorothioate isomer in the presence of Mg^{2+} suggests that it too is not directly coordinated with a metal cofactor during cleavage;[18] however, outer sphere coordination with either R_p or S_p phosphate oxygen is still possible.

The classic model of RNA catalysis is supplied by bovine pancreatic RNase. The numerous similarities between RNA catalysis by this RNase and the hairpin ribozyme suggest a common basic mechanism. This protein cleaves RNA in a sequence specific manner using an in-line attack mechanism.[19] The 2'-OH is deprotonated by His-12, and then is available for nucleophilic attack on the phosphorus. The resulting trigonal bipyramid contains both attacking and leaving groups at axial positions. The cleavage results in products with 5'-OH (leaving group) and 2',3'-cyclic phosphate termini. In the case of RNase, the trigonal bipyramidal intermediate is thought to be stabilized by interactions between Lys-41 and a non-bridging phosphate oxygen.[20] This particular role may be filled in the hairpin ribozyme by a hexahydrated Mg^{2+} or $Co(NH_3)_6^{3+}$ complex.[18] Hexahydrated Mg^{2+} has been shown to coordinate to phosphate oxygens in yeast tRNA[Phe],[21] and cobalt hexaammine has been shown to coordinate to a non-bridging phosphate oxygen in the stabilization of a Z-DNA structure.[22] The fact that the 2'-OH of A10 is directly across from the cleavage site and that it is

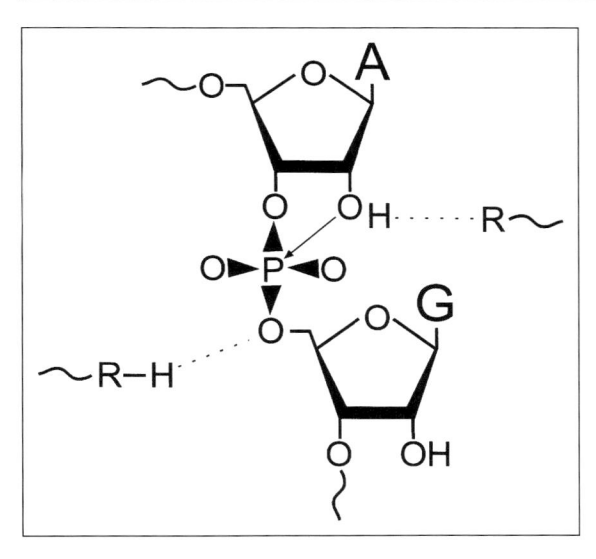

Fig. 2.2. Mechanism of catalysis by the hairpin ribozyme. Direct involvement of metals in the catalytic step is not the case. Rather, functional groups on the ribozyme/substrate complex itself are likely to participate in the catalytic step.

Table 2.1. Unimolecular rate constants and pK_a values for cleavage of the hairpin ribozmyme

Metal	k (min⁻¹)	pK_a
Mg^{2+}	1.8 ± 0.2	11.4
Ca^{2+}	3.6 ± 0.7	12.8
Sr^{2+}	2.2 ± 0.4	13.3
Ba^{2+}	2.2 ± 0.7	13.5

critical to catalysis, is particularly significant in light of this possible role for the metal. Given the fact that As_5 can accommodate any base identity and retain substantial catalytic activity,[23] it seems likely that this base is oriented outside of the base stacking system of helix 2. The cleavage site could therefore be positioned closer to nucleotide A10, facilitating the formation of a binding pocket for a hydrated metal. The pocket would consist of outer sphere coordination sites, including the 2'-OH of A10, the cleavage site non-bridging phosphate oxygen, and possibly N^3 of A10. Additional coordination sites are likely to be supplied by functional groups in loops 2 and 4 in the folded ribozyme-substrate structure (Fig. 2.2).

Since deprotonation of the 2'-OH in the case of RNase A is carried out by a histidine, and obviously no such histidine exists in the ribozyme, the question arises: What deprotonates the 2'-OH in the hairpin ribozyme? In the hammerhead, it has been suggested that deprotonation is mediated by a partially hydrated metal cofactor in the reaction. This same hypothesis is not supported in the hairpin ribozyme, since a variety of metals support high cleavage rates regardless of the differing pK_a values of their hydrated complexes (Table 2.1). The answer to this question is even more difficult to ascertain given the fact that the pH optimum of the reaction has not been reached. Consequently, no significant pK_a has been determined. The deprotonation may occur by action of an RNA functional group or a solvent molecule whose pKa has been perturbed by the molecular environment created by folding of the hairpin ribozyme.

It appears that at least two metal binding sites are used for cleavage by the hairpin ribozyme in its active structure. Evidence suggesting this is as follows:
1. two cofactors support cleavage when either one alone could not;[24] and
2. the sigmoidal shape of the curve showing cleavage reaction rate as a function of Mg^{2+} concentration, indicative of multiple binding sites (see ref. 25 and Siwkowski, unpublished data).

To date, however, it has not been definitively determined exactly how many binding sites exist.

Generally, metals have been proposed to serve two different roles in ribozyme-mediated catalysis; structural and catalytic.[26,27] The role the metal plays in catalysis by the hairpin ribozyme has been suggested to be structural rather than catalytic. The finding that hexaammine cobalt chloride supports cleavage by the hairpin ribozyme in the absence of other metals suggests that the metal normally carries out its role as a fully hydrated complex, thereby working through outer sphere interactions with its coordinated waters rather than through an inner sphere mechanism.[18] Outer sphere coordination between Mg^{2+} and a phosphodiester is strongly favored over inner sphere complex formation from a thermodynamic standpoint.[28] The $Co(NH_3)_6^{3+}$ complex stabilizes an RNA helix junction structure and, albeit to a lesser degree than Mg^{2+}, tertiary structure.[29] Given the high pK_a of the coordinated amine groups with hexaammine cobalt chloride, as well as the slow ligand exchange rate, it seems unlikely that the complex can promote the deprotonation of the 2'-OH, which is likely to be the first step of the cleavage reaction pathway. These findings point to the metal serving a structural role in the formation of the transition state structure; however, a possible catalytic role, wherein the metal coordinates to a phosphate oxygen to prepare the phosphorus for nucleophilic attack, cannot be entirely excluded.

Using a cis-cleaving ribozyme (Fig. 2.3b), kinetic cleavage rate constants supported by Mg^{2+}, Ca^{2+}, Sr^{2+}, and Ba^{2+} were all very similar (Table 2.1). These results show rate of cleavage is independent of the ionic radius or coordination number of the metal cofactor. Furthermore, the cleavage rate constant is not dependent on the pK_a of the hydrated metal. While Mn^{2+} supports cleavage, Co^{2+} does not, nor does Li^+, Na^+, K^+, or Cs^+. This pattern is very similar to that reported for a class of proposed structural sites in the *Tetrahymena* ribozyme,[27] further supporting the concept that the metal serves to stabilize structure in the hairpin ribozyme.

The importance of inter-domain interactions for catalysis is particularly clear when reviewing the evidence obtained from several groups—all showing that catalytic rate is dependent on the distance between the 5' end of the substrate and the 3' end of the ribozyme. A series of linkers, each consisting of a different number of bases, when joining the 3' end of the ribozyme to the 5' end of the substrate (Fig. 2.3c), corresponded directly to increased levels of circularization (i.e., ligation) with increasing linker length.[4] When 1,3-propanediol phosphate units for nucleotide residues were used as linker units, similar results were obtained.[6] When the method was revised to retain the linker between the 3' end of the ribozyme and the 5' end of the substrate and the removal of the bond between ribozyme positions A15 and C16, along with the addition of a single additional base 5' to C16 (Fig. 2.3d), the results were consistent wherein catalysis was dependent on linker length.[14]

A hairpin ribozyme was constructed in which the two domains were attached in the opposite manner as that found in the native structure, where the two domains are joined by formation of a new helix containing variable-length linkers between the 5' end of the ribozyme and the 3' end of the cytidine immediately preceding loop 3 (Fig. 2.3e).[8] In this particular construct, the substrate region and ribozyme region containing loop 2 are separate RNAs, so that the final cleavage reaction is trimolecular. The same pattern associating increasing linker length with increasing cleavage rate was observed. The domains can be totally separated (Fig. 2.3f) and, when the reaction has high concentrations of the RNA comprising the domains, cleavage rates were obtained which were similar to those of the standard bimolecular reaction between hairpin ribozyme and substrate (Fig. 2.3a).[30]

Using a slightly different construct (Fig. 2.3g), this ability to obtain cleavage activity when physically separated domains were combined was again demonstrated.[31] When linkers of varying lengths were inserted between A14 and A15, a different trend from the previous studies was observed. With the exception of an increase in activity accompanying the insertion of a single nucleotide, the cleavage levels associated with remaining linker lengths followed the basic trend of increasing linker length causing lower cleavage activity. This result suggested that close restraint of one domain to the other facilitated cleavage rather than decreasing it as was seen in the previous studies.

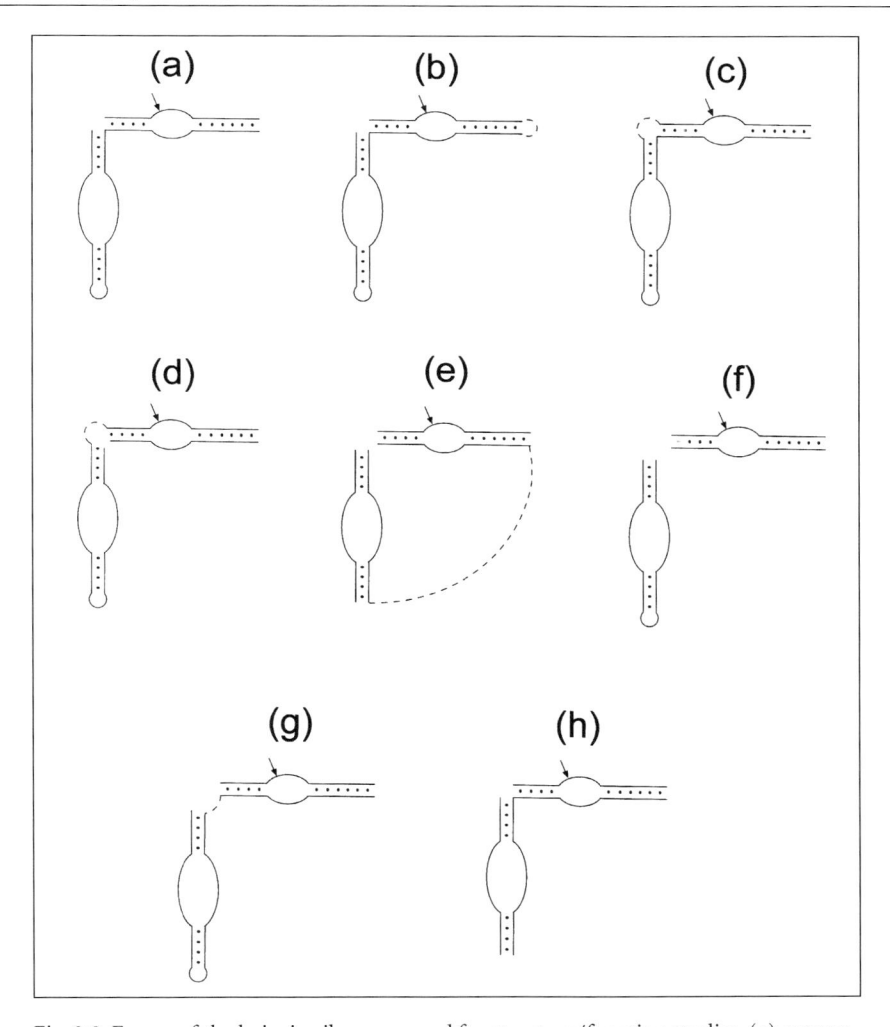

Fig. 2.3. Forms of the hairpin ribozyme used for structure/function studies. (a) conventional form for bimolecular trans reactions;[5] (b) cis-cleaving form with 3' end of substrate linked to 5' end of ribozyme;[7] (c) 5' end of substrate linked to 3' end of ribozyme;[6] (d) 5' end of substrate linked to 3' end of ribozyme with break at A15;[14] (e) construct of Komatsu et al, 1995;[8] (f) domain I and domain II are separate;[30,31] (g) with a linker placed at A15;[31] (h) Tripartite construct used for functional group studies.[13,25,33]

Complexes between 3' cleavage products and ribozymes are much stronger than predicted from simple helix association,[12] suggesting that the remainder of the molecule is contributing to stabilization of the binding—perhaps by folding over at the hinge region.[32] Such a folding at A15 would allow helices 2 and 4 to interact and perhaps contribute to the stabilization. The exact nature of these interactions is unknown; however, it is reasonable to expect that critical tertiary interactions could also occur between any or all of the required loop regions. It is very likely that components of loops 1, 2, 4, and 5 interact in some way. The interactive groups could be any of the six required positions in these loops.[7,23]

The study of specific functional group requirements has done much to explain the catalytic mechanism, as well as structure. When the role of 2'-OH groups was analyzed, there were four positions, A10, G11, A24, and C25, where substitution with either a 2'-H or 2'-O-methyl resulted in drastic reductions in cleavage rate.[33] Phosphorothioate substitutions on the hairpin ribozyme revealed that, while there are three positions which accompany a modest reduction in cleavage (5' to A7, A9, and A10), no phosphorothioate substitution within the ribozyme appears to prevent cleavage.[34]

Another form of functional group substitution study, base substitution, determined the secondary structure of the hairpin ribozyme. This method has been employed using two different schemes, each with success. These are mutational analysis and in vitro selection. Mutation analysis, wherein base substitutions are made precisely, has the advantage of being able to directly interrogate the molecule regarding the importance of a specific base identity. The second scheme, in vitro selection, has the potential advantage of allowing one to rapidly scan for more globally significant interactions, but its interpretation is often difficult. It has greater potential utility for co-variation of multiple sites wherein each site is randomly mutagenized and then selected by an in vitro method. However, randomization of approximately 15 bases in a given experiment is the upper limit, since it is necessary to produce a reasonable number of each sequence variant in a reaction. Additionally, with increasing numbers of bases randomized, larger numbers of selected sequences have to be analyzed, particularly when selection conditions are stringent. This is true because, under very strong selection pressures, only the most active sequences will be retained to a high degree. Both of these schemes have been used to locate the base pairs in the helical regions of the ribozyme-substrate complex. The seventeen Watson-Crick base pairs in the structure were all originally identified by mutagenesis[3,5] while the 18th base pair found, the A:G pair in helix 4, was originally identified by in vitro selection and then confirmed by mutagenesis.[7,35]

Both direct mutagenesis and in vitro selection have been successful in identifying key bases in the loop regions.[7,23,35] However, no covariations have been identified to date between any of the four required loops. Mutational analysis data show that there are six base positions in the ribozyme-substrate complex which, when mutated to any of the non-native variants, result in cleavage rates below the lower limit of detection. These are ribozyme base positions G8, A22, A23, C25, and A38, as well as substrate base position Gs6.[7,23] The remaining base positions show varying sensitivities to change with respect to their supporting cleavage.

The five required ribozyme bases are involved either in structure or in the catalytic event itself—exactly which is at present unknown. The required substrate base, Gs6, the base immediately 3' of the cleavage site, has an exocyclic amino group which is absolutely required for cleavage and may have particular significance to the catalytic structure at the cleavage site.[36]

With the advent of the more exotic RNA phosphoramidites, the determination of requirements for specific functional groups other than merely base or 2'-OH moieties was possible. Two studies that exemplify this manner of investigation examined functional groups in the loop regions of the hairpin ribozyme.[13,25] These studies have been helpful in suggesting important sites within nucleotide residues of the RNA where key interactions may occur. The use of propyl linkers as well as abasic substitutions at specific positions within the molecule have also been used to demonstrate the relative unimportance of several positions as well. When combined with mutational analysis data, these studies have gone far in suggesting sites used in secondary and possible tertiary interactions.

Conclusions

The hairpin ribozyme, while in the class of ribozymes which carry out cleavage to yield 2',3'-cyclic phosphate and 5'-OH termini, has a structure and mechanism unique among all known ribozymes. It alone is capable of facile ligation and it has excellent catalytic parameters. Substrate recognition occurs by formation of two helices, helix 1 and helix 2. Helix 1 is of variable length and helix 2 is fixed at 4 bp. The scissile phosphate is at the ApG in the substrate where the G is required and is part of a preferred BN*GUC sequence.[5] The catalytic reaction itself likely occurs without the direct involvement of a multivalent cation—again a unique aspect of the hairpin ribozyme.

References

1. Gerlach WL, Buzayan JM, Schneider IR et al. Satellite tobacco ringspot virus RNA: Biological activity of DNA clones and their in vitro transcripts. Virology 1986; 151:172-185.
2. Hampel A, Tritz R. RNA catalytic properties of the minimum (-)sTRSV sequence. Biochemistry 1989; 28:4929-4933.
3. Hampel A, Tritz R, Hicks M et al. 'Hairpin' catalytic RNA model: Evidence for helices and sequence requirement for substrate RNA. Nucleic Acids Res 1990; 18:299-304.
4. Feldstein P, Bruening G. Catalytically active geometry in the reversible circularization of 'mini-monomer' RNAs derived from the complementary strand of tobacco ringspot virus satellite RNA. Nucleic Acids Res 1993; 21:1991-1998.
5. Anderson P, Monforte J, Tritz R. Mutagenesis of the hairpin ribozyme. Nucleic Acids Res 1994; 22:1096-1100.
6. Komatsu Y, Koizumi M, Nakamura H et al. Loop-size variation to probe a bent structure of a hairpin ribozyme. J Am Chem Soc 1994; 116:3692-3696.
7. Siwkowski A, Shippy R, Hampel A. Analysis of hairpin ribozyme base mutations in loops 2 and 4 and their effects on cis-cleavage in vitro. Biochemistry 1997; 36:3930-3940.
8. Komatsu Y, Kanzaki I, Ohtsuka E. Enhanced folding of hairpin ribozymes with replaced domains. Biochemistry 1996; 35:9815-9820.
9. Buzayan JM, Gerlach WL, Bruening G. Non-enzymatic cleavage and ligation of RNAs complementary to a plant virus satellite RNA. Nature 1986; 323:349-353.
10. Buzayan JM, Hampel A, Bruening G. Nucleotide sequence and newly formed phosphodiester bond of spontaneously ligated satellite tobacco ringspot virus RNA. Nucleic Acids Res 1986; 14:9729-9743.
11. DeYoung MB, Siwkowski AM, Lian Y et al. Catalytic properties of hairpin ribozymes derived from chicory yellow mottle virus and arabis mosaic virus satellite RNAs. Biochemistry 1995; 34:15785-15791.
12. Hegg LA, Fedor MJ. Kinetics and thermodynamics of intermolecular catalysis by hairpin ribozymes. Biochemistry 1995; 34:15813-15828.
13. Schmidt S, Beigelman L, Karpeisky A et al. Base and sugar requirements for RNA cleavage of essential nucleoside residues in internal loop B of the hairpin ribozyme: Implications for secondary structure. Nucleic Acids Res 1996; 24:573-581.
14. Komatsu Y, Kanzaki I, Koizumi M et al. Modification of primary structures of hairpin ribozymes for probing active conformations. J Mol Biol 1995; 252:296-304.
15. Buzayan JM, Feldstein PA, Bruening G et al. RNA mediated formation of a phosphorothioate diester bond. Biochem Biophys Res Commun 1988; 156:340-347.
16. van Tol H, Buzayan JM, Feldstein PA et al. Two autolytic processing reactions of a satellite RNA proceed with inversion of configuration. Nucleic Acids Res 1990; 18:1971-1975.
17. Chowrira BM, Burke JM. Binding and cleavage of nucleic acids by the 'hairpin' ribozyme. Biochemistry 1991; 30:8518-8522.
18. Hampel A, Cowan JA. A unique mechanism for RNA catalysis: The role of metal cofactors in hairpin ribozyme cleavage. Chemistry and Biology 1997; 4:513-517.
19. Usher DA, Erenrich ES, Eckstein F. Geometry of the first step in the action of ribonuclease A. Proc Nat Acad Sci 1972; 69:115-118.

20. Fersht A. The structures and mechanisms of selected enzymes. In: Enzyme Structure and Mechanism. 2nd ed. New York: W.H. Freeman and Co., 1984:389-452.
21. Saenger W. Principles of Nucleic Acid Structure. Cantor CR, ed. New York: Springer-Verlag, 1984:331-349.
22. Gessner RV, Quigley GJ, Wang AH-J et al. Structural basis for stabilization of Z-DNA by cobalt hexaammine and magnesium cations. Biochemistry 1985; 24:237-240.
23. Shippy R, Siwkowski A, Hampel A. Mutational analysis of loops 1 and 5 of the hairpin ribozyme. Biochemistry 1998; 37:564-578.
24. Chowrira BM, Berzal-Herranz A, Burke JM. Ionic requirements for RNA binding, cleavage, and ligation by the hairpin ribozyme. Biochemistry 1993a; 32:1088-1095.
25. Grasby JA, Mersmann K, Singh M et al. Purine functional groups in essential residues of the hairpin ribozyme required for catalytic cleavage of RNA. Biochemistry 1995; 34:4068-4076.
26. Guerrier-Takada C, Haydock K, Allen L et al. Metal ion requirements and other aspects of the reaction catalyzed by M1 RNA, the RNA subunit of ribonuclease P from Escherichia coli. Biochemistry 1986; 25:1509-1515.
27. Grosshans CA, Cech TR. Metal ion requirements for sequence-specific endoribonuclease activity of the tetrahymena ribozyme. Biochemistry 1989; 28:6888-6894.
28. Cowan JA. Biological chemistry of magnesium ion with physiological metabolites, nucleic acids, and drug molecules. In: Cowan JA, ed. The Biological Chemistry of Magnesium. New York: VCH Publishers, Inc., 1995:185-209.
29. Laing LG, Gluick TC, Draper DE. Stabilization of RNA structure by Mg ions: Specific and non-specific effects. J Mol Biol 1994; 237:577-587.
30. Butcher SE, Heckman JE, Burke JM. Reconstitution of hairpin ribozyme activity following separation of functional domains. J Biol Chem 1995; 270:29648-29651.
31. Shin C, Choi JN, Song SI et al. The loop B domain is physically separable from the loop A domain in the hairpin ribozyme. Nucleic Acids Res 1996; 24:2685-2689.
32. Walter NG, Burke JM. Real-time monitoring of hairpin ribozyme kinetics through base-specific quenching of fluorescein-labeled substrates. RNA 1997; 3:392-404.
33. Chowrira BM, Berzal-Heranz A, Keller CF et al. Four ribose 2'-hydroxyl groups essential for catalytic function of the hairpin ribozyme. J Biol Chem 1993b; 268:19458-19462.
34. Chowrira BM, Burke JM. Extensive phosphorothioate substitution yields highly active and nuclease-resistant hairpin ribozymes. Nucleic Acids Res 1992; 20:2835-2840.
35. Siwkowski A, Humphrey M, DeYoung MB, Hampel A. Screening for important base identities in the hairpin ribozyme by in vitro selection for cleavage. BioTechniques 1998; 24:278-284.
36. Chowrira BM, Berzal-Herranz A, Burke JM. Novel guanosine requirement for catalysis by the hairpin ribozyme. Nature 1991; 354:320-322.

CHAPTER 3

Biochemistry of Hepatitis Delta Virus Catalytic RNAs

N. Kyle Tanner

Introduction

Hepatitis delta virus (HDV) is a unique human pathogen with a world-wide distribution. It is associated with a high incidence of fulminant hepatitis and premature death, although the severity of the disease varies widely depending on the geographic location (reviewed in refs. 1-5). HDV is a satellite virus of hepatitis B (HBV), but HDV is completely unrelated to its helper virus. It requires the coat proteins encoded by HBV for encapsulation and formation of infectious particles, but infection and replication occur independently. HDV is a unique mammalian virus, but it does share a number of features with certain pathogens found in plants: the viroids and viroid-like satellite viruses (reviewed in refs. 6, 7). These features include a single-stranded RNA genome, an RNA-dependent rolling-circle mode of replication, and the ability of the isolated RNA to self-cleave in vitro. The self-cleaving reaction is probably used in vivo to process the intermediates generated during rolling-circle replication into unit-length progeny (Fig. 3.1). However, unlike the hammerhead and hairpin (paper clip) motifs found in the plant viruses, the sequences constituting the HDV self-cleaving domains are unique, and they form an entirely different catalytic motif. This review will summarize the characteristics of the HDV self-cleaving domains, show how they can be converted into trans-cleaving ribozymes, and discuss how the properties of the catalytic domains can be exploited for developing therapeutic or prophylactic agents.

Properties of HDV

To better understand the catalytic domains, it is first useful to briefly discuss some general properties of the virus (reviewed in refs. 1-5). A cartoon of the viral life cycle is shown in Figure 3.1. HDV consists of a circular, single-stranded RNA strand of about 1700 nucleotides (nt). The RNA has a high content of guanines and cytidines (60%), and it is capable of making extensive intramolecular base pairs (~70%) to form a long rod-shaped structure that is visible by electron microscopy (Fig. 3.2).[8,9] The infectious genomic (-) strand is found in large excess over the complementary antigenomic (+) strand, which is a replicative intermediate. Small quantities of linear dimer and trimer molecules are also found, which is consistent with a rolling-circle mechanism of replication. No DNA intermediates are evident, and replication is most likely due to an RNA-dependent activity of the host's RNA pol II.[10-12] Unlike the plant viruses, HDV expresses a protein (HDAg) from a single open reading frame (ORF). Early in infection, this is a 195 amino acid (aa) protein (small

Ribozymes in the Gene Therapy of Cancer, edited by Kevin J. Scanlon and Mohammed Kashani-Sabet.
©1998 R.G. Landes Company.

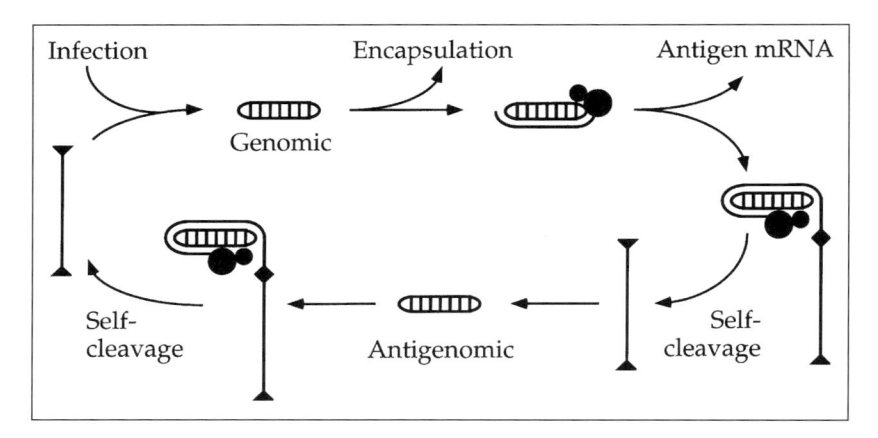

Fig. 3.1. Cartoon for HDV replication. The virion enters the cell as a circular genomic strand within a nucleoprotein complex (not shown). This is transported to the nucleus, and the circular RNA serves as a template for a host-derived, RNA-dependent, RNA polymerase (most likely RNA pol II). The small antigen protein, and perhaps other host-specific factors, is required for replication, and it is perhaps associated with the polymerase. Linear multimers are generated that are site-specifically cleaved at the catalytic domains (shown as diamonds). These are then ligated by an unknown mechanism to form the closed-circular antigenomic strand, which similarly acts as a template for rolling-circle replication. The genomic strand is used to express the HDAg mRNA. Late in infection, the closed-circular genomic strand, as a nucleoprotein complex with the HDAg proteins, is encapsulated with the coat proteins of HBV. The catalytic domains are not shown within the circular forms for clarity.

HDAg) that is required for replication (reviewed in ref. 4). Later in infection, a specific RNA editing event eliminates a stop codon and extends the ORF by 19 aa (refs. 13, 14 and references therein). The large HDAg inhibits replication and promotes encapsulation. Both the large and small HDAg will stimulate self-cleavage in transfected cells, but they are not required for activity (ref. 15 and references therein). The small HDAg has some homology to a human transcription factor,[16] although there is some dispute over the significance of this.[17]

The genomic and antigenomic RNAs have self-cleaving activity. The antigenomic catalytic domain is located just downstream of the HDAg ORF (Fig. 3.2), and it is close to one end of the predicted rod-shaped structure. The genomic self-cleaving domain is located in a position that is juxtaposed to the antigenomic domain in this structure; that is, the antisense of the antigenomic domain has extensive complementarity to the genomic domain sequence (Fig. 3.2). Hence, the two catalytic domains are similar—but not identical—in sequence. The integrity of both the genomic and antigenomic ribozymes is required for replication in transfected cells (see below). However, some mutations within the catalytic domains, which otherwise do not affect catalytic activity, block replication of HDV in transfected cells.[18] Thus, sequences within the catalytic domains are important for other roles in the viral life cycle besides self-cleavage. An intact antigenomic catalytic domain stabilizes the 3' transcript after cleavage at the polyadenylation site (ref. 19 and references therein).

Properties of the Catalytic Domains

The catalytic domains of HDV have been the subject of extensive analyses. This material is reviewed in detail elsewhere,[20-22] so I will limit myself here to summarizing the characteristics and incorporating some recent observations. The minimum sequence required

Fig. 3.2. Features within the HDV RNA. (a) shows the genomic RNA as a closed-circular, rod-shaped structure. Intramolecular base pairing is not shown for clarity. The genomic RNA is the template for transcribing the HDAg mRNA. Early in infection, a 195 aa ORF is expressed. Late in infection, an RNA editing event eliminates a stop codon and extends the ORF by 19 aa. The position of the polyadenylation signal is as indicated. The antigenomic catalytic domain is just downstream of the ORF. (b) is an enlargement of one end of the rod-shaped structure showing the sequence details of the catalytic domains and flanking elements. This folding was done according to ref. 20 and the HDV numbering is according to ref. 9. Note that other variations of this folding are possible and that there is no experimental evidence for this particular structure. The catalytic domains are in juxtaposition to each other within this structure; that is, the genomic domain has extensive complementarity to the antisense sequence of the antigenomic domain.

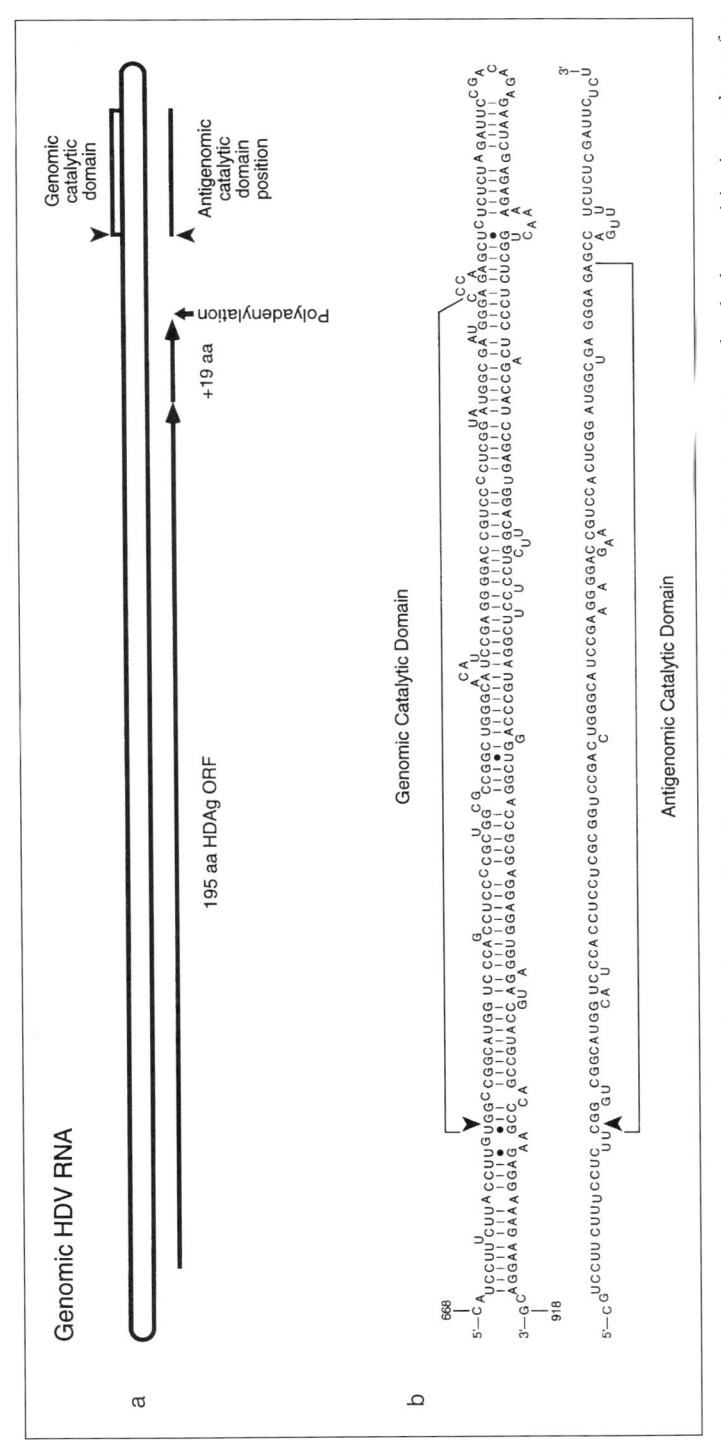

for optimum catalytic activity consists of one nt 5' and 84 nt 3' to the cleavage site for both the genomic and antigenomic domains. Slightly shorter constructs retain activity, but they are less reactive and less stable to denaturants. Constructs with longer 3' extensions are also often less reactive, apparently because they form competing interactions that are inhibitory. High temperatures and/or denaturants are needed to melt out these interactions and partially restore activity. However, strain comparisons and experiments with trans-cleaving forms indicate that a small number of additional 3' sequences may be beneficial (see below). Sequences 5' to the +1 nt (relative to the cleavage site) will enhance the activity of some constructs, although the mechanism for this is still unclear.[23,24] The minimum sequence requirement 5' to the cleavage site is a characteristic also shared by the catalytic domain isolated from the *Neurospora* VS RNA, but it is clear that the catalytic domains are not the same (ref. 25 and references therein).

A number of secondary structure models have been proposed (reviewed in refs. 20, 22), but it now generally agreed that the pseudoknot model, first presented by Been and coworkers,[26,27] best fits the experimental data for both the genomic and antigenomic domains (Fig. 3.3), and it will form the basis for my further discussions. This structure consists of two helical regions (I, II) and two hairpins (III, IV; nomenclature of ref. 26). The sequences forming helix II are discontinuous and they constitute the pseudoknot interaction. For comparison, other secondary structure models generally agree with the general character of helix I and hairpin IV. Moreover, many of the models form hairpin III with some minor alterations of the folding. However, none of the other models form helix II. Rather, these sequences are generally shown interacting with sequences 5' to the cleavage site.

The secondary structure models of HDV have been extensively tested by site-specific mutagenesis, chemical probing, enzymatic digestion and analog substitution (reviewed in refs. 20-22). Unfortunately, these data are often very difficult to analyze and compare because of differences in the constructs and methods of analysis. As admonished by Uhlenbeck,[28] mutations within structured RNAs can have unanticipated effects. For HDV, many mutations affect both the reaction rate and the ability of the catalytic domains to fold into active structures. Analyses that measure the time it takes for half the material to react inevitably incorporate the rate of the reaction plus the time it takes for misfolded molecules to assume an active conformation. The catalytic domains of HDV seem to be particularly prone to misfolding, even with constructs containing the wild type sequence, and widely different interpretations of some of the data have resulted. My laboratory distinguished between these two different phenomena by measuring the reaction rates at early times and by comparing these rates at different reaction temperatures.[29] Higher temperatures increase the conformational flexibility of RNA and thereby facilitate the formation of active molecules. This is reflected in the reaction profiles at the different temperatures. Nevertheless, despite these difficulties, the various analyses are largely consistent with the pseudoknot model.

Additional studies were made to determine the spatial relationships of the different nucleotides. Bravo et al[30] used deoxy-4-thiouracil-substituted substrates in a trans-cleaving construct of the antigenomic catalytic domain (see Fig 3.5a). The 4-thiouracil is activated by long UV light, and it forms crosslinks with nucleotides in close proximity. They found crosslinks between the -1 and -2 positions and C24, G28 and C76 (numbering for cis-cleaving construct). Likewise, Rosenstein and Been[31] used a photo-activatable azidophenacyl group tethered to the phosphate at the cleavage site in a similar system and in a cis-cleaving system. They obtained crosslinks within junction IV/II, the 5' half of helix III and within loop III, showing that these regions are in close proximity. Oddly, the in trans form gave a somewhat different crosslinking pattern than the in cis form. Lead-cleavage studies also indicate that these regions are close together in tertiary space.[32] Recent mutagenic data indicate that

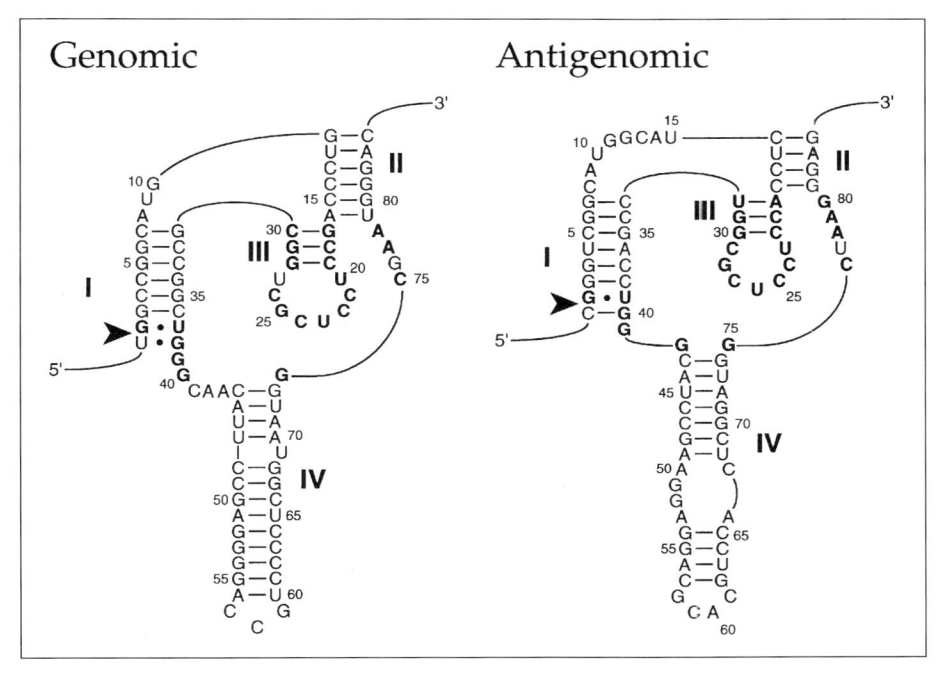

Fig. 3.3. The pseudoknot secondary-structure models of the catalytic domains. The minimal sequence requirements for optimal activity are shown. Numbering is relative to the cleavage site and nomenclature is according to refs. 26, 27. The cleavage sites are indicated by arrowheads. Nucleotides that are important for catalytic activity are indicated in bold.

G41 and G75 in the antigenomic domain are probably stacked at the base of hairpin IV, and they may form non Watson-Crick base pairs.[33] Similar interactions are possible for G40 and G74 in the genomic domain, but the data for this are still inconclusive.[33] Probing with Fe(II)-EDTA, which is sensitive to exposed ribose functionalities, shows that the junction regions I/IV and IV/II, and loop III are largely protected from the solvent.[31] This result is consistent with phosphorothiolate-interference studies.[34] Ethidium bromide and time-resolved fluorescence spectroscopy indicate that the secondary structure of the antigenomic domain is highly structured even in 95% formamide at 25°C.[35] In the same vein, NMR studies of a model RNA designed to mimic the antigenomic hairpin III, with helix II coaxially stacked at its base, show that the structure is particularly stable, and that it forms unusual interactions.[36]

Strain Comparisons

Phylogenetic comparisons are a powerful technique for elucidating important sequences involved in secondary and tertiary interactions in RNA.[6,37,38] However, since the genomic and antigenomic HDV RNAs are the sole examples of the pseudoknot catalytic motif, this methodology might be expected to be of limited use. Fortunately, this is not the case. Like many RNA viruses, HDV has a very high frequency of mutations during replication, and there is significant sequence variability between different isolates. Currently, there are three classified genotypes of the virus (ref. 39 and reference therein). Genotype I is the most widespread, and it is associated with a range of clinical symptoms, from very mild to severe.

Genotype II is less widespread, and it is associated with a mild form of the disease. It is 88.5 to 95.6% similar to genotype I.[40] In contrast, genotype III, which also has a limited distribution, is associated with a particularly severe form of the disease.[41] It is more divergent from the other two genotypes and shares only 61 to 80% similarity.[40,41] A phylogenetic tree was derived for much of this sequence data.[42]

Sequence alignments of the catalytic domains were made previously,[20,22] and they support the pseudoknot model as shown in Figure 3.4. However, additional sequences were added to the databases since these publications. These data largely confirm the previous interpretations, but they provide some additional information. This material is summarized in Figure 3.4. However, I should state that the events leading to the changes within highly variable regions are unknown. Sequence alignments are therefore based on the simplest interpretation of the data that involve the fewest alterations. Recent data provide evidence for slightly different interpretations of the variability within hairpin IV and the 3' flanking sequences than previously shown.[20,22] Nevertheless, despite the high degree of isolate variability, it is clear that the core sequences of the catalytic domains are strongly conserved. Most of the changes occur within hairpin IV, which mutagenic data indicate to be very malleable. These changes rearrange but do not alter the general characteristics of the structure.

For convenience in the further discussions, genomic sequences will be indicated as (-) and the antigenomic as (+). The equivalent nucleotides G76(-) and U77(+) were shown to be alterable by site-specific mutagenesis and the substitution of an A or C at this position is not surprising.[43,44] The A78G(+) change is unexpected since changing this position to a uridine, or the equivalent A77U(-), significantly reduces activity in vitro.[43,44] However, a purine substitution may be better tolerated. U23C(-) and the equivalent U26C(+) maintain the pyrimidine character of the loop, which is consistent with the mutagenic data (reviewed in refs. 20, 22). The more extensive alterations of the genomic loop III sequence in the Lai et al isolate[45] (k) are somewhat surprising, and they may reflect an artifact; nevertheless, they make the spatial relationship of the sequence more like that found in the antigenomic loop. As previously noted,[20] the sequence variability of the different isolates is consistent with stem II forming and with its elongation by one nucleotide for the genomic domain (generally) and five nt for the antigenomic domain (always). Finally, the 3' flanking sequence gives a suggestion for the enormous potential for variability within the HDV sequence. The fact that the 5' flanking sequences show less variability could reflect the importance of these sequences in catalytic activity as previously proposed.[23,24] However, it is probable that they are important for other aspects of the viral life cycle.

Data Summary

The experimental data and sequence comparisons are consistent with the pseudoknotted structure as shown in Figure 3.3. Helix I, helix II and hairpin IV are mostly structural elements in which the sequences can be altered as long as the structural features are maintained. There are some sequence requirements around the cleavage site in helix I, and this will be discussed in more detail in the section on trans-cleaving ribozymes. Helix III is also a structural element, but it has sequence-specific requirements. It is most likely coaxially stacked with helix II, rather than with helix I; as discussed below, this is needed to maintain the spatial relationship of the loop III sequences relative to the catalytic site. The single-stranded regions loop III, junction I/IV, and junction IV/II have specific sequence requirements and together with helices I and III they probably form the catalytic core of the ribozyme. They may be involved in chelating the divalent cation(s) and orienting the scissile linkage.

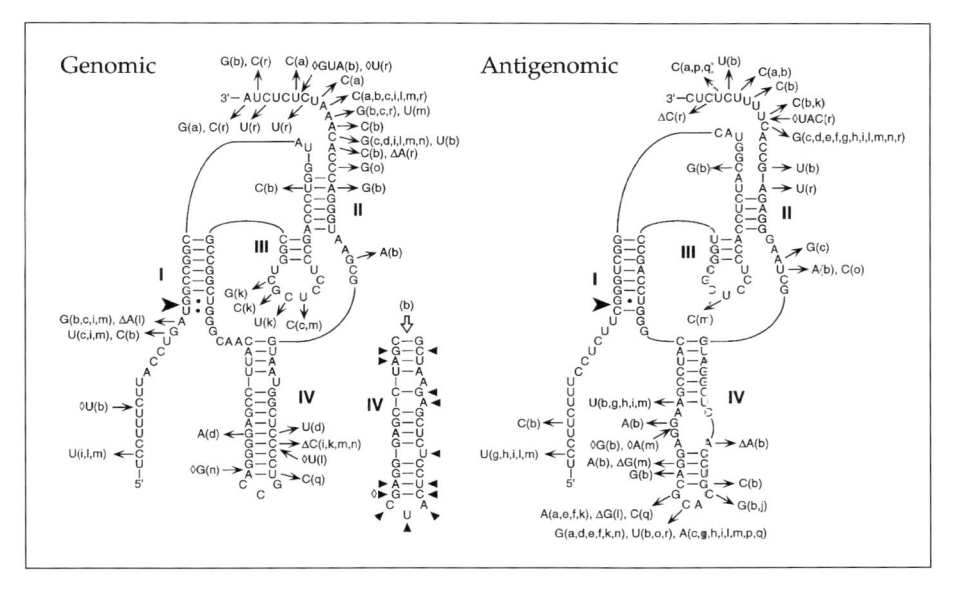

Fig. 3.4. Sequence variability of HDV isolates. The primary sequences are those most commonly found. These sequences were isolated from woodchuck (which had passed through chimpanzee and human),[78] human,[79] chimpanzee,[80] Central African Republic isolate passed through woodchuck,[81] North American (14 clones),[82] Italian isolate passed through chimpanzee (origin of HDV used to infect woodchucks),[78,9] and from several French patients.[78,83] Note that while the sequence of isolates was the same in the region shown, they varied at other positions. Positions of sequence variability are as shown: ◊ indicates insertions; Δ indicates deletions. However, in highly variable regions (helix IV and the 3' flanking sequence) of some isolates, the nature of the changes are unclear. The changes shown represent the simplest interpretation that is consistent with the alignment of all the strains. The parentheses indicate the isolate: (a) human US-2;[41] b) northern South American Peru-1;[41] (c) South Pacific island of Nauru;[84] (d) Taiwan;[85] (e) Japan, patient M (9/20/86);[86] (f) Japan, patient M (7/6/89);[86] (g) Japan, patient S (7/18/83);[86] (h) Japan, patient S (8/6/87);[86] (i) Japan;[87] (j) woodchuck;[88] (k) human;[45] (l) Lebanon;[89] (m) Taiwan strain Taiwan 3;[40] (n) central China;[90] (o) patient from southern California;[82] and (p), (q), (r) three patients from Los Angeles.[85] Hairpin IV is redrawn in the case of the Peru-1 isolate for the genomic sequence to clarify the nature of the changes (indicated by the wedges). Microheterogeneity (quasi-species) within clones is not shown because of uncertainty as to the source of the difference.

A three-dimensional model of the genomic ribozyme was derived from these data with an interactive graphical computer.[44] This model brings helix I, loop III, junction I/IV and junction VI/II into close proximity, and it has helix II and hairpin IV pointing off from the catalytic core. A similar model was also made for the antigenomic strand.[30] A different model was proposed for the antigenomic model based on the axehead secondary structure.[46] This model is similar to the previous two models, but it is more open and junction IV/II follows a different pathway. However, recent data are largely consistent with the pseudoknot three-dimensional model. Crosslinking studies with photo-activatable agents close to the scissile linkage show the close proximity of loop III and junction IV/II to the cleavage site.[30,31] Fe(II)-EDTA protection[31] and phosphorothiolate interference[34] experiments also indicate that these regions are protected from the solvent, as predicted by the model. However, details of the model need to be refined. The crosslinking studies of Been and Rosenstein[31] and biophysical studies of Kolk et al[36] indicate that the loop III sequence has a slightly different orientation with respect to the cleavage site. Moreover, junction I/IV is more protected than expected from the model.[31] Clearly additional studies are needed to further clarify the spatial relationships of the different elements.

Self-Cleavage Reaction

The catalytic requirements for HDV were reviewed in detail previously;[20-22] I will simply summarize that information here and add some recent information. Like all catalytic RNAs, HDV has an absolute requirement for a divalent cation, such as Mg^{2+}, Ca^{2+} or Mn^{2+}. Very low concentrations (< 0.1 mM) of these cations are sufficient to cleave optimized constructs. Monovalent cations do not support the reaction. Circular dichroism measurements indicate that there are three bound Mg^{2+}, although this was done with a three-strand construct (Fig. 3.5f) that required 100 mM Mg^{2+} for optimum activity.[47]

Like the other self-cleaving RNAs, the reaction generates products with 2',3-cyclic phosphates and 5' hydroxyls. A 2' deoxyribose at the scissile linkage blocks cleavage.[48] Previous work showed that the reaction was independent of pH from 5.0 to 9.0, but recent experiments show a linear increase of the reaction rate with increasing pH from 4.0 to 6.0, with a pH optimum around 7.0 to 7.5.[47,49] This latter result is more consistent with what one would expect if the observed reaction rate actually corresponds to the chemical cleavage step. The temperature optimum is around 55°C to 65°C for constructs near the optimal size.[20] Phosphorothiolate substitutions have also been made at the scissile linkage.[34,49] A pro-R_p phosphorothiolate is poorly cleaved, and it is not recovered by using Mn^{2+}. The pro-S_p phosphorothiolate was slightly less reactive than the normal linkage. These results suggest that Mg^{2+} does not interact directly with the pro-R oxygen.[49] A similar result was also recently obtained for the hammerhead ribozyme.[50]

Previous studies indicated that the catalytic domains also catalyze a ligation reaction, which might be used to generate the circular templates used in replication and encapsulation (Fig. 3.1).[51,52] However, in one case this was shown to be an artifact of the assay conditions[53,54] and in the other the reaction conditions were not physiological and an equal proportion of both 2',5' and 3',5' linkages was formed.[52] Currently, the best indication is that the RNAs are circularized by a host-encoded ligase.[55,56]

Biological Relevance

Recently, a number of experiments were conducted to determine the biological relevance of the catalytic domains in the life cycle of the virus. Mutations that disrupt catalytic activity in vitro will similarly block replication of the virus in cell culture.[56,18] Moreover, shortening the rod-shaped structure to within a few nt of the 3' ends of the catalytic domains reduces replication to barely detectable levels.[57] Additional studies have also looked at the cleavage activity independent of viral replication.[18] These studies indicate that catalytic activity is essential for replication, but that sequence alterations that maintain self-cleavage activity are not always sufficient to maintain replication. Hence, the sequences within the catalytic domains play other roles in the life cycle of the virus besides self-cleavage. This may account for the high degree of sequence conservation within the catalytic domains, which is in contrast to the flexibility revealed by the mutagenesis experiments. Finally, mutations were made and tested in cell culture to distinguish among three common HDV secondary structure models.[18] These experiments show that the sequences defining the pseudoknot structure are required for activity and that this structure is used in vivo.

Since the self-cleaving domains are regenerated with the ligation of the linear progeny, the catalytic activity of HDV must be regulated in some fashion during the viral life cycle to prevent inappropriate cleavage of the template or encapsulated RNA. A model was pro-

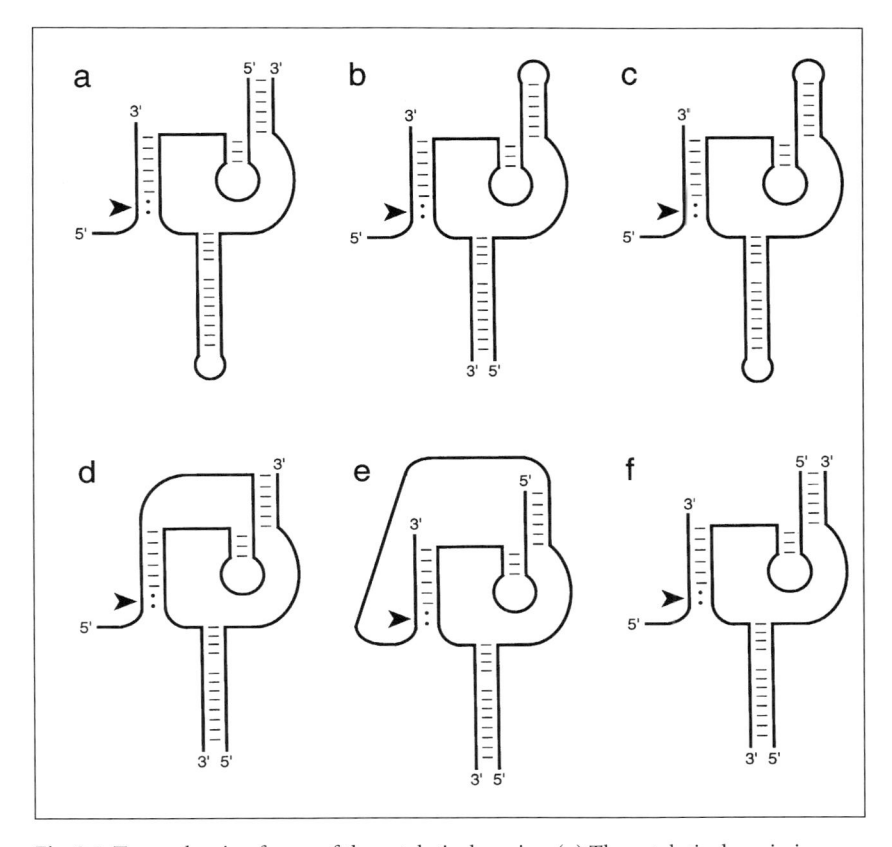

Fig. 3.5. Trans-cleaving forms of the catalytic domains. (a) The catalytic domain is separated within junction I/II. This is the most commonly used form, and it was originally designed by Been and coworkers.[26,27] (b) is a variant where the transcriptional start and stop have been circularly permuted.[48,66] (c) is a completely closed circular ribozyme that was constructed with the aid of a permuted catalytic intron.[66] (d) This construct was originally designed based on the ax head secondary structure,[23] but it is equally applicable to the pseudoknot model. (e) is a variant of (d) where the transcriptional start and stop sites are circularly permuted.[64] (f) is a trans-cleaving form made from three separate strands.[63,47] Genomic, antigenomic and synthetic sequences are used (see text and Table 3.1).

posed (ref. 58 and references therein) where the rod-shaped structure of the HDV RNA (Fig. 3.2) sequesters the catalytic domain sequences and prevents formation of the active structure. However, during replication the catalytic domain rapidly forms and cleaves the precursor before these interactions occur. According to this model, the dimer and trimer molecules found in vivo are dead-end replication products that are blocked for self-cleavage. Evidence for this model is that constructs containing sequences that are complementary to the catalytic domain (attenuators), which are either HDV-derived 3' to the catalytic domain or artificial (5' or 3' to the catalytic domain), are processed to circular products in human hepatoma cells.[55] They are not processed (self-cleaved or ligated) in vitro. The HDV-encoded HDAg enhances cleavage, but it is not necessary.[15] These results indicate that host-encoded proteins, in conjunction with the attenuator sequence, participate in regulating the catalytic activity. Moreover, constructs containing attenuators are properly processed in mammalian cells but not in yeast or *Escherichia coli*, which give results similar to those obtained in vitro.[55] Thus, the factor(s) is (are) probably mammalian-specific. An intriguing observation in this light is the sequence similarity between the genomic catalytic domain and human 7S RNA.[59]

Trans-Cleaving Activity

As with the other catalytic RNAs, the cis-cleaving activity of HDV can be converted into a trans-cleaving activity by dividing the catalytic domain into separate "substrate" and "ribozyme." I put these in quotations because both are required for the formation of the active structure and because there are many ways of making such constructs. Hence, the substrate is defined as the molecule that is cleaved and the ribozyme is the unaltered, reusable component. Figure 3.5 shows different variants of the HDV ribozymes, which are applicable for both the genomic and the antigenomic forms. It is clear that a number of variants are possible. The catalytic domains have been successfully divided within junction I/II (Fig. 3.5a,b,c)[48,60-62] and within loop IV (Fig. 3.5d,e).[23,62] It is also possible to make a construct, consisting of three separate strands, that is divided in both regions (Fig. 3.5f).[47,63] In some instances, at least, molecules can be separated at the 3' extremity of loop III,[64] although cleaving within loop III would normally be expected to eliminate activity.[63,65] It is not possible to separate the molecule within junctions II/III, III/I, I/IV and IV/II.[63-65] Separation within helix IV is possible, but constructs separated within helix I or II are less effective (Lescure and Tanner, unpublished data).[64] The transcription starts and stops can be circularly permuted within these structures (Fig. 3.5b,e).[60,64,66] A particularly intriguing variant takes advantage of permuted exon-intron sequences within a self-splicing group I intron to generate a completely closed-circular molecule (Fig. 3.5c).[66] This molecule is resistant to nucleases found in serum[66] and recently it was successfully generated within *E. coli*.[67]

A comparison of the catalytic properties of these constructs is shown in Table 3.1. Care must be exercised in evaluating this table because the details of the individual constructs vary substantially. Many of the constructs have an artificial hairpin IV, some have an abbreviated stem II and others are hybrid constructs containing sequence elements from both the genomic and antigenomic domains. Moreover, no distinction is made between single turnover (ribozyme saturating) and multiple turnover (substrate saturating) conditions. The latter can be 10-fold less than the former, which probably reflects rate-limiting product release.[48] Association constants are shown, where available, but they are consistent with the values expected for Watson-Crick base pairing between the substrate and ribozyme. Up to 12-fold turnover was obtained with various hybrid constructs at physiological temperatures.[66] However, these were obtained using Ca^{2+} as the divalent cation; Mg^{2+} was less effective.

The most frequently used designs of the trans-cleaving ribozymes are variants of constructs separated within junction I/II (Fig. 3.5a,b,c), where the substrate consists of an 8 nucleotide sequence that binds to the ribozyme to form helix I. There are minimal sequence requirements for this construct (see below), and product release is not expected to be as limiting as in the other constructs. On the other hand, a target site of 7 to 8 nt is of limited specificity. Unfortunately, as discussed below, it is not yet possible to extend helix I. Moreover, making base pairs between sequences 5' to the -1 nucleotide and junction I/IV are strongly inhibitory (Lescure and Tanner, unpublished data).[22] In contrast, ribozymes separated within loop IV contain extensive base pairs (Fig. 3.5d). However, in this case the substrate has many of the conserved nucleotides, and these are unlikely to be found in a targeted RNA. The circularly permuted variant (Fig. 3.5e) reduces the number of conserved nt within the substrate, but it imposes other limitations.

Table 3.1. Comparison of trans-cleaving ribozymes

Construct*	Cleavage Rate (k_{obs})	Turnover	Conditions
(a) Genomic[65]	0.022 min^{-1} (1.7 min^{-1})[‡]	ND	pH 7.1, 37°C, 1 mM MgCl$_2$
(a) Genomic[49,68]	~1.90 min^{-1}	ND	pH 7.4, 37°C, 10 mM MgCl$_2$
(a) Genomic[63]	ND	ND	pH 8.0, 37°C, 10 mM MgCl$_2$
(a) Antigenomic[48]	~2.8 min^{-1}	6-fold	pH 8.0, 55°C, 10 mM MgCl$_2$
(a) Antigenomic[61]	ND	ND	55°C, 10 mM MgCl$_2$
(a) Hybrid[60]	1.5 min^{-1}	6-fold	pH 8.0, 37°C, 10 mM MgCl$_2$
(a) Hybrid[66]	~0.25 min^{-1} (~5-fold)[°]	~12-fold	pH 8.0, 37°C, 10 mM CaCl$_2$
(a) Selected[68]	2.45 min^{-1}	ND	pH 7.4, 37°C, 10 mM MgCl$_2$
(b) Hybrid[60]	0.52 min^{-1}	3-fold	pH 8.0, 37°C, 10 mM MgCl$_2$
(b) Hybrid[66]	~0.25 min^{-1} (~3.5-fold)[°]	~12-fold	pH 8.0, 37°C, 10 mM CaCl$_2$
(c) Hybrid[66]	0.29 min^{-1} (~3-fold)[°]	~12-fold	pH 8.0, 37°C, 10 mM CaCl$_2$
(d) Genomic[62]	0.011 min^{-1}	ND	pH 7.2, 50°C, 12 mM MgCl$_2$
(d) Genomic/Antigenomic[23]	ND	ND	pH 7.5, 50°C, 5 mM MgCl$_2$
(e) Hybrid[64]	0.66 min^{-1}	6-fold	pH 7.5, 50°C, 12 mM MgCl$_2$
(e) Hybrid[91]	0.17 min^{-1} (0.98 min^{-1})[‡]	8-fold (3-fold)[‡]	pH 7.5, 50°C, 12 mM MgCl$_2$
(f) Genomic[63]	ND	ND	pH 8.0, 37°C, 10 mM MgCl$_2$
(f) Hybrid[47]	~0.09 min^{-1} (0.38 min^{-1})[#]	ND	pH 8, 37°C, 10 mM MgCl$_2$

* the letters in parentheses refer to the constructs shown in Figure 3.5. 'Hybrid' is a combination of genomic and antigenomic sequences, and it generally contains a synthetic hairpin IV. 'Selected' is an in vitro selected sequence.
‡, longer helix II; °, turnover in the presence of 10 mM MgCl$_2$; #, reaction in 100 mM MgCl$_2$.

In general, the antigenomic sequence is more effective than the genomic sequence as a trans-cleaving ribozyme. The reasons for this are unclear, but it appears to reflect the greater propensity of the genomic catalytic domain to misfold or for the substrate to bind in a nonproductive fashion (Lescure and Tanner, unpublished data). Interestingly, in vitro selection experiments of a randomly mutagenized genomic sequence yields a construct that is very similar to the antigenomic sequence.[68] For this reason, many workers combined different sequence elements from the two domains to make HDV hybrids. These normally have the antigenomic helix I and loop III, and the genomic helix II, helix III, junction I/IV, and junction IV/II. Hairpin IV often consists of a shorter artificial sequence. Extending helix II will enhance the catalytic rate of at least some constructs (Table 3.1).[65,68]

While not all possible basepair combinations have been tested, it appears there are few sequence requirements for helix I other than that basepairing is maintained and that the helix is 7 base pairs long. There is little evidence for a base pair at the -1 position, although it is reasonable to expect that the -1 nt is constrained in some fashion for cleavage to occur. Extending the helix or shortening it drastically reduces activity.[44,69] Watson-Crick base pairs are preferred and G-U base pairs at positions other than the +1 position are inhibitory.[20,69] The -1 nucleotide preference is C = U>A>>G for the antigenomic[43] and U>C>A>>G for the genomic,[70] although except for G the differences are not large. The +1 position is preferably a purine with a pyrimidine base pair (G-U>A-C>G-C>A-U for the antigenomic[43] and G-U>G-C>A-U for the genomic).[70] Interestingly, a G-C base pair was obtained at the +1 position in the in vitro selection experiments.[68] In the same set of in vitro selection experiments, a variant catalytic domain was isolated that cleaves between +1 and +2 when there is a U-G, G-G or A-G base pair at the +1 position.[70] This phenomenon is unique for the selected construct, so its significance is unclear. The mechanism for this aberrant cleavage site is unknown, but this construct may be useful in elucidating the characteristics of the catalytic core.

Applications

The applications of the trans-cleaving forms of HDV are rather limited to date. Researchers generally do not publish their failed experiments, so it is unclear how often the trans-cleaving ribozymes have been tested. However, to my knowledge there is no successful application of the various trans-cleaving forms in vivo or in cell culture. This may reflect the difficulty of obtaining effective ribozymes at physiological temperatures. Effective, in this case, means both high activity and turnover. The major problem seems to be maintaining the ribozyme element in a conformation that is both competent for binding the substrate and functional for catalysis. Fortunately, people are devising clever ways of reducing these problems, and future constructs may suffer less from these problems. This bodes well for their future use in vivo.

However, because of the minimum sequence requirements 5' to the cleavage site, the cis-cleaving form has found a number of applications. It is used to trim the ends of in vitro transcribed RNAs to generate discrete products for biophysical studies.[71] Likewise, it is used to release ribozymes that are synthesized as part of a long transcript, and the HDV ribozyme was compared with the hammerhead and hairpin as releasing elements for processing ribozyme cassettes generated in vitro and in cell culture.[72] Finally, it seems to be a popular tool amongst negative-strand RNA virologists for generating the discrete ends of cDNA transcripts in vivo that are required for replication.[73-76]

Moreover, since the HDV pathogen is a serious health problem and since the catalytic domains are essential for replication, the HDV ribozymes are potential targets themselves for therapeutic agents. Some antibiotics are effective inhibitors of catalytic activity in vitro at μmolar concentrations.[32] Although there is little evidence that these agents are equally effective in vivo, they nevertheless provide the basis for combinatorial screenings to isolate forms that may prove effective.[77] Antisense oligonucleotides are also effective inhibitors of catalytic activity in vitro (Thill, Crain-Denoyelle and Tanner, unpublished data) and in cell culture (Sureau, unpublished data).

Concluding Remarks

Catalytic RNAs are widely found in plants, bacteria, bacteriophage and lower eukaryotes. However, HDV is the only ribozyme found in man, and its catalytic activity is probably optimized for this cellular environment. Indeed, as described above, the self-cleaving reaction of HDV is regulated only within mammalian cells. Moreover, the HDV virion can be a vector for delivering the ribozyme to the intended cell. While earlier constructs were uninspiring, recent trans-cleaving ribozymes show high activity and turnover under physiological conditions. With the aid of the three-dimensional model, it may be possible to further optimize the activity and to design constructs with greater sequence specificity. There is still much to learn about the HDV catalytic domains.

Acknowledgments

I am grateful to Patrick Linder and to members of the Department of Medical Biochemistry for their support. I thank Josette Banroques for checking through the text. This work was supported, in part, with a grant from the Roche Research Foundation.

References

1. Taylor JM. Human hepatitis delta virus. Curr Top Microbiol Immunol 1991; 168:141-166.
2. Taylor JM. The structure and replication of hepatitis delta virus. Annu Rev Microbiol 1992; 46:253-276.
3. Lai MM. Molecular biologic and pathogenetic analysis of hepatitis delta virus. J Hepatol 1995; 22:127-131.
4. Lai MMC. The molecular biology of hepatitis delta virus. Annu Rev Biochem 1995; 64:259-286.
5. Poisson F, Roingeard P, Goudeau A. The hepatitis delta virus: A singular replication. M S-Med Sci 1995; 11:1379-1387.
6. Symons RH. Small catalytic RNAs. Annu Rev Biochem 1992; 61:641-671.
7. Symons RH. Plant pathogenic RNAs and RNA catalysis. Nucleic Acids Res 1997; 25:2683-2689.
8. Kos A, Dijkema R, Arnberg AC et al. The hepatitis delta (δ) virus possesses a circular RNA. Nature 1986; 323:558-560.
9. Wang KS, Choo QL, Weiner AJ et al. Structure, sequence and expression of the hepatitis delta (δ) viral genome [published erratum appears in Nature 1987; 328:456]. Nature 1986; 323:508-514.
10. MacNaughton TB, Gowans EJ, McNamara SP et al. Hepatitis delta antigen is necessary for access of hepatitis delta virus RNA to the cell transcriptional machinery but is not part of the transcriptional complex. Virology 1991; 184:387-390.
11. Fu TB, Taylor J. The RNAs of hepatitis delta virus are copied by RNA polymerase II in nuclear homogenates. J Virol 1993; 67:6965-6972.
12. Beard MR, MacNaughton TB, Gowans EJ. Identification and characterization of a hepatitis delta virus RNA transcriptional promoter. J Virol 1996; 70:4986-4995.
13. Casey JL, Gerin JL. Hepatitis D virus RNA editing: Specific modification of adenosine in the antigenomic RNA. J Virol 1995; 69:7593-7600.
14. Polson AG, Bass BL, Casey JL. RNA editing of hepatitis delta virus antigenome by dsRNA-adenosine deaminase. Nature 1996; 380:454-456.
15. Jeng KS, Su PY, Lai MM. Hepatitis delta antigens enhance the ribozyme activities of hepatitis delta virus RNA in vivo. J Virol 1996; 70:4205-4209.
16. Brazas R, Ganem D. A cellular homolog of hepatitis delta antigen: Implications for viral replication and evolution. Science 1996; 274:90-94.
17. Long M, de Souza SJ, Gilbert W. Delta-interacting protein A and the origin of hepatitis delta antigen. Science 1997; 276:824-825.
18. Jeng KS, Daniel A, Lai MM. A pseudoknot ribozyme structure is active in vivo and required for hepatitis delta virus RNA replication. J Virol 1996; 70:2403-2410.
19. Hsieh SY, Yang PY, Chu CM et al. Role of the ribozyme of hepatitis delta virus on the transcription after polyadenylation. Biochem Biophys Res Commun 1994; 205:864-871.
20. Tanner NK. The catalytic RNAs from hepatitis delta virus: Structure, function and applications. In: Dinter-Gottlieb G, ed. The Unique Hepatitis Delta Virus. Austin: R.G. Landes, 1995:11-31.

21. Been MD. Cis- and trans-acting ribozymes from a human pathogen, hepatitis delta virus. Trends Biochem Sci 1994; 19:251-256.
22. Been MD, Wickham GS. Self-cleaving ribozymes of hepatitis delta virus RNA. Eur J Biochem 1997; 247:741-753.
23. Branch AD, Robertson HD. Efficient trans cleavage and a common structural motif for the ribozymes of the human hepatitis delta agent. Proc Natl Acad Sci USA 1991; 88:10163-10167.
24. Gottlieb PA, Prasad Y, Smith JB et al. Evidence that alternate foldings of the hepatitis delta RNA confer varying rates of self-cleavage. Biochemistry 1994; 33:2802-2808.
25. Beattie TL, Collins RA. Identification of functional domains in the self-cleaving Neurospora VS ribozyme using damage selection. J Mol Biol 1997; 267:830-840.
26. Perrotta AT, Been MD. A pseudoknot-like structure required for efficient self-cleavage of hepatitis delta virus RNA. Nature 1991; 350:434-436.
27. Rosenstein SP, Been MD. Evidence that genomic and antigenomic RNA self-cleaving elements from hepatitis delta virus have similar secondary structures. Nucleic Acids Res 1991; 19:5409-5416.
28. Uhlenbeck OC. Keeping RNA happy. RNA 1995; 1:4-6.
29. Thill G, Vasseur M, Tanner NK. Structural and sequence elements required for the self-cleaving activity of the hepatitis delta virus ribozyme. Biochemistry 1993; 32:4254-4262.
30. Bravo C, Lescure F, Laugaa P et al. Folding of the HDV antigenomic ribozyme pseudoknot structure deduced from long-range photocrosslinks. Nucleic Acids Res 1996; 24:1351-1359.
31. Rosenstein SP, Been MD. Hepatitis delta virus ribozymes fold to generate a solvent-inaccessible core with essential nucleotides near the cleavage site phosphate. Biochemistry 1996; 35:11403-11413.
32. Rogers J, Chang AH, von Ahsen U et al. Inhibition of the self-cleavage reaction of the human hepatitis delta virus ribozyme by antibiotics. J Mol Biol 1996; 259:916-925.
33. Been MD, Perrotta AT. Optimal self-cleavage activity of the hepatitis delta virus RNA is dependent on a homopurine base pair in the ribozyme core. RNA 1995; 1:1061-1070.
34. Jeoung YH, Kumar PK, Suh YA et al. Identification of phosphate oxygens that are important for self-cleavage activity of the HDV ribozyme by phosphorothioate substitution interference analysis. Nucleic Acids Res 1994; 22:3722-3727.
35. Duhamel J, Liu DM, Evilia C et al. Secondary structure content of the HDV ribozyme in 95% formamide. Nucleic Acids Res 1996; 24:3911-3917.
36. Kolk MH, Heus HA, Hilbers CW. The structure of the isolated, central hairpin of the HDV antigenomic ribozyme: Novel structural features and similarity of the loop in the ribozyme and free in solution. EMBO J 1997; 16:3685-3692.
37. Kirsebom LA. RNase P—a 'Scarlet Pimpernel.' Mol Microbiol 1995; 17:411-20.
38. Saldanha R, Mohr G, Belfort M et al. Group I and group II introns. FASEB J 1993; 7:15-24.
39. Shakil AO, Hadziyannis S, Hoofnagle JH et al. Geographic distribution and genetic variability of hepatitis delta virus genotype I. Virology 1997; 234:160-167.
40. Lee CM, Changchien CS, Chung JC et al. Characterization of a new genotype II hepatitis delta virus from Taiwan. J Med Virol 1996; 49:145-154.
41. Casey JL, Brown TL, Colan EJ et al. A genotype of hepatitis D virus that occurs in northern South America. Proc Natl Acad Sci USA 1993; 90:9016-9020.
42. Krushkal J, Li WH. Substitution rates in hepatitis delta virus. J Mol Evol 1995; 41:721-726.
43. Perrotta AT, Been MD. Core sequences and a cleavage site wobble pair required for HDV antigenomic ribozyme self-cleavage. Nucleic Acids Res 1996; 24:1314-1321.
44. Tanner NK, Schaff S, Thill G et al. A three-dimensional model of hepatitis delta virus ribozyme based on biochemical and mutational analyses. Curr Biol 1994; 4:488-498.
45. Lai ME, Mazzoleni AP, Porru A et al. Unpublished 1995; accession number X85253.
46. Branch AD, Polaskova JA. 3-D models of the antigenomic ribozyme of the hepatitis delta agent with eight new contacts suggested by sequence analysis of 188 cDNA clones. Nucleic Acids Res 1995; 23:4180-4189.
47. Sakamoto T, Tanaka Y, Kuwabara T et al. Properties of hepatitis delta virus ribozyme, which consists of three RNA oligomer strands. J Biochem Tokyo 1997; 121:1123-1128.

48. Perrotta AT, Been MD. Cleavage of oligoribonucleotides by a ribozyme derived from the hepatitis delta virus RNA sequence. Biochemistry 1992; 31:16-21.
49. Fauzi H, Kawakami J, Nishikawa F et al. Analysis of the cleavage reaction of a trans-acting human hepatitis delta virus ribozyme. Nucleic Acids Res 1997; 25:3124-3130.
50. Zhou DM, Kumar PKR, Zhang LH et al. Ribozyme mechanism revisited: Evidence against direct coordination of a Mg^{2+} ion with the pro-R oxygen of the scissile phosphate in the transition state of a hammerhead ribozyme-catalyzed reaction. J Am Chem Soc 1996; 118:8969-8970.
51. Wu HN, Lai MM. Reversible cleavage and ligation of hepatitis delta virus RNA. Science 1989; 243:652-654.
52. Sharmeen L, Kuo MY, Taylor J. Self-ligating RNA sequences on the antigenome of human hepatitis delta virus. J Virol 1989; 63:1428-1430.
53. Rosenstein SP, Been MD. Self-cleavage of hepatitis delta virus genomic strand RNA is enhanced under partially denaturing conditions. Biochemistry 1990; 29:8011-8016.
54. Wu HN, Lai MM. RNA conformational requirements of self-cleavage of hepatitis delta virus RNA. Mol Cell Biol 1990; 10:5575-5579.
55. Lazinski DW, Taylor JM. Intracellular cleavage and ligation of hepatitis delta virus genomic RNA: Regulation of ribozyme activity by cis-acting sequences and host factors. J Virol 1995; 69:1190-1200.
56. Macnaughton TB, Wang YJ, Lai MM. Replication of hepatitis delta virus RNA: Effect of mutations of the autocatalytic cleavage sites. J Virol 1993; 67:2228-2234.
57. Wu TT, Netter HJ, Lazinski DW et al. Effects of nucleotide changes on the ability of hepatitis delta virus to transcribe, process, and accumulate unit-length, circular RNA. J Virol 1997; 71:5408-5414.
58. Lazinski DW, Taylor JM. Regulation of the hepatitis delta virus ribozymes: To cleave or not to cleave? RNA 1995; 1:225-233.
59. Negro F, Gerin JL, Purcell RH et al. Basis of hepatitis delta virus disease? Nature 1989; 341:111.
60. Been MD, Perrotta AT, Rosenstein SP. Secondary structure of the self-cleaving RNA of hepatitis delta virus: Applications to catalytic RNA design. Biochemistry 1992; 31: 11843-11852.
61. Prasad Y, Smith JB, Gottlieb PA et al. Deriving a 67-nucleotide trans-cleaving ribozyme from the hepatitis delta virus antigenomic RNA. Antisense Res Dev 1992; 2:267-277.
62. Wu HN, Wang YJ, Hung CF et al. Sequence and structure of the catalytic RNA of hepatitis delta virus genomic RNA. J Mol Biol 1992; 223:233-245.
63. Lescure F, Blumenfeld M, Thill G et al. Trans cleavage of RNA substrates by an HDV-derived ribozyme. Prog Clin Biol Res 1993; 382:99-108.
64. Lai YC, Lee JY, Liu HJ et al. Effects of circular permutation on the cis-cleavage reaction of a hepatitis delta virus ribozyme: Application to trans-acting ribozyme design. Biochemistry 1996; 35:124-131.
65. Kawakami J, Yuda K, Suh YA et al. Constructing an efficient trans-acting genomic HDV ribozyme. FEBS Lett 1996; 394:132-136.
66. Puttaraju M, Perrotta AT, Been MD. A circular trans-acting hepatitis delta virus ribozyme. Nucleic Acids Res 1993; 21:4253-4258.
67. Puttaraju M, Been MD. Circular ribozymes generated in *Escherichia coli* using group I self-splicing permuted intron-exon sequences. J Biol Chem 1996; 271:26081-26087.
68. Nishikawa F, Kawakami J, Chiba A et al. Selection in vitro of trans-acting genomic human hepatitis delta virus (HDV) ribozymes. Eur J Biochem 1996; 237:712-718.
69. Wu HN, Lee JY, Huang HW et al. Mutagenesis analysis of a hepatitis delta virus genomic ribozyme. Nucleic Acids Res 1993; 21:4193-4199.
70. Nishikawa F, Fauzi H, Nishikawa S. Detailed analysis of base preferences at the cleavage site of a trans-acting HDV ribozyme: A mutation that changes cleavage site specificity. Nucleic Acids Res 1997; 25:1605-1610.

71. Ferre-D'Amare AR, Doudna JA. Use of cis- and trans-ribozymes to remove 5' and 3' heterogeneities from milligrams of in vitro transcribed RNA. Nucleic Acids Res 1996; 24:977-978.
72. Chowrira BM, Pavco PA, McSwiggen JA. In vitro and in vivo comparison of hammerhead, hairpin, and hepatitis delta virus self-processing ribozyme cassettes. J Biol Chem 1994; 269:25856-25864.
73. Bridgen A, Elliott RM. Rescue of a segmented negative-strand RNA virus entirely from cloned complementary DNAs. Proc Natl Acad Sci USA 1996; 93:15400-15404.
74. Conzelmann KK, Schnell M. Rescue of synthetic genomic RNA analogs of rabies virus by plasmid-encoded proteins. J Virol 1994; 68:713-719.
75. Sidhu MS, Chan J, Kaelin K et al. Rescue of synthetic measles virus minireplicons: Measles genomic termini direct efficient expression and propagation of a reporter gene. Virology 1995; 208:800-807.
76. Pattnaik AK, Ball LA, LeGrone AW et al. Infectious defective interfering particles of VSV from transcripts of a cDNA clone. Cell 1992; 69:1011-1020.
77. Mei HY, Cui M, Sutton ST et al. Inhibition of self-splicing group I intron RNA: High-throughput screening assays. Nucleic Acids Res 1996; 24:5051-5053.
78. Deny P, Zignego AL, Rascalou N et al. Nucleotide sequence analysis of three different hepatitis delta viruses isolated from a woodchuck and humans. J Gen Virol 1991; 72:735-739.
79. Houghton M, Wang K-S, Choo Q-L et al. Hepatitis delta diagnostics and vaccines, their preparation and use. Patent 1988; EP 0251575-A1.
80. Kos T, Molijn A, van Doorn LJ et al. Hepatitis delta virus cDNA sequence from an acutely HBV-infected chimpanzee: Sequence conservation in experimental animals. J Med Virol 1991; 34:268-279.
81. Langon T, Pichoud C, Jamard C et al. Analysis of a hepatitis delta virus (HDV) isolate from the Central African Republic. Unpublished 1997; accession number AJ000558.
82. Makino S, Chang MF, Shieh CK et al. Molecular cloning and sequencing of a human hepatitis delta (δ) virus RNA. Nature 1987; 329:343-346.
83. Saldanha JA, Thomas HC, Monjardino JP. Cloning and sequencing of RNA of hepatitis delta virus isolated from human serum. J Gen Virol 1990; 71:1603-1606.
84. Chao YC, Chang MF, Gust I et al. Sequence conservation and divergence of hepatitis delta virus RNA. Virology 1990; 178:384-392.
85. Chao YC, Lee CM, Tang HS et al. Molecular cloning and characterization of an isolate of hepatitis delta virus from Taiwan. Hepatology 1991; 13:345-352.
86. Imazeki F, Omata M, Ohto M. Heterogeneity and evolution rates of delta virus RNA sequences. J Virol 1990; 64:5594-5599.
87. Imazeki F, Omata M, Ohto M. Complete nucleotide sequence of hepatitis delta virus RNA in Japan. Nucleic Acids Res 1991; 5439.
88. Kuo MY, Goldberg J, Coates L et al. Molecular cloning of hepatitis delta virus RNA from an infected woodchuck liver: Sequence, structure, and applications. J Virol 1988; 62:1855-1861.
89. Lee CM, Bih FY, Chao YC et al. Evolution of hepatitis delta virus RNA during chronic infection. Virology 1992; 188:265-273.
90. Liu S, Yi Y, Cong X et al. Molecular cloning and sequencing of a hepatitis delta antigen-coding cDNA from China. Ping Tu Hsueh Pao 1994; 9:15-22.
91. Lee CB, Lai YC, Ping YH et al. The importance of the helix 2 region for the cis-cleaving and trans-cleaving activities of hepatitis delta virus ribozymes. Biochemistry 1996; 35:12303-12312.

Section II
Expression and Delivery of Ribozymes

CHAPTER 4

Exogenous Delivery of Ribozymes

Mark A. Reynolds

Introduction

Hammerhead ribozymes are trans-acting, RNA-based molecules that specifically cleave target mRNA transcripts in the absence of protein-based cofactors or enzymes.[1,2] Over the past several years, considerable progress has been made in our laboratories toward the development of these molecules as therapeutic agents.[3] Chemically-modified (stabilized) hammerhead ribozymes are highly resistant to nuclease degradation while retaining catalytic cleavage rates that are similar to their parent, unmodified (all-ribo) versions.[4] These stabilized ribozymes specifically inhibit smooth muscle cell proliferation in culture,[5] prevent cytokine-stimulated (interleukin-1) expression of stromelysin mRNA in a rabbit-knee osteoarthritis model[6] and inhibit VEGF-stimulated angiogenesis in a rat cornea model.[7] For the two in vivo studies just listed, a single administration of the ribozyme in a saline vehicle permitted sufficient tissue trafficking and cellular uptake for activity to be observed in a dose-dependent manner.

The ability to observe pharmacodynamic effects with free (saline) ribozyme formulations in vivo is very important, since it provides us with a baseline for comparing alternative delivery technologies. Although the field of exogenous ribozyme delivery is still relatively new, there is a wealth of information pertaining to the delivery of antisense oligonucleotides and DNA that may be directly applicable to ribozymes. While this chapter will focus primarily on the exogenous delivery of synthetic hammerhead ribozymes, many of the drug delivery systems described below may also be applicable to plasmid-based ribozyme expression vectors.[8-10]

While local delivery of ribozymes is now emerging as clinically viable, sustained-release delivery systems offer the potential for enhanced potency and/or less frequent dosing. Furthermore, the development of drug carriers for systemic delivery would bring this technology to a much greater number of human diseases, including cancer.

Tissue Culture Studies

The study of cellular uptake in tissue culture is probably not applicable to in vivo pharmacokinetic modeling. For example, cell culture studies typically require drug carriers such as cationic lipids for uptake and efficacy,[11,12] whereas in vivo studies have shown that antisense oligonucleotides[13-19] and ribozymes[6,7,20] are efficacious in the absence of any carrier. Nevertheless, cell culture studies are an important first step toward identifying lead ribozymes against a given target sequence. Such studies have indicated that oligonucleotides enter cells primarily via pinocytotic or endocytotic mechanisms.[21-24] When fluorescent-tagged oligonucleotides are used, they can be observed inside the cell in the form of punctate

Ribozymes in the Gene Therapy of Cancer, edited by Kevin J. Scanlon and Mohammed Kashani-Sabet.
©1998 R.G. Landes Company.

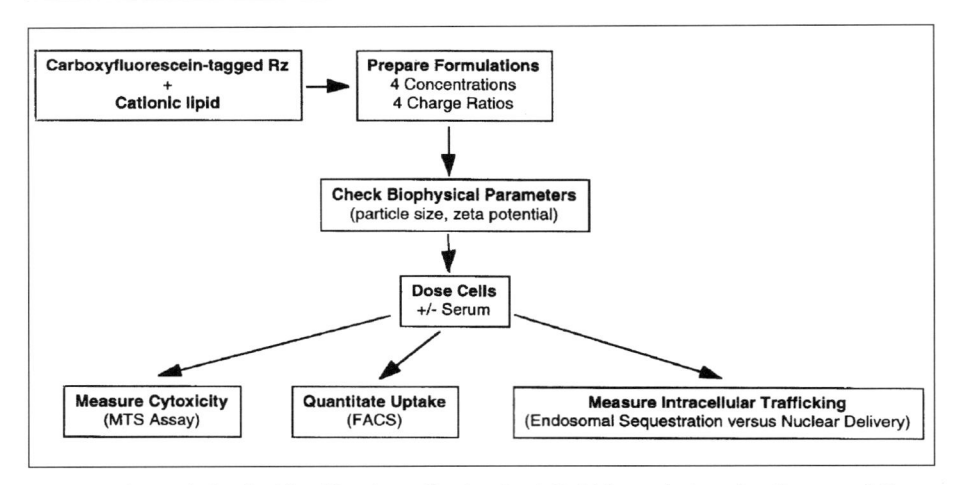

Fig. 4.1. Schematic for the identification of lead cationic lipid formulations for ribozyme delivery to a given cell type. A similar scheme can be used with other carriers (e.g., polycations, positively charged nanoparticles, etc.).

(presumably endosomal) bodies. Since the targets for antisense oligonucleotides and ribozymes reside in the cytoplasm and nucleus, many laboratories have focused on drug carriers that can mediate endosome release.

In order to identify lead formulations for ribozyme delivery in tissue culture, we have developed a screening method using fluorescent-tagged ribozymes that examines total cellular uptake, subcellular trafficking and cytotoxicity (Fig. 4.1). Microinjection experiments with fluorescent-tagged ribozyme show fairly rapid trafficking from the cytoplasm to the nucleus of the cell (typically within about 5 min after injection, unpublished data). Similar observations have been reported for antisense oligonucleotides.[25,26] Thus, we use nuclear fluorescence as a measure of the ability of a formulation to promote endosomal release. Total cellular uptake can be estimated by fluorescence activated cell sorting (FACS) analysis, using standardized fluorescent microbeads for calibration. This is a convenient method for estimating the efflux of ribozymes over time following a single treatment (Fig. 4.2). Finally, the cytotoxicity of the drug carrier/ribozyme complex is an important parameter that can be conveniently measured by colorimetric metabolic activity analysis (e.g., MTS assay). We find that drug carrier/ribozyme formulations can usually be optimized to reduce cytotoxicity (e.g., by varying the charge ratios in the case of cationic carriers).

Cationic Lipids

Cationic lipids are amphiphiles that contain a positively charged head group, for binding polynucleotides through charge interactions, and a hydrophobic domain capable of associating with membranes or lipid bilayers. A considerable number of these compounds have been described for the transfection of DNA plasmids,[27-29] oligonucleotides[11,12,30,31] and ribozymes.[5] Typically, cationic lipids are mixed with a fusogenic lipid such as dioleoyl phosphatidylethanolamine (DOPE), which is thought to promote endosome release.[32] It appears that cationic lipid complexes must enter the endosomal pathway for fusion to occur, and that binding to the cell surface is not sufficient for cytoplasmic release.[33,34] Perhaps one reason why so many different cationic lipids have been described is that lipids which work well for one cell type do not always work for another. Panels of cationic lipids have been described that enable the researcher to identify an optimal formulation for a given cell type.[29]

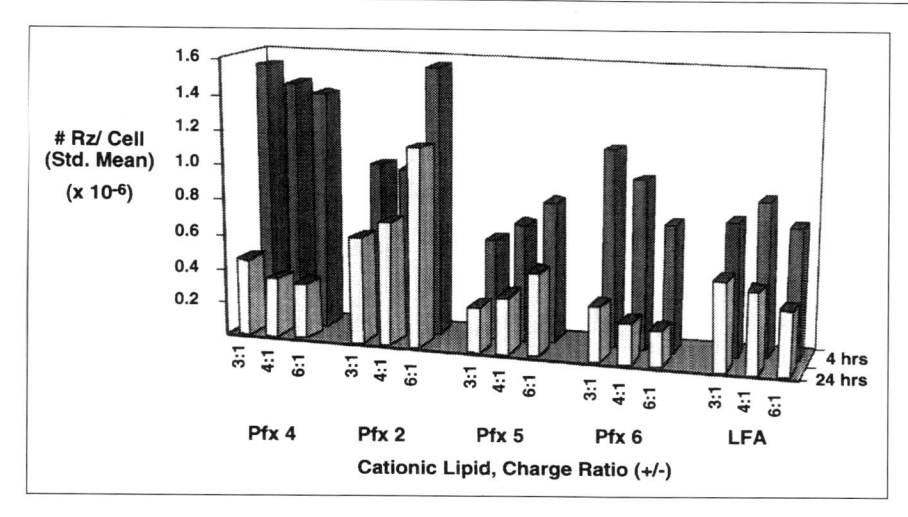

Fig. 4.2. Ribozyme delivery to human aortic smooth muscle cells in culture. Cells were treated with cationic lipid formulations as indicated, containing carboxyfluorescein-labeled ribozyme, for 4 h in serum-free media. For the t = 4 h timepoint, the cells were washed and assayed immediately for ribozyme internalization (based on fluorescence) using a FACScan instrument (Bectin-Dickinson). For the t = 24 h timepoint, the cells were washed and then incubated in serum-containing media for 20 h prior to analysis. The mean number of ribozymes internalized per cell was determined using fluorescent microbead standards for calibration (Molecular Probes, Inc.).

In our hands, the identification of lead cationic lipid reagents and the method by which they are complexed with ribozymes are equally important. For example, the charge ratio (+/−, molar ratio of cationic lipid to phosphodiester bonds) can dramatically affect the physical properties of the complex, as can the choice of cell culture media to use (Table 4.1). Cationic lipid/ribozyme complexes have a tendency to aggregate in solution, particularly in the presence of some types of cell culture media, which may adversely affect cellular uptake. The charge ratio can also affect the ability of the complex to get taken up by cells and to release the packaged ribozymes into the cytoplasm and nucleus (Fig. 4.3). Methods for characterizing and optimizing cationic lipid formulations have been described.[35] In particular, it is important to determine the size distribution of the complexes over time, since this is a measure of the tendency for a given lipid:ribozyme combination to aggregate during the treatment regimen.

Polycations

Polycations that have been used for oligonucleotide and DNA plasmid delivery include polylysines, polyethylenimine and polyamidoamine (PAMAM) dendrimers. These compounds condense polynucleotides to form small particles that are taken up by cells either through pinocytotic or endocytotic mechanisms.

Polylysines are known to promote cellular uptake, but lack an endosome-release mechanism. Various ligands such as transferrin,[36,37] glycosyl moieties[38] and folate[39,40] have been conjugated to polylysine to promote receptor-mediated uptake. In this case, it is important that the polylysine/oligonucleotide complexes are small (i.e., <120 nm) in order to enter clathrin-coated pits on the cell surface. Folate-conjugated polylysine has been used to deliver ribozyme multimers with some success.[40] Adenovirus[41,42] and fusogenic peptides[43] have

Table 4.1. Optimization of LipofectAMINE™:ribozyme formulations[a]

a) Effect of different culture media[b]

	T = 15 min		T = 2 h	
Media	Mean Diam. (nm)	Polydispersity	Mean Diam. (nm)	Polydispersity
IMDM	250	0.152	311	0.191
DMEM	639	0.392	3601	0.464
OptiMEM	694	0.432	3676	0.292

b) Effect of different charge ratios[c]

Charge Ratio	Mean Diam. (nm)	Polydispersity
2:1	1503	0.364
4:1	154	0.127
6:1	107	0.110
8:1	106	0.158

[a] LipofectAMINE™ was purchased from Life Technologies Inc. A stabilized hammerhead ribozyme was used having the sequence 5'-u$_s$u$_s$u$_s$u$_s$ccc*u* GAuGaggccgaaaggccGaaAuucucB-3', where lowercase letters refer to 2'-*O*-methyl modified bases; capital letters refer to unmodified ribonucleotides; s = phosphorothioate linkages; ***u*** = 2'-C-allyl modified uridine; B = inverted abasic residue. Samples were analyzed in a Malvern Zetasizer 4 laser light scattering device.
[b] 20 µM lipid concentration, room temperature.
[c] IMDM media, 20 µM lipid concentration, T = 15 min.

been coupled with polylysine formulations to enhance endosome release. A combination of receptor-ligands and fusogenic molecules may be required for optimal delivery. Major disadvantages of such formulations include their complexity and high cost.

Polyethylenimine (PEI) is an inexpensive reagent that has been shown to transfect plasmid DNA into cells with high efficiency.[44] Since endosomes are known to be acidic, it has been proposed that PEI becomes further protonated inside the endosome, resulting in an osmotic pressure gradient that promotes endosome release. PAMAM dendrimers are well-defined, uniform polymers that have also been shown to mediate DNA transfection and deliver oligonucleotides in cell culture.[45,46] We have tested both of these compounds with fluorescently-labeled ribozymes according to the protocol outlined in Figure 4.1, and have observed high levels of nuclear fluorescence for each reagent (typically >70% of the cells in a field for a given cell type, unpublished results).

pH-Sensitive Liposomes

A number of investigators have employed liposomes for the delivery of antisense oligonucleotides[47-52] and ribozymes[53,54] in cell culture. Most of this work has been conducted with small unilamellar vesicles (SUVs), which can be prepared in a size range sufficient for cellular uptake via endocytosis (<200 nm). Two principal drawbacks to this approach are:
1. low encapsulation efficiencies (typically <20%); and
2. the absence of an endosome-release mechanism.

Thus, the majority of internalized liposomes deliver their nucleic acid payload to the lysosome, rather than enabling release into the cytoplasm and nucleus.[51] pH-sensitive liposomes were developed to enhance endosome release by incorporating lipids with protonatable

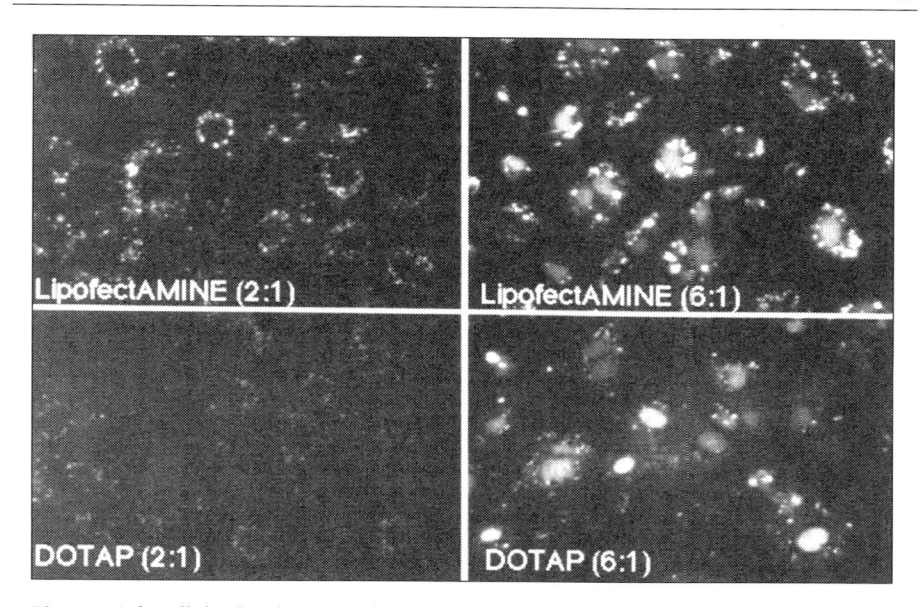

Fig. 4.3. Sub-cellular localization of internalized ribozymes. HeLa cells were treated with cationic lipid formulations, containing carboxyfluorescein-labeled ribozyme, for 2 h in serum-free media. The cells were washed and then examined by epifluorescence microscopy using a Nikon N200 microscope (40x objective) hooked up to a Hitachi HV-C20 CCD camera. The data was stored and processed using Adobe Photoshop.

head groups (e.g., oleic acid[51] and cholesterylhemisuccinate, or CHEMS[55]) together with a fusogenic lipid such as phosphatidylethanolamine. This approach enhances the cellular uptake and efficacy of antisense oligonucleotides in tissue culture.[48-50,52,53,55-61] Such studies have not yet been reported for ribozyme delivery.

Devices

Electroporation has been used in selected cases to deliver DNA plasmids and oligonucleotides into cells in culture.[62,63] A biolistic device (Gene Gun™, Bio-Rad Corporation) has recently been made available for research applications. When fully optimized, such devices could eventually offer some advantages compared to cationic lipids, e.g., by providing more general delivery protocols that can be applied to a variety of different cell types. At the present time, however, their utility is somewhat limited, since it is very difficult to achieve high levels of delivery without considerable cell death.

Localized Delivery In Vivo

There is considerable evidence in the literature that antisense oligonucleotides are active in vivo when administered as free (saline vehicle) formulations. Studies conducted in our laboratories have shown that stabilized hammerhead ribozymes are also active when administered locally as saline solutions. For example, a 2'-O-methyl modified ribozyme containing 2'-amino substitutions at U4 and U7 and five unmodified ribonucleotides was designed against stromelysin mRNA and evaluated in a rabbit knee arthritis model.[6] Intraarticular injections gave a dose-dependent inhibition of new stromelysin mRNA synthesis, stimulated by introduction of IL-1. A similar ribozyme targeted to the *flt*-1 VEGF

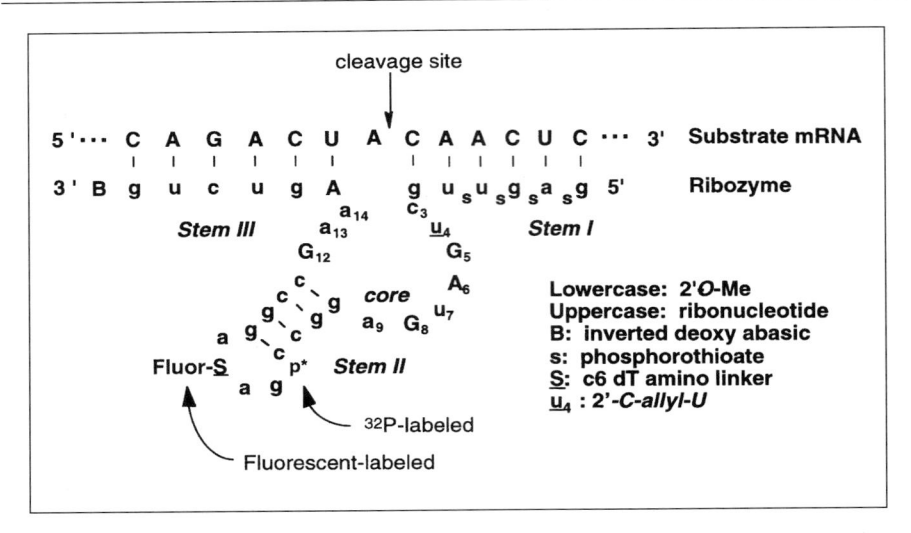

Fig. 4.4. Structure of a stabilized hammerhead ribozyme used in our laboratory for biodistribution experiments. As indicated in the figure, the ribozyme can be modified with either (a) an internal [^{32}P]-label (contains a 2'-O-methyl A residue in place of S); or (b) a fluorescent-label (non-radioactive).

receptor inhibited VEGF-stimulated neovascularization in a rat corneal implant model.[7] In this case, the ribozyme was delivered via an intracorneal implant and also by sub-conjunctival injection into the limbus. In one report from another laboratory, a 2'-O-allyl-modified hammerhead ribozyme containing five unmodified ribonucleotides showed good inhibition of amelogenin expression following a single injection into the jaw of newborn mice.[20]

These data suggest that the rate limiting steps for cellular uptake and trafficking of ribozymes in vivo are different from those observed in tissue culture. We have employed radiolabeled and fluorescently-labeled ribozymes to measure biodistribution and cellular uptake in vivo (Fig. 4.4). For radiolabeling, we typically use a kinase/ligation reaction that inserts an internal ^{32}P-phosphodiester bond in the Stem II region.[6] For fluorescent-labeling, we insert an aminolinker-modified base in the Stem II region and couple with N-hydroxysuccinimide-activated fluorescent probes (Molecular Probes, Inc.). Our data indicate that hammerhead ribozymes can transport into tissue and enter cells following localized administration as free (saline) solutions.

Trafficking of Free Ribozyme After Localized Administration

Intraarticular

The biodistribution of [^{32}P]-labeled ribozyme following a single intraarticular injection in rabbit knees has been described.[6] Tissues were harvested at 4 and 24 h post-administration in one experiment and at 1, 3 and 7 d post-administration in a second experiment. Synovial tissue was harvested and the amounts of total ribozyme accumulation were determined by scintillation counting. The percentage of intact (non-catabolized) ribozyme was determined by polyacrylamide gel electrophoresis. Peak concentrations of ribozyme accumulation were observed at 24 h, with approximately a 4-fold drop in synovial radioactivity at 7 d. The 4 h samples showed fully intact ribozyme (no ribozyme catabolites were observed); and the 24 h samples showed 80-90% intact ribozyme. Autoradiographic analysis of synovial tissue sections taken at 24 h indicated most of the ribozyme to be intracellular. This was confirmed subsequently using tetramethylrhodamine-labeled ribozyme (Fig. 4.5). Epifluorescence images showed most of the intracellular fluorescence to be in the form of punctate (presumably endosomal) bodies at 4 h, with more diffuse cytoplasmic fluorescence after 24 h. This data indicates that endosomal release of ribozymes in vivo may occur more rapidly than is typically observed in cell culture.

Intraocular

We have developed ribozymes targeting the VEGF receptors *flt*-1 and KDR as potential anti-angiogenic agents. A rat cornea implant model was developed to demonstrate the anti-angiogenic potential of these ribozymes.[7] A tetramethylrhodamine-labeled ribozyme was used to observe trafficking from the implant toward the targeted vascular endothelial cells of the pericorneal plexus. As shown in Figure 4.6, the ribozyme can indeed passage from the implant toward the targeted tissue and enter cells surrounding blood vessels. We conclude that tissue distribution and cellular uptake are not rate-limiting for hammerhead ribozymes in this model.

Delivery Systems for Localized Administration

Although very limited data is available at this time, it appears that ribozymes can traffic into tissue and enter target cells when administered locally. Drug delivery systems can potentially enhance ribozyme efficacy following localized administration. Such systems protect the encapsulated ribozyme from catabolic breakdown and provide sustained-release into surrounding tissues. The selection of lead drug delivery systems for preclinical development depends on the indication and route of administration. Again, biodistribution studies can be used for this screening process using fluorescent and/or radiolabeled ribozymes, provided that an adequate animal model is available.

Biodegradable polymers

Biodegradable polymers have been employed extensively for protein and peptide delivery.[64] Poly(L-lactic acid) (PLA) matrices have been shown to provide sustained-release for antisense oligonucleotides.[65] These materials also protect the encapsulated oligonucleotide from degradation in the presence of serum. Microbeads of PLA and poly(L-lactic-co-glycolic) acid (PLGA) can be prepared for localized administrations via a variety of different routes (e.g., intraarticular, intraocular, intratumoral, subcutaneous, etc.).

In our laboratory, we have found that modified hyaluronic acid and carboxymethylcellulose (Sepragel™ Bioresorbable Gel, Genzyme Corporation) is well-suited for intraarticular delivery of ribozymes.[66] Radiolabeled ribozyme was formulated in Sepragel™ and tested for biodistribution in the hind legs of male New Zealand rabbits following a single intraarticular injection. In vitro release studies showed an initial burst of ribozyme release over the first several hours (8-15%), followed by a more linear sustained release over the next three days (20-45%). A comparison of ribozyme accumulation in synovial tissue for free (saline) versus Sepragel™ formulation is shown in Table 4.2.

Nanoparticles

Polyalkylcyanoacrylate nanoparticles have been described for the delivery of antisense oligonucloctides via subcutaneous injection.[67] The oligonucleotides are adsorbed onto the surface of these particles via ionic interactions. The resulting complexes offer significant protection from nuclease degradation, even for unmodified oligonucleotides.[68] Biodistribution studies have shown that these particles rapidly accumulate in the liver

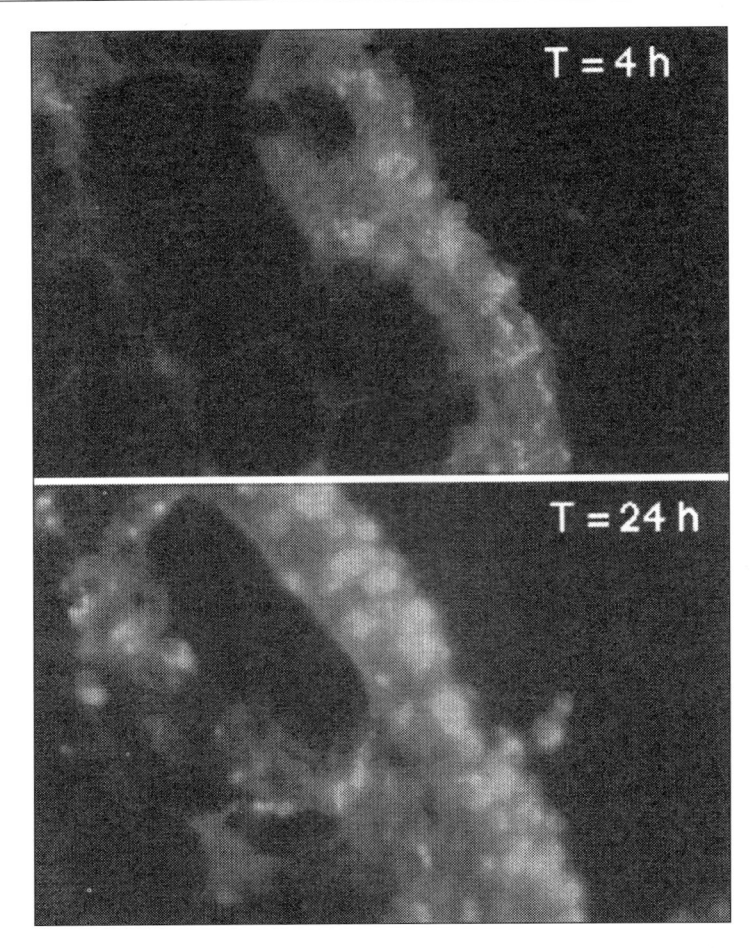

Fig. 4.5. Biodistribution of tetramethylrhodamine-labeled ribozyme in the rabbit knee synovium. Female New Zealand rabbits were treated with the ribozyme (50 µM in saline vehicle) by intraarticular injection. At the times indicated, the tissue was harvested and analyzed by epifluorescence microscopy. The intraarticular space is shown at the top right. Internalized ribozyme occurs in synoviocytes and is shown to passage below the surface layer and around fat cells. At t = 4 h, the intracellular fluorescence is predominantly punctate (presumably endosomes and lysosomes); at t = 24 h the fluorescence is more diffuse (presumably cytoplasmic).

Exogenous Delivery of Ribozymes 49

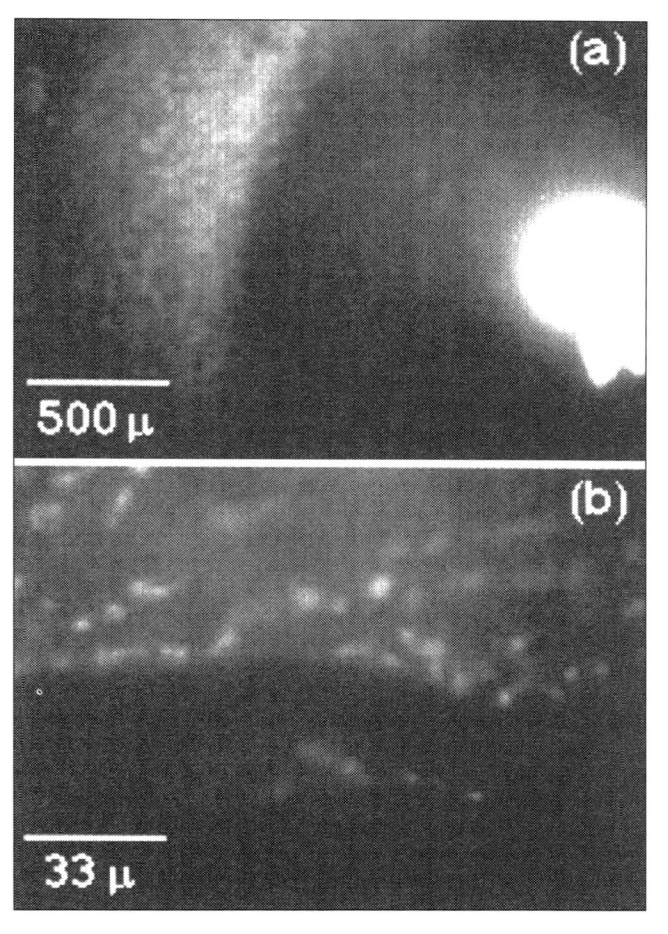

Fig. 4.6. Biodistribution of tetramethylrhodamine-labeled ribozyme in the rat cornea. A sterile nitrocellulose filter disc (0.5 mm diameter) was soaked in a solution containing the ribozyme and then surgically implanted into the cornea of a male Sprague-Dawley rat, approximately 3 mm from the pericorneal plexus. The tissue was then examined by epifluorescence microscopy approximately 24 post-implantation.

following intravenous administration in mice.[69] Thus, these drug carriers may be less well-suited for systemic delivery than for local delivery.

A novel type of nanoparticle that gives high encapsulation of oligonucleotides has recently been described, the SupraMolecular BioVector (SMBV).[70] These particles contain a positively charged polysaccharide core surrounded by a lipid bilayer consisting of phosphatidylcholine and cholesterol. Encapsulation is achieved by incubating the oligonuceotide with SMBV approximately 10°C below the phase-transition temperature of the outer membrane bilayer. SMBV nanoparticles protect oligonucleotides from nuclease degradation and enhance cell uptake in tissue culture.

Iontophoresis

Iontophoretic devices are available through a variety of different manufacturers for topical delivery of small molecules, peptides and proteins.[71-73] One such device is also being developed for gene transfer (E-TRANS™, Alza Corporation).

A recent study showed that a 2'-O-methyl modified hammerhead ribozyme containing a 2'-C-allyl modification at U4 and five unmodified ribonucleotides can be delivered locally into pig coronary arteries using an iontophoretic porous balloon catheter (e-Med,

Table 4.2. Biodistribution of [^{32}P]-labeled stabilized hammerhead ribozyme to rabbit knee synovium following intraarticular administration of saline or Sepragel^{TM} vehicle[a]

Formulation	Tissue	# Knees	Ribozyme delivered (ng/mg tissue)*
T = 24 Hrs			
Saline	Synovium	8	146 ± 51
Sepragel™ (Med)	Synovium	8	266 ± 79
T = 72 Hrs			
Saline	Synovium	6	82 ± 29
Sepragel™ (Med)	Synovium	6	190 ± 54

[a] Male New Zealand White Rabbits (3-4 kg) were anesthetized with ketamine-HCl and injected intraarticularly with about 200 x 10^6 cpm of [^{32}P]-internally labeled ribozyme together with unlabeled ribozyme corresponding to a total dose of 100 μg in a volume of 250 μl. At the indicated timepoints, tissues were harvested and total ratioactivity was determined by scintillation counting.

Inc.).[74] [^{3}H]-labeled ribozyme was prepared by exchange with tritiated water.[75] Arteries were treated according to the iontophoretic catheter manufacturer's recommendations and then sacrificed at various timepoints. Tissues were harvested and the amount of tritium accumulation in artery tissue was determined by scintillation counting (Table 4.3). Tetramethylrhodamine-labeled ribozyme was delivered similarly and shown to occur intracellularly based on epifluorescence and confocal microscopy measurements (data not shown).

Systemic Delivery

To date, there are no published pharmacodynamic studies of stabilized hammerhead ribozymes administered systemically. However, recent advances in large-scale oligonucleotide synthesis have made it possible to initiate such experiments. It is anticipated that this work will eventually enable stabilized ribozymes for the treatment of systemic diseases, including inflammatory diseases and cancers.

Plasma Pharmacokinetics of Stabilized Hammerhead Ribozymes

Plasma pharmacokinetic parameters were recently described in a rat model for a stabilized hammerhead ribozyme, containing 2'-O-allyl ribonucleotides except for eight unmodified ribonucleotides in the catalytic core.[76] 5'-carboxyfluorescein-labeled ribozyme was administered via a single tail vein injection at approximately 1.25 mg/kg. Intact ribozyme and ribozyme catabolites were quantitated after tissue digestion and processing by polyacrylamide gel electrophoresis. The tissue biodistribution data showed almost complete endonucleolytic cleavage after 48 h, presumably within the unmodified GAAA region. A biphasic plasma clearance profile was observed, with a distribution half life of 12 min and an elimination half life of 6.5 h.

Plasma pharmacokinetic studies have been conducted in our laboratory with a 2'-O-methyl modified hammerhead ribozyme containing a 2'-C-allyl sugar at the U4 position and five unmodified ribonucleotides in the catalytic core.[77] Plasma clearance profiles have been determined in mice following single bolus intravenous doses of up to 30 mg/kg. The plasma elimination half life in the mouse for this modified ribozyme is around 30 min. The major routes of elimination appear to be via renal filtration and catabolism. Thus, although

Table 4.3. Iontophoretic Delivery of [³H]-labeled stabilized ribozyme to pig coronary arteries[a]

Artery	Rz Remaining in the Tissue (per Wet Tissue Weight)		
	30 min	1 day	3 days
LAD	48 ng/mg	4.4 ng/mg	2.2 ng/mg
LCX	Untreated	3.2 ng/mg	2.4 ng/mg
RCA	37 ng/mg	Untreated	Untreated

[a] Juvenile domestic pigs (~25 kg) were anesthetized and the coronary arteries were instrumented under aseptic conditions via a femoral artery approach, under fluoroscopic guidance. Immediately after balloon angioplasty in each epicardial arterial segment the balloon catheter was removed and exchanged for the iontophoretic porous balloon catheter (e-Med, Inc.). The device was used according to the manufacturer's specifications to deliver the test oligonucleotide to each specified artery. One of the three arteries per heart (LAD, LCX or RCA) was left untreated for use as a control. Tissues were harvested at the times indicated and total radioactivity was determined by scintillation counting.

chemically modified ribozymes are highly stable in vitro in the presence of human serum, they are catabolized in vivo to some extent.

In both studies, stabilized ribozymes appear to be eliminated from plasma at much faster rates compared to phosphorothioate (PS) modified antisense oligonucleotides. Rat plasma half lives for PS oligonucleotides have been determined to be in the range of 34-53 h.[78-80] PS oligonucleotides are known to bind plasma proteins,[81] which presumably leads to longer plasma clearance profiles and protection from nuclease degradation. It is possible that ribozymes bind plasma proteins to a lesser extent and/or are more exposed to catabolic enzymes in plasma.

Drug Delivery Systems for the Systemic Administration of Ribozymes

A variety of approaches currently being investigated for the systemic delivery of antisense oligonucleotides may also be applicable to hammerhead ribozymes. Additionally, technologies being studied for non-viral gene transfer may also be suitable for ribozyme expression vectors. While many different routes of administration have been considered (i.e., intraperitoneal, oral, pulmonary, intravenous), most of our studies have been done via the intravenous route, since this gives complete and nearly instantaneous plasma exposure.

Bioconjugates

One potential method for increasing plasma circulation half life of a ribozyme is to increase its lipophilicity. For example, aliphatic moieties such as cholesterol have been conjugated to PS oligonucleotides and examined for biodistribution in the mouse.[82] Such modifications promote binding to low-density lipoproteins in the plasma, thereby preventing renal filtration and enhancing delivery to certain target organs such as the liver.[83] In one study, conjugation of cholesterol to an antisense PS oligonucleotide enhanced its biological activity in vivo.[84] One of the potential drawbacks to this approach is that the lipophilic moiety can adversely affect intracellular trafficking, causing the oligonucleotide to become sequestered in membrane compartments and preventing it from finding its intended mRNA target. Cleavable linkers have been proposed to release the oligonucleotide from its lipophilic carrier once inside the cell. For example, disulfide bonds can be cleaved after intracellular delivery with disulfide reductases or glutathione.[85] Biodegradable ester bonds have also been employed for release of a lipophilic 5'-palmitoyl moiety from an antisense oligonucleotide.[86]

Cationic lipids

Cationic lipids have been studied for systemic gene transfer.[31,50,51,87-91] As in the case of tissue culture studies, these compounds are thought to enhance transfection by promoting cell uptake and endosome release. However, blood components such as the complement system can associate with (opsonize) cationic lipid/DNA complexes, leading to rapid clearance by the mononuclear phagocytotic system (MPS).[92] Thus, many studies have shown high levels of exogenous gene expression in the lung, liver and spleen, yet it is unclear whether these genes are capable of reaching their intended target cells (e.g., Kupfer cells versus hepatocytes in the liver). The detailed physical analysis and optimization of cationic lipid/DNA complexes is leading toward improved transfection efficiencies, particularly for pulmonary delivery, (e.g., for the treatment of cystic fibrosis[93]). Nevertheless, further improvements will be useful to provide cationic lipid formulations that can be more effectively administered systemically and accumulate in target tissues such as metastatic cancers.

We have examined a simple cationic lipid formulation of 1,2-dioleoyl-3-trimethylammonium propane (DOTAP) with a 2'-O-methyl-modified hammerhead ribozyme containing a 2'-C-allyl modification at U4 and five unmodified ribonuclesides in the catalytic core.[94] One-to-one charge ratio formulations (positively charged lipid to phosphodiester bond) were made with [^{32}P]-labeled ribozyme and administered to BALB/c mice via a tail vein injection. Major organs were dissected at various timepoints, digested and quantitated by liquid scintillation counting. Aliquots were also analyzed by polyacrylamide gel electrophoresis to determine intact ribozyme and ribozyme catabolites. Representative data are shown in Figure 4.7. Unlike plasmid biodistribution data that is based on expression, these data indicate directly the tissue exposure of the ribozyme. Thus, cationic lipid formulations are capable of enhancing the tissue biodistribution of stabilized hammerhead ribozymes when administered systemically. However, ribozyme catabolism is observed in the tissues, although more rapid catabolism is seen in animals treated with the ribozyme in saline vehicle alone (no drug carrier). The plasma clearance profile for this DOTAP/ribozyme complex is shown in Figure 4.8. As anticipated, plasma clearance is fairly rapid, consistent with the tendency for cationic lipid/polynucleotide particles to become opsonized and removed by MPS tissues.

Long-circulating liposomes

Surface-modified (long-circulating) liposomes have emerged as powerful tools for modulating the pharmacokinetic profiles, resulting in increased therapeutic windows and/or new label indications for existing drugs such as doxorubicin (e.g., Kaposi's sarcoma) and amphotericin B (e.g., systemic fungal infections).[95-98] These modified liposomes are resistant to opsonization, thereby enabling them to circulate for long periods of time in the blood. This property enhances the ability of the encapsulated drug to get delivered to its intended target tissue. In particular, long-circulating liposomes have been found to selectively accumulate by extravasation into solid tumor tissue.[99-101] Thus, long-circulating liposomes may be particularly well-suited for use with novel, cytostatic antitumor drugs that are designed to inhibit angiogenesis.

Since the early 1970s, biodistribution studies of conventional liposomes following intravenous administration have shown rapid elimination from plasma into MPS tissues.[102] The various types of modifications that have been applied to enhance liposome circulation times have been reviewed elsewhere.[103,104] Examples include the incorporation of monosialoganglioside (GM1), sphingomyelin (SM) and phosphatidylinositol (PI). More recently, the

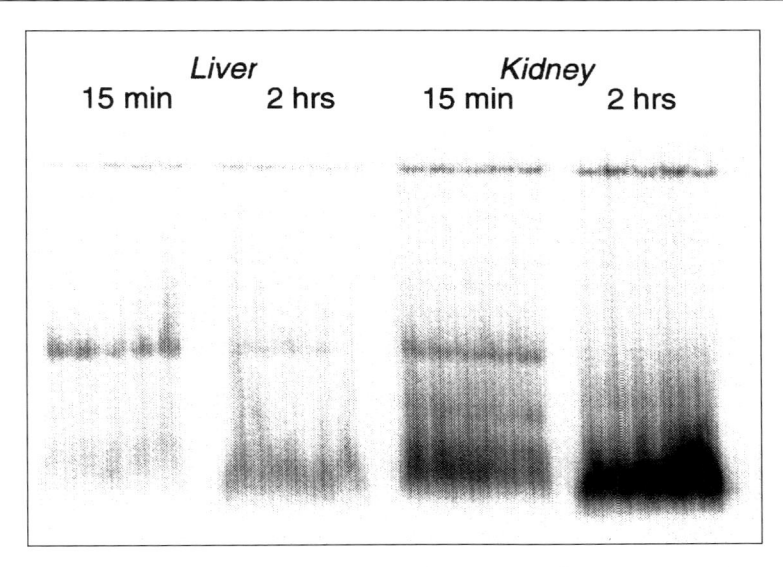

Fig. 4.7. Biodistribution of [^{32}P]-labeled ribozyme in Balb/c mice. A DOTAP-ribozyme formulation (1:1 charge ratio, containing 1-5 x 10^5 cpm of [^{32}P]-labeled ribozyme, 3 μmole total lipid dose) was administered via a single bolus tail vein injection. At the times indicated, animals were euthanized by CO$_2$ asphyxiation and then perfused with normal saline through the heart until the liver was cleared of blood (5-10 ml). The tissue samples were then pulverized or homogenized and digested with proteinase K-containing buffer (0.5% SDS/100 mM NaCl/10 mM Tris (pH 8.0)/25 mM EDTA/135 μg/ml proteinase K) at 50°C for 1 hour. Aliquots were removed and assayed for radioactivity using a Packard Model 2500 scintillation analyzer. Then, an equal volume of gel loading buffer (95% formamide/0.05% bromophenol blue/20 mM EDTA) was added and samples were electrophoresed on a 20% polyacrylamide/7 M urea/1 x TBE gel. Bands corresponding to intact ribozyme and ribozyme catabolites were detected and quantitated using a Molecular Dynamics Model 425E PhosphorImager.

incorporation of polymer-modified lipids have been used, particularly poly(ethylene glycol) (or PEG). PEG-modified lipids have been extensively studied in numerous liposome formulations and are now commercially available for research use. Theoretical calculations have shown that PEG polymers form a "brush" or steric barrier on the surfaces of liposomes.[103,105] PEG-modified liposomes are resistant to protein binding, and thereby are resistant to opsonization and removal from the blood by RES tissues.

The application of long-circulating liposome technology to gene transfer is currently being investigated in a number of laboratories, although few accounts have been described in the literature. Considerations for optimal delivery include methods to enhance encapsulation. Encapsulation efficiency is particularly important for ribozymes, which are still fairly costly to synthesize.

We have investigated several prototype liposome formulations for their effects on the biodistribution of stabilized hammerhead ribozymes in a murine Lewis lung carcinoma model.[106] [^{32}P]-labeled ribozyme was encapsulated by the reverse-evaporation method,[107] extruded to approximately 100 nm diameter using a Lipex extrusion device (Vancouver,

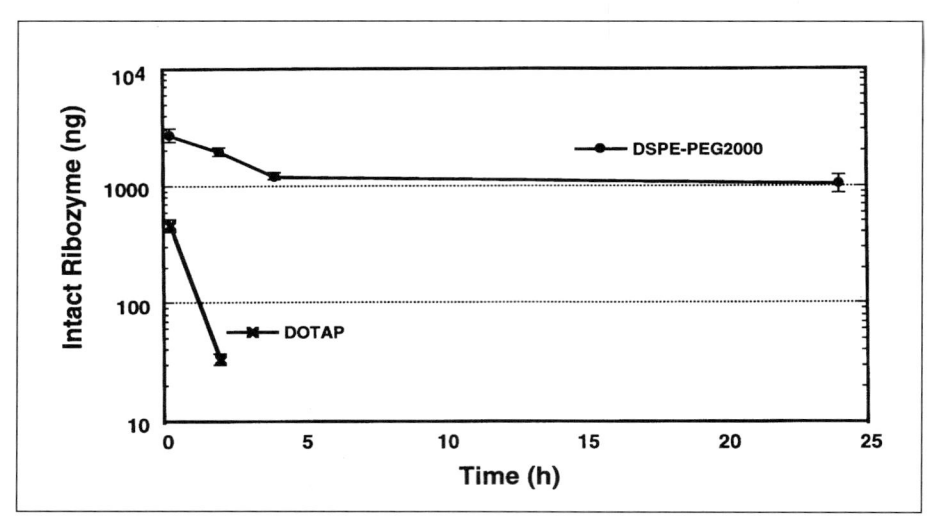

Fig. 4.8. Plasma distribution profiles for lipid-ribozyme formulations in Balb/c mice. DOTAP = simple cationic lipid complex of DOTAP and ribozyme (1:1 charge ratio); DSPE-PEG2000 = ribozyme encapsulated in liposomes containing egg yolk phosphatidylcholine, cholesterol, DOTAP and 1,2-disteroyl-phosphatidylethanolamine-PEG2000. Animals received a single dose of approximately 1 mg/kg ribozyme (containing 1-5 x 10^6 cpm [^{32}P]-labeled ribozyme, 3 μmol total lipid) via tail vein injection. At the indicated timepoints, animals were euthanized by CO$_2$ asphyxiation and blood was sampled from the heart. Total radioactivity was determined by scintillation counting and intact ribozyme was determined by PAGE analysis as described in Figure 4.7. Each data point represents the standard mean of n = 5 animals.

Canada), and purified by size-exclusion chromatography through Sepharose CL-4B. Intact ribozyme was determined by polyacrylamide gel electrophoresis, as described above. Typical plasma profiles are given in Figure 4.8. The most favorable formulation, based on plasma clearance data, was a liposome composition containing EYPC/Chol/DOTAP/DSPE-PEG2000. The cationic lipid DOTAP was included to enhance ribozyme encapsulation. According to our data, PEG-lipids are capable of masking the surface to protein binding, even in the presence of cationic lipids, thereby permitting enhanced encapsulation and long-circulating properties to be achieved simultaneously.

Bioerodible polymers

In a recent study, bioerodible polymer microspheres were shown to offer an oral delivery route for plasmid DNA.[108] The microbeads, consisting of poly(fumaric acid:sebacic acid), poly(FA:SA), were formulated with a DNA plasmid containing a bacterial gene for β-galactosidase. Rats fed the DNA-containing microspheres showed β-galactosidase expression in the small intestine and liver. Micrographs showed that the microparticles can traverse through the mucosal epithelium and follicle-associated epithelium. Such technologies may allow the oral delivery of oligonucleotides and ribozymes.

Future Applications

The technologies just described are only a small subset of the available drug delivery systems that may be applied to stabilized hammerhead ribozymes. It is anticipated that more data will become available in the near future as the cost of ribozyme production decreases due to current efforts in large-scale synthesis. Some of these systems may also be applied to stabilized ribozyme expression vectors.

Although the results from our preliminary pharmacokinetic studies are indicative of a fairly rapid plasma clearance profile for stabilized hammerhead ribozymes, it is anticipated that continuous infusion may lead to improved plasma and tissue biodistributions. Studies are currently in progress using sustained-delivery devices for intravenous, intraperitoneal, and intratracheal administration.

Targeted liposomes (immunoliposomes) are being developed for more selective delivery to diseased tissues.[109] For example, sterically stabilized anti-HER2 immunoliposomes have been designed for targeting to human breast cancers.[110] While such approaches have been shown to work in vitro, selective targeting in vivo remains to be demonstrated.

I am particularly intrigued by the possibility of applying long-circulating liposome technologies to ribozyme delivery. Based on similar studies, it appears likely that long-circulating liposomes may enhance ribozyme delivery to tumor tissue, and possibly to other neovascularized tissues such as occur in various inflammatory diseases. One of the key issues currently being addressed is ribozyme release, i.e., its ability to escape from the drug carrier and traffic into surrounding tissue and cells. As illustrated above, we have already generated data indicating that ribozymes can enter cells in vivo in the absence of any drug carrier. The utility of a drug carrier for ribozyme delivery relies on its ability to enhance tissue exposure and also to promote cellular uptake either directly or indirectly through sustained release. There is some evidence that liposomes are more rapidly degraded in tumor tissue compared to normal tissue, resulting in greater drug release in the former case.[111] Thus, long-circulating liposomes may be particularly well suited for exogenous ribozyme delivery in treating disseminated cancers. We are currently investigating this possibility in our laboratory using fluorescent-labeled ribozymes and histological examination with confocal microscopy.

References

1. Usman N, Beigelman L, McSwiggen JA. Hammerhead ribozyme engineering. Curr Opin Struct Biol 1996; 6:527-533.
2. Usman N, Stinchcomb DT. Design, synthesis, and function of therapeutic hammerhead ribozymes. Nucleic Acids Mol Biol 1996; 10:243-264.
3. Christoffersen RE, Marr JJ. Ribozymes as human therapeutic agents. J Med Chem 1995; 38(12):2023-37.
4. Beigelman L, McSwiggen JA, Draper KG et al. Chemical modification of hammerhead ribozymes. J Biol Chem 1995; 27:25702-25708.
5. Jarvis TC, Alby LJ, Beaudry AA et al. Inhibition of vascular smooth muscle cell proliferation by ribozymes that cleave c-*myb* mRNA. RNA 1996; 2:419-428.
6. Flory CM, Pavco PA, Jarvis TC et al. Nuclease-resistant ribozymes decrease stromelysin mRNA levels in rabbit synovium following exogenous delivery to the knee joint. Proc Natl Acad Sci USA 1996; 93(2):754-8.
7. Cushman C, Escobedo J, Parry TJ et al. Ribozyme inhibition of VEGF-mediated endothelial cell proliferation in cell culture and VEGF-induced angiogenesis in a rat corneal model. Angiogenesis Inhibitors and other novel therapeutic strategies for Ocular Diseases of Neovascularization. Boston, MA: IBC USA Conferences, 1996.
8. Thompson JD, Macejak D, Couture L, Stinchcomb DT. Ribozymes in gene therapy. Nature Med 1995; 1(3):277-8.
9. Ohkawa J, Taira K. Possibility for gene therapy by ribozyme RNA. Igaku no Ayumi 1995; 175(9):638-41.
10. Wong-Staal F. Ribozyme gene therapy for HIV infection intracellular immunization of lymphocytes and CD34+ cells with an anti-HIV-1 ribozyme gene. Adv Drug Delivery Rev 1995; 17(3):363-8.

11. Bennett CF, Chiang M-Y, Chan H et al. Cationic lipids enhance cellular uptake and activity of phosphorothioate antisense oligonucleotides. Mol Pharmacol 1992; 41:1023-33.
12. Bennett CF, Chiang M-Y, Chan H, Grimm S. Use of cationic lipids to enhance the biological activity of antisense oligonucleotides. J Liposome Res 1993; 3(1):85-102.
13. Dean NM, McKay R. Inhibition of protein kinase C-α expression in mice after systemic administration of phosphorothioate antisense oligodeoxynucleotides. Proc Natl Acad Sci USA 1994; 91:11762-11766.
14. Dean N, McKay R, Miraglia L et al. Inhibition of growth of human tumor cell lines in nude mice by an antisense oligonucleotide inhibitor of protein kinase C-α expression. Cancer Res 1996; 56:3499-3507.
15. Haller H, Dragun D, Miethke A et al. Antisense oligonucleotides for ICAM-1 attenuate reperfusion injury and renal failure in the rat. Kidney Interntl 1996; 50:473-480.
16. Monia BP, Johnston JF, Geiger T, Muller M, Fabbro D. Antitumor activity of a phosphorothioate antisense oligodeoxynucleotide targeted against C-raf kinase. Nature Med 1996; 2:668-675.
17. Nyce JW, Metzger WJ. DNA antisense therapy for asthma in an animal model. Nature 1997; 385:721-725.
18. Rubenstein M, Mirochnik Y, Chou P, Guinan P. Antisense oligonucleotide intralesional therapy for human PC-3 prostate tumors carried by athymic nude mice. J Surgical Oncol 1996; 62:194-200.
19. Yazaki T, Ahmad S, Chahlavi A et al. Treatment of glioblastoma U-87 by systemic administration of an antisense protein kinase C-α phosphorothioate oligodeoxynucleotide. Molecular Pharmacol 1996; 50:236-242.
20. Lyngstadaas SP, Risnes S, Sproat BS, Thrane PS, Prydz HP. A synthetic, chemically stabilized modified ribozyme eliminates amelogenin, the major translation product in developing mouse enamel in vivo. EMBO J 1995; 14:5224-5229.
21. Nakai D, Seita T, Tetsuya T et al. Cellular uptake mechanism for oligonucleotides: Involvement of endocytosis in the uptake of phosphodiester oligonucleotides by a human colorectal adenocarcinoma cell line, HCT-15. J Pharmacol and Exp Ther 1996; 278:1362-1372.
22. Beltinger C, Saragovi HU, Smith RM et al. Binding, uptake, and intracellular trafficking of phosphorothioate-modified oligodeoxynucleotides. J Clin Invest 1995; 95:1814-1823.
23. Shoji Y, Akhtar S, Periasamy A, Herman B, Juliano RL. Mechanism of cellular uptake of modified oligodeoxynucleotides containing methylphosphonate linkages. Nucleic Acids Res 1991; 19(20):5543-5550.
24. Stein CY, Tonkinson JL, Zhang L-M et al. Dynamics of the internalization of phosphodiester oligodeoxynucleotides in HL60 cells. Biochemistry 1993; 32:4855-4861.
25. Fisher TL, Terhorst T, Cao X, Wagner RW. Intracellular disposition and metabolism of fluorescently-labeled unmodified oligonucleotides microinjected into mammalian cells. Nucleic Acids Res 1993; 21:3857-3865.
26. Leonetti JP, Mechit N, Degols G, Gagnor C, Lebleu B. Intracellular distribution of microinjected AS oligonucleotides. Proc Natl Acad Sci USA 1991; 88:2702-2706.
27. Remy J-S, Sirlin C, Vierling P, Behr J-P. Gene transfer with a series of lipophilic DNA-binding molecules. Bioconjugate Chem 1994; 5:647-654.
28. van der Woude I, Wagenaar A, Meekel AAP et al. Novel pyridinium surfactants for efficient, nontoxic in vitro gene delivery. Proc Natl Acad Sci USA 1997; 94:1160-1165.
29. Griffiths T, Russell M, Froning K et al. The PerFect(TM) lipid optimizer kit for maximizing lipid-mediated transfection of eukaryotic cells. BioTechniques 1997; 22(5):982-988.
30. Capaccioli S, DiPasqual G, Mini E, Mazzei T, Quattrone A. Cationic lipids improve antisense oligonucleotide uptake and prevent degradation in cultured calls and in human serum. Biochem Biophys Res Commun 1993; 197:818-25.
31. Lappalainen K, Urtti A, Jääkeläinen I, Syrjänen K, Syrjänen S. Cationic liposomes mediated delivery of antisense oligonucleotides targeted to HPV 16 E7 mRNA in CaSki cells. Antiviral Res 1994; 23:119-30.

32. Farhood H, Serbina N, Huang L. The role of dioleoyl phosphatidylethanolamine in cationic liposome mediated gene transfer. Biochim Biophys Acta 1995; 1235:289-295.
33. Zabner J, Fasbender AJ, Moninger T, Poellinger KA, Welsh MJ. Cellular and molecular barriers to gene transfer by a cationic lipid. J Biol Chem 1995; 270:18997-19007.
34. Wrobel I, Collins D. Fusion of cationic liposomes with mammalian cells occurs after endocytosis. Biochim Biophys Acta 1995; 1995:296-304.
35. Eastman S, Siegel C, Tousignant J, Smith A, Cheng S, Scheule R. Biophysical characterization of cationic lipid: DNA complexes. Biochim Biophys Acta 1997; 1325:41-62.
36. Wagner E, Cotten M, Mechtler K, Kirlappos H, Birnstiel ML. DNA-binding transferrin conjugates as functional gene-delivery agents: Synthesis by linkage of polylysine or ethidium homodimer to the transferrin carbohydrate moiety. Bioconjugate Chem 1991; 2:226.
37. Wagner E, Cotten M, Foisner R, Birnstiel ML. Transferrin-polycation-DNA complexes: The effect of polycations on the structure of the complex and DNA delivery to cells. Proc Natl Acad Sci USA 1991; 88:4255-4259.
38. Erbacher P, Roche A, Monsigny M, Midoux P. glycosylated polylysine/DNA complexes: Gene transfer efficiency in relation with the size and the sugar substitution level of glycosylated polylysines and with the plasmid size. Bioconjugate Chem 1995; 6:401-410.
39. Citro G, Szcylik C, Ginobbi P, Zupi G, Calabretta B. Inhibition of leukaemia cell proliferation by folic acid-polylysine-mediated introduction of c-*myb* antisense oligodeoxynucleotides into HL-60 cells. Proc Natl Acad Sci USA 1993:463-467.
40. Leopold LH, Shore SK, Newkirk TA, Reddy RMV, Reddy EP. Multi-unit ribozyme-mediated cleavage of bcr-abl mRNA in myeloid leukemias. Blood 1995; 85(8):2162-70.
41. Curiel DT, Agarwal S, Wagner E, Cotten M. Adenovirus enhancement of transferrin-polylysine-mediated gene delivery. Proc Natl Acad Sci USA 1991; 88:8850-4.
42. Wagner E, Zatloukal K, Cotten M et al. Coupling of adenovirus to transferrin-polylysine/DNA complexes greatly enhances receptor-mediated gene delivery and expression of transfected genes. Proc Natl Acad Sci USA 1992; 89:6099-6103.
43. Plank C, Oberhauser B, Mechtler K, Koch C, Wagner E. The influence of endosome-disruptive peptides on gene transfer using synthetic virus-like gene transfer systems. J Biol Chem 1994; 269:12918-12924.
44. Boussif O, Lezoualc'h F, Zanta MA et al. A versatile vector for gene and oligonucleotide transfer into cells in culture and in vivo: Polyethyenimine. Proc Natl Acad Sci USA 1995; 92:7297-7301.
45. Bielinska A, Kukowska-Latallo JF, Johnson J, Tomalia DA, Baker JRJ. Regulation of in vitro gene expression using antisense oligonucleotides or antisense expression plasmids transfected using starburst PAMAM dendrimers. Nucleic Acids Res 1996; 24:2176-2182.
46. Haensler J, Szoka FCJ. Polyamidoamine cascade polymers mediate efficient transfection of cells in culture. Bioconjugate Chem 1993; 4:372-379.
47. Leonetti JP, Machy P, Degols G, Lebleu B, Leserman L. Antibody-targeted liposomes containing oligodeoxyribonucleotides complementary to viral RNA selectively inhibit viral replication. Proc Natl Acad Sci USA 1990; 87:2448-51.
48. Ropert C, Malvy C, Couvreur P. Inhibition of the Friend retrovirus by antisense oligonucleotides encapsulated in liposomes: Mechanism of action. Pharm Res 1993; 10:1427-33.
49. Zelphati O, Zon G, Leserman L. Inhibition of HIV-1 Replication in cultured cells with antisense oligonucleotides encapsulated in immunoliposomes. Antisense Res Dev 1993; 3:323-38.
50. Thierry AR, Dritshilo A. Intracellular availability of unmodified, phosphorothioated and liposomally encapsulated oligodeoxynucleotides for antisense activity. Nucleic Acids Res 1992; 20(21):5691-5698.
51. Staubinger RM, Papahadjopoulos D. Liposomes as carriers for intracellular delivery of nucleic acids. Methods Enzymol 1983; 101:512-527.
52. Thierry AR, Rahman A, Dritshilo A. Liposomal delivery as a new approach to transport of antisense oligonucleotides. In: Izant RP, ed. Gene Regulation: Biology of Antisense RNA and DNA. New York: Raven Press, Ltd., 1992:147-161.
53. Chonn A, Cullis PR. Recent advances in liposomal drug-delivery systems. Current Opinion Biotechnol 1995; 6:698-708.

54. Sullivan SM. Liposome-mediated uptake of ribozymes. METHODS: A Companion to Methods in Enzymology 1993; 5:61-66.
55. Chu C-J, Dijkstra J, Lai M-Z, Hong K, Szoka F. Efficiency of cytoplasmic delivery by pH-sensitive liposomes to cells in culture. Pharm Res 1990; 7(8):824-834.
56. Connor J, Yatvin M, Huang L. pH-sensitive liposomes: Acid-induced liposome fusion. Proc Natl Acad Sci USA 1984; 81:1715-1718.
57. Collins D, Litzinger D, Huang L. Structural and functional comparisons of pH-sensitive liposomes composed of phosphatidylethanolamine and three different diacylsuccinylglycerols. Biochim Biophys Acta 1989; 1025:234-242.
58. Ropert S, Lavignon M, Dubernet C, Couvreur P, Malvy C. Oligonucleotides encapsulated in pH sensitive liposomes are efficient toward Friend retrovirus. Biochem Biophys Res Commun 1992; 183:879-85.
59. Straubinger R. pH-Sensitive liposomes for delivery of macromolecules into cytoplasm of cultured cells. Methods Enzymol 1993; 221:361-376.
60. Wang S, Lee RJ, Cauchon G, Gorenstein DG, Low PS. Delivery of antisense oligonucleotides against the human epidermal growth factor receptor into cultured KB cells with liposomes conjugated to folate via polyethylene glycol. Proc Natl Acad Sci USA 1995; 92:3318-3322.
61. Loke SL, Stein C, Zhang X, Avigan M, Cohen J, Neckers LM. Delivery of c-*myc* antisense phosphorothioate oligodeoxynucleotides to hematopoietic cells in culture by liposome fusion: Specific reduction in c-*myc* protein expression correlates with inhibition of cell growth and DNA synthesis. Current Topics in Microbiol and Immunol 1988; 141:282-289.
62. Bergan R, Connell Y, Fahmy B, Neckers L. Electroporation enhances c-myc antisense oligodeoxynucleotide efficacy. Nucleic Acids Res 1993; 21:3567-3573.
63. Rabinowitz J, Magnuson T. Independent gene targeting by coelectroporation of multiple vectors. Anal Biochem 1995; 228:180-182.
64. Gombotz W, Pettit D. Biodegradable polymers for protein and peptide drug delivery. Bioconjugate Chem 1995; 6:332-351.
65. Lewis KJ, Irwin WJ, Akhtar S. Biodegradable poly(L-lactic acid) matrices for the sustained delivery of antisense oligonucleotides. J Controlled Release 1995; 37:173-183.
66. Min J, Bouhana K, Jensen K et al. Sepragel(TM) enhances the biodistribution of hammerhead ribozymes in a rabbit knee model of osteoarthritis. 1996 (manuscript in preparation).
67. Schwab B, Chavany C, Duroux I et al. Antisense oligonucleotides adsorbed to polyalkylcyanoacrylate nanoparticles specifically inhibit mutated Ha-*ras*-mediated cell proliferation and tumorigenicity in nude mice. Proc Natl Acad Sci USA 1994; 91:10460-10464.
68. Chavany C, Saison-Behmoaras T, Le Doan T et al. Adsorption of oligonucleotides onto polyisohexylcyanoacrylate nanoparticles protects them against nucleases and increases their cellular uptake. Pharm Res 1994; 11:1370-1378.
69. Nakada Y, Fattal E, Foulquier M, Couvreur P. Pharmacokinetics and biodistribution of oligonucleotides adsorbed onto poly(isobutylcyanoacrylate) nanoparticles after intravenous administration in mice. Pharm Res 1996; 13:38-43.
70. Berton M, Sixou S, Kravtzoff R et al. Improved oligonucleotide uptake and stability by a new drug carrier, the SupraMolecular Bio Vector (SMBV). Biochim Biophys Acta 1997; 1355:7-19.
71. Green PG. Iontophoretic delivery of peptide drugs. J Controlled Release 1996; 41:33-48.
72. Sage BH Jr. Insulin iontophoresis. Pharm Biotechnol 1997; 10:319-341.
73. Singh J, Bhatia KS. Topical iontophoretic drug delivery: pathways, principles, factors, and skin irritation. Med Res Rev 1996; 16:285-296.
74. Robinson KA, Chronos NAF, Kleinman ME et al. Local delivery of c-*myb* ribozymes to coronary arteries of pigs using an iontophoretic catheter. 1997 (manuscript in preparation).
75. Graham MJ, Freier SM, Crooke RM, Ecker DJ, Maslova RN, Lesnik EA. Tritium labeling of antisense oligonucleotides by exchange with tritiated water. Nucleic Acids Res 1993; 21:3737-3743.

76. Desjardins JP, Sproat BS, Beijer B et al. Pharmacokinetics of a synthetic, chemically modified hammerhead ribozyme against the rat cytochrome P-450 3A2 mRNA after single intravenous injections. J Pharmacol Exp Ther 1996; 278(3):1419-1427.
77. Sandberg JA, Agrawal A, Bouhana K et al. Pharmacokinetics of an anti-FLT ribozyme (RPI.4610) in normal and tumor bearing mice after daily bolus or continuous intravenous infusion. Oligonucleotide & Gene Therapy Based Antisense Therapeutics with New Application for Genomics. San Diego, CA: IBC USA Conferences, 1997.
78. Cossum PA, Truong L, Owxens SR, Markham PM, Shea JP, Crooke S. Pharmacokinetics of a ^{14}C-labeled phosphorothioate oligonucleotide ISIS 2105 after intradermal administration in rats. J Pharmacol Exp Ther 1994; 269:89-94.
79. Agrawal S, Temsamani J, Galbraith W, Tang JY. Pharmacokinetics of antisense oligonucleotides. Clin Pharmacokinet 1995; 28:7-16.
80. Iversen PL, Mata J, Tracewell WG, Zon G. Pharmacokinetics of an antisense phosphorothioate oligodeoxynucleotide against rev from human immunodeficiency virus type 1 in the adult male rat following single injections and continuous infusion. Antisense Res Devel 1994; 4:43-52.
81. Bennet CF, Dean N, Ecker DJ. Pharmacology of antisense therapeutic agents. In: Agrawal S, ed. Methods in Molecular Medicine: Antisense Therapeutics. Totowa, NJ: Humana Press, 1994:13-46.
82. Crooke S, Graham M, Zuckerman J et al. Pharmacokinetic properties of several novel oligonucleotide analogs in mice. Journal Pharmacol Exp Ther 1996; 277(2):923-937.
83. Firestone RA. Low-density lipoprotein as a vehicle for targeting antitumor compounds to cancer cells. Bioconjugate Chem 1994; 5:105-113.
84. Desjardins J, Mata J, Brown T et al. Cholesterol-conjugated phosphorothioate oligodeoxynucleotides modulate CYP2B1 expression in vivo. J Drug Targeting 1995; 2:477-485.
85. Boutorine AS, Kostina EV. Reversible covalent attachment of cholesterol to oligodeoxynucleotides for studies of the mechanisms of their penetration into eucaryotic cells. Biochimie 1993; 75:34-41.
86. Polushin NN, Cohen JS. Antisense pro-drugs: 5'-ester oligodeoxynucleotides. Nucleic Acids Res 1994; 22:5492-5496.
87. Thierry AR, Rabinovich P, Peng B et al. Characterization of liposome-mediated gene delivery: Expression, stability and pharmacokinetics of plasmid DNA. Gene The 1997; 4:226-287.
88. Liu Y, Mounkes LC, Liggitt HD et al. Factors influencing the efficiency of cationic liposome-mediated intravenous gene delivery. Nature Biotechnol 1997; 15:167-173.
89. Liu Y, Liggitt D, Zhong W et al. Cationic liposome-mediated intravenous gene delivery. J Biol Chem 1995; 270(42):24864-24870.
90. Thierry AR, Lunardi-Iskandar Y, Bryant JL et al. Systemic gene therapy: Biodistribution and long-term expression of a transgene in mice. Proc Natl Acad Sci USA 1995; 92:9742-9746.
91. Stewart MJ, Plautz GE, Del Buono L et al. Gene transfer in vivo with DNA-liposome complexes: Safety and acute toxicity in mice. Human Gene Ther 1992; 3:267-275.
92. Plank C, Mechtler K, Szoka FJ, Wagner E. Activaton of the complement system by synthetic DNA complexes: A potential barrier for intravenous gene delivery. Human Gene Ther 1996; 7:1437-1446.
93. Lee E, Marshall J, Siegel C et al. Detailed analysis of structures and formulations of cationic lipids for efficient gene transfer to the lung. Human Gene Ther 1996; 7:1701-1717.
94. Sandberg JA, Min JJ, Jensen KL et al. Lipid-based carriers enhance biodistribution and efficacy of an anti-angiogenic ribozyme in a murine Lewis lung carcinoma model. 1998 (submitted).
95. Hartsel S, Bolard J. Amphotericin B: New life for an old drug. Trends Pharmacol Sci 1996; 17:445-449.
96. Janknegt R. Liposomal formulations of cytotoxic drugs. Support Care Cancer 1996; 4:298-304.

97. Leenders AC, de Marie S. The use of lipid formulations of amphotericin B for systemic fungal infections. Leukemia 1996; 10:1570-1575.
98. Working PK, Dayan AD. Pharmacological-toxicological expert report CAELIX(TM) (Stealth(TM) Liposomal Doxorubicin HCl). Human & Experimental Toxicol 1996; 15:752-785.
99. Wu N, Da D, Rudoll T, Needham D, Whorton A, Dewhirst M. Increased microvascular permeability contributes to preferential accumulation of stealth liposomes in tumor tissue. Cancer Res 1993; 53:3765-3770.
100. Unezaki S, Murayama K, Hosoda J-I et al. Direct measurement of the extravasation of polyethyleneglycol-coated liposomes into solid tumor tissue by in vivo florescence microscopy. Intl J Pharm 1996; 144:11-17.
101. Lasic DD, Papahadjopoulos D. Liposomes revisited. Science 1995; 267:1275-1276.
102. Hwang KJ, Beaumier PL. Partial interaction of liposomes with the biological milieu. In: Gregoriadis G, ed. Liposomes as Drug Carriers—Recent Trends and Progress. New York: Wiley, 1988:19-34.
103. Lasic DD, Needham D. The "stealth" liposome: A prototypical biomaterial. Chemical Reviews 1995; 95(8):2601-2627.
104. Woodle M. Surface-modified liposomes: Assessment and characterization for increased stability and prolonged blood circulation. Chem Phys Lipids 1993; 64:249-262.
105. Torchilin VP, Omelyanenko VG, Papisov MI et al. Poly(ethylene glycol) on the surface: On the mechanism of polymer-coated liposome longevity. Biochim Biophys Acta 1994; 1195:11-20.
106. Min J, Jensen K, Bouhana K et al. Long-circulating liposomes enhance the pharmacokinetics of hammerhead ribozymes in a murine Lewis lung cancer model. 1997 (manuscript in preparation).
107. Szoka F, Papahadjopolous D. Procedure for preparation of liposomes with large internal aqueous space and high capture by reverse-phase evaporation. Proc Natl Acad Sci USA 1978; 75(9):4194-4198.
108. Mathiowitz E, Jacob JS, Jong YS et al. Biologically erodible microspheres as potential oral drug delivery systems. Nature 1997; 386:410-414.
109. Allen T, Moase E. Therapeutic opportunities for targeted liposomal drug delivery. Adv Drug Del Rev 1996; 21:117-133.
110. Kirpotin D, Park JW, Hong K et al. Sterically stabilized anti-HER2 immunoliposomes: Design and targeting to human breast cancer cells in vitro. Biochemistry 1997; 36:66-75.
111. Wu NZ, Braun RD, Gaber MH et al. Simultaneous measurement of liposome extravasation and content release in tumors. Microcirculation 1997; 4(1):83-101.

CHAPTER 5

Novel RNA Motif (Dimeric Minizyme) Capable of Cleaving L6 *BCR-ABL* Fusion (b2a2) mRNA with High Specificity

Tomoko Kuwabara, Masaki Warashina and Kazunari Taira

Introduction

The hammerhead ribozyme is one of the smallest RNA enzymes. Because of its small size and potential utility as an antiviral agent, it has been extensively investigated in terms of the mechanism of its action and possible applications in vivo. It was first recognized as the sequence motif responsible for self-cleavage (cis action) in the satellite RNAs of certain viruses.[1] The putative consensus sequence required for activity has three duplex stems and a conserved "core" of two non-helical segments, plus an unpaired nucleotide at the cleavage site. The trans-acting hammerhead ribozyme consists of an antisense section (stem I and stem III) and a catalytic domain with a flanking stem/loop II section.[2,3] Such RNA motifs can cleave oligoribonucleotides at specific sites (most effectively at GUC).[4-8] Because of its small size and potential utility as an anti-virus agent, this ribozyme has been extensively investigated in terms of the mechanism of its action and possible applications in vivo.[9-26] For such applications, it is clearly necessary to direct the ribozyme specifically to the cellular RNA target of interest.

Chronic myelogenous leukemia (CML) is a clonal myeloproliferative disorder of hematopoietic stem cells associated with the Philadelphia chromosome.[27] The reciprocal chromosomal translocation t(9; 22) (q34; q11) can be subdivided into two types: K28 translocations and L6 translocations. They result in the formation of the *BCR-ABL* fusion gene, which encodes two types of mRNA: b3a2 (consisting of *bcr* exon 3 and *abl* exon 2) and b2a2 (consisting of the *bcr* exon 2 and *abl* exon 2) (Fig. 5.1).[28-33] Both of these mRNAs are translated into a protein of 210 kDa (p210[BCR-ABL]) which is unique to the malignant cell phenotype.[34]

For the design of ribozymes that will disrupt chimeric RNAs, it is necessary to target the junction sequence. Otherwise, normal mRNAs that share part of the chimeric RNA sequence would also be cleaved by the ribozyme, with resultant damage to the host cells. In the case of the *BCR-ABL* chimeric RNA sequence b3a2, a potential ribozyme-cleavage site, a GUU triplet, is located three nucleotides upstream from the chimeric junction. A conventionally designed hammerhead ribozyme might be expected to specifically cleave the abnormal mRNA generated from K28 translocations. Indeed, several such examples have been

Ribozymes in the Gene Therapy of Cancer, edited by Kevin J. Scanlon and Mohammed Kashani-Sabet.
©1998 R.G. Landes Company.

Fig. 5.1. *BCR-ABL* translocations and fusion mRNAs. The two types of chromosomal translocation—K28-type (upper panel) and L6-type (lower panel)—that are associated with CML and the corresponding fusion mRNAs are depicted. Dotted lines connecting *bcr* and *abl* exons indicate alternative splicing pathways.

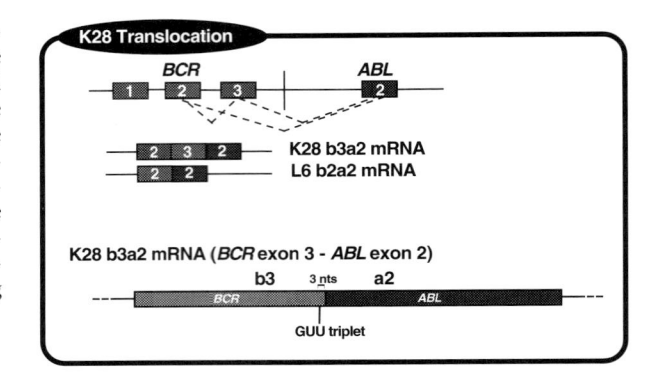

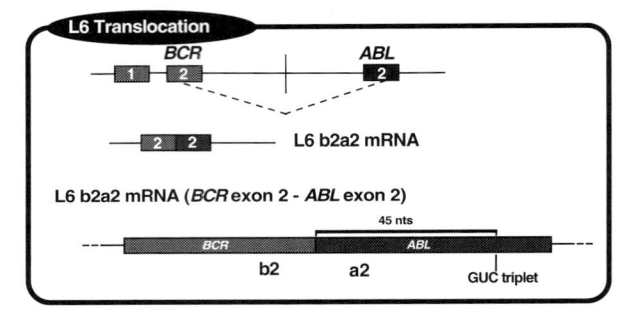

reported.[35-43] By contrast, in the case of the b2a2 sequence, which results from L6 translocations, as well as some K28 translocations, there are no triplet sequences that are potentially cleavable by hammerhead ribozymes within two or three nucleotides from the *BCR-ABL* junction.[44] In designing ribozymes that might cleave b2a2 mRNA, we must be sure to avoid cleavage of the normal *abl* mRNA itself.

Recently, we discovered a novel motif in a minizyme, a hammerhead ribozyme with short oligonucleotide linkers instead of stem/loop II.[45] Our previous study demonstrated that a minizyme with high-level activity forms a dimeric structure with a common stem II. Because of their dimeric structure, heterodimeric minizymes are capable of recognizing two independent sequences. We wondered whether it would be possible to design a novel heterodimeric minizyme that would form a catalytically competent structure only in the presence of the L6 *BCR-ABL* (b2a2) mRNA junction, by the use of one of the substrate-recognition sequences as the recognition arm of an active heterodimeric minizyme.

Since we were interested in cleaving b2a2 mRNA, we compared the specificity and catalytic activity of conventional hammerhead ribozymes and our novel heterodimeric minizyme with respect to the cleavage of *BCR-ABL* chimeric L6 (b2a2) mRNA.

Current Research

Minizymes

The hammerhead ribozyme is a small and versatile nucleic-acid molecule which can cleave RNA at specific sites. In its most useful form, it consists of a substrate-binding region (stem I and stem III) and a catalytic domain with a flanking stem-loop II region (Fig. 5.2A). In attempts to identify functional groups and to elucidate the role of the stem II region,

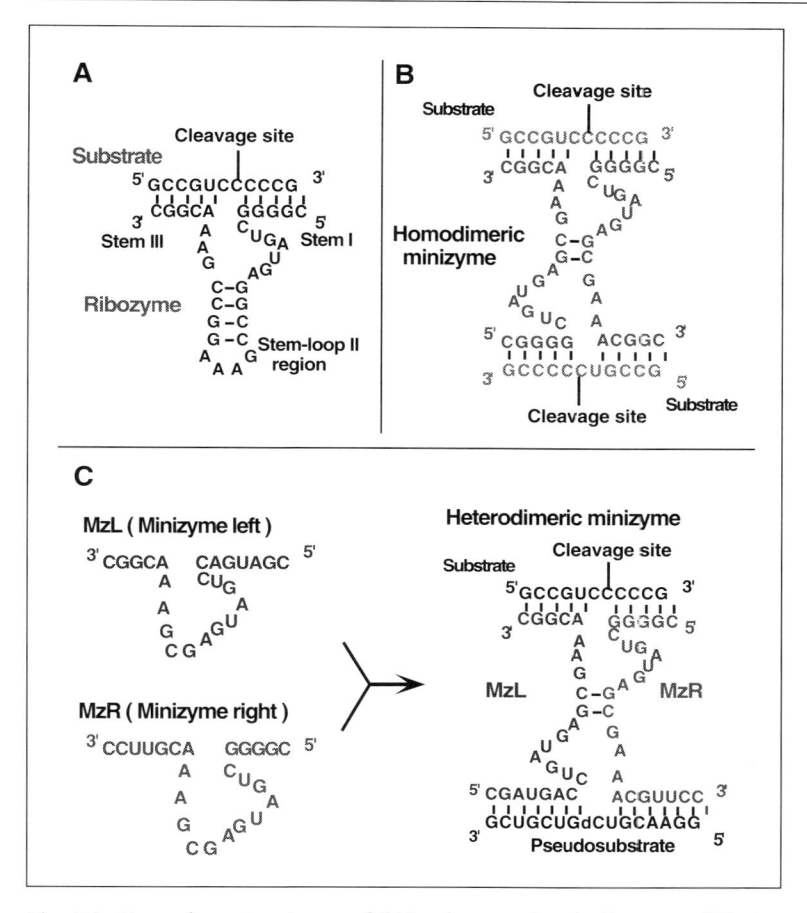

Fig. 5.2. Secondary structures of (A) a hammerhead ribozyme, (B) the homodimeric minizyme and (C) the heterodimeric minizyme used in a previous study.[45] In the case of the heterodimeric minizyme, the heterodimer (MzL-MzR) can generate two different binding sites: One is complementary to the sequence of a substrate, the other is complementary to an uncleavable pseudosubstrate. Only after the formation of the heterodimer could the substrate be cleaved.

various modifications and deletions have been made in this region.[46-52] Such minizymes are smaller versions of hammerhead ribozymes in which the stem-loop II region has been replaced by a short linker. They can, therefore, be synthesized more economically and chemical modifications can be made more easily. For the application of such enzymes as therapeutic agents for the treatment of infectious diseases and cancer, minizymes seem to be particularly attractive. However, activities of originally synthesized minizymes were two to three orders of magnitude lower than those of the parental hammerhead ribozymes, a result that led to the suggestion that minizymes might not be suitable as gene-inactivating reagents.[51] Thus, original minizymes were considered to be crippled structures and attracted minimal interest because of their extremely low activity, as compared to that of the full-sized ribozyme.

Fig. 5.3. The effect of the concentrations of the pseudosubstrate on the cleavage activity of the heterodimeric minizyme. (A) Time courses of cleavage activity of the heterodimeric minizyme in various concentrations of the pseudosubstrate (PsS): open square, 0 M; closed circle, 200 nM; open circle, 500 nM; triangle, 750 nM; closed square, 1 μM. (B)The effect of the concentrations of the pseudosubstrate on V_0 (min^{-1}).

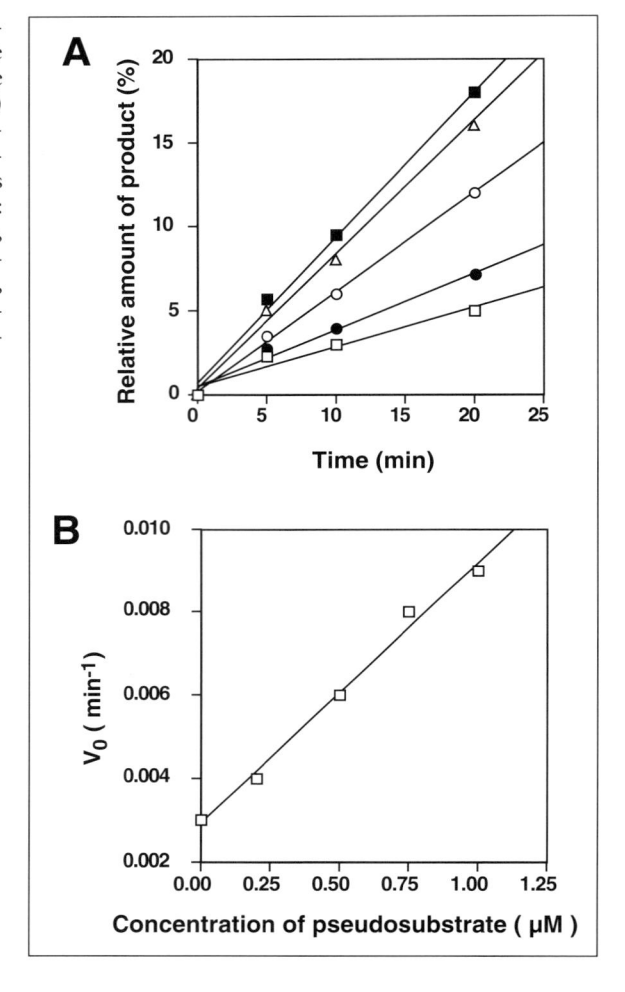

We later found that some minizymes have cleavage activity nearly identical to that of the wild type hammerhead ribozyme.[45] In the case of the active minizymes, the linker sequences were palindromic, so that two minizymes were capable of forming a dimeric structure with a common stem II (Fig. 5.2B). The activity of the homodimeric minizyme (a dimer with two identical binding sequences) depends on Mg^{2+} ions, and interactions with the substrates also stabilize the dimeric structures.[45,53,54] Figure 5.3 shows the dependence of cleavage activities of the MzL-MzR heterodimeric minizyme (a dimer with two different binding sequences, Fig. 5.2C) on concentrations of a pseudosubstrate. Since the dimer formation is essential for the cleavage reaction of the minizyme, the cleavage activity increases linearly by the addition of a pseudosubstrate. This kinetic study of the heterodimeric minizyme indicates that the active form of the minizyme is clearly a dimer. Since this novel RNA motif, a dimeric minizyme, has two substrate-binding regions and two catalytic domains, it was possible to construct dimeric minizymes that would cleave a target substrate at two sites simultaneously.[55] The cleavage activity and the stability of dimeric minizymes increased with increases in number of G-C pairs in the common stem II region of the dimeric minizyme.[55]

Cleavage of BCR-ABL mRNA by Conventional Ribozymes

In the sequence of *BCR-ABL* chimeric L6 (b2a2) mRNA, there are no triplet sequences that are potentially cleavable by hammerhead ribozymes within two or three nucleotides from the *BCR-ABL* junction. In the sequence of b2a2, ribozyme-cleavage sites in the vicinity of the *BCR-ABL* junction are located 7, 8, 9, and 19 nucleotides away from the junction. A GUC triplet, which is generally most susceptible to cleavage by hammerhead ribozymes, is also located 45 nucleotides from the junction. For the design of ribozymes that will disrupt chimeric RNAs, it is necessary to target the junction sequence. If such a GUC triplet was selected as a cleavage site of ribozymes, normal *abl* mRNA that shares part of the abnormal *BCR-ABL* RNA sequence would also be cleaved by the ribozyme, with resultant damage to the host cells (Fig. 5.4A). In designing ribozymes that might cleave b2a2 mRNA, we must be sure to avoid cleavage of the normal *abl* mRNA itself.

Previous attempts have involved a combination of a long antisense arm and the ribozyme sequence.[56,57] In the previous studies, long antisense sequences of about 10 to 30 nucleotides in length, which could bind to and cover the junction region for some distance from the cleavage sites, were connected to one of the binding sites of hammerhead ribozymes (81-mer, 41-mer and 52-mer Rzs) (Fig. 5.4B). The lengths of annealing arms are important for the activity of ribozymes because they influence the efficiency, as well as the specificity, of the cleavage reaction. In the case of a ribozyme that is directed against two non-contiguous sequences, the specificity is particularly important if we are to avoid nonspecific cleavage of normal mRNAs. Among the conventional ribozymes depicted in Figure 5.4B, which were designed to cleave L6 *BCR-ABL* chimeric mRNA specifically, the 52-mer Rz and the 41-mer Rz had long binding arms, in the stem III region, of 20 and 12 nucleotides, respectively. In the case of the 81-mer Rz, the binding arm was 50 nucleotides in length in the stem III region and was connected to the ribozyme sequence by a 13-nucleotide spacer sequence that was non-complementary to the substrate, to achieve greater flexibility of binding.[56] The 52-mer Rz was designed to cleave the L6 *BCR-ABL* mRNA at the UUC triplet located 9 nts 3' of the junction.[57] The 41-mer Rz was designed to cleave the substrate at the CUU triplet located 8 nts 3' of the junction. The 81-mer Rz was designed to cleave the substrate at the GUA triplet located 19 nts 3' of the junction. According to a published report, the 81-mer and 41-mer Rzs should have enhanced specificity for the chimeric b2a2 mRNA substrate. However, according to other studies, it seems that hammerhead ribozymes have cleavage ability even if the binding arm is as little as three nucleotides in length. As can be seen from Figure 5.4B, the binding region of these antisense-type ribozymes to the normal *abl* mRNA sequence consisted of at least six base pairs. Therefore, we could not exclude the possibility that such ribozymes might bind non-specifically to and cleave the normal *abl* mRNA just as they specifically cleave the *BCR-ABL* (b2a2) mRNA. Moreover, longer substrate-binding arms might lower the rate of dissociation from the substrate, with a resultant reduction in the ribozyme-turnover rate. Therefore, we synthesized ribozymes (81-mer, 41-mer, and 52-mer Rzs in Fig. 5.4B) that were identical to those in the literature and re-examined their specificities.

Comparison of the Specificities of Conventional Hammerhead Ribozymes and Novel Dimeric Minizymes with Respect to the Cleavage of BCR-ABL Chimeric L6 (b2a2) mRNA

Since a minizyme with high-level activity forms a dimeric structure with a common stem II,[45,53-55] it has two independent substrate-binding regions. Therefore, we decided to

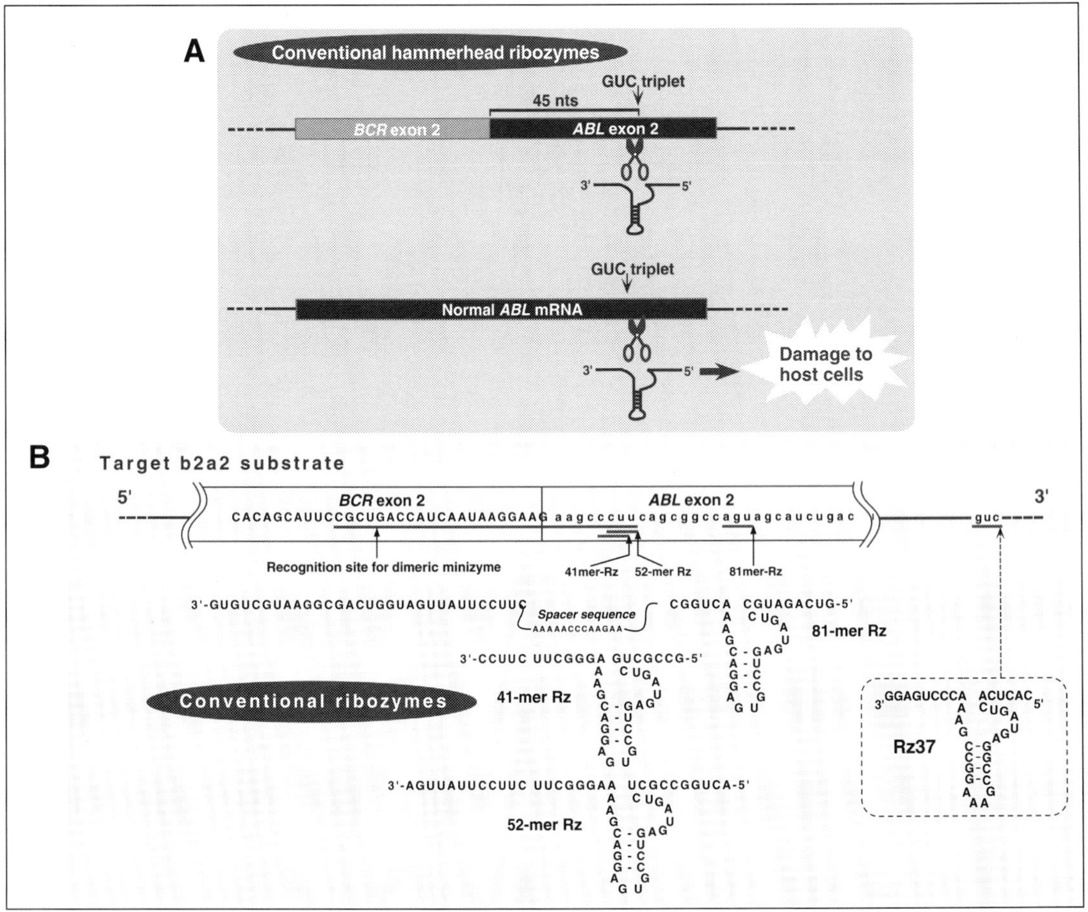

Fig. 5.4. Cleavage of normal and/or abnormal RNAs by conventional ribozymes. The control ribozyme (Rz37), which targets the same site as the dimeric minizyme on L6 b2a2 mRNA, is expected to cleave not only the abnormal chimeric BCR-ABL mRNA but also the normal *abl* mRNA since the cleavage site is located far from the *BCR-ABL* junction (upper panel). Nucleotide sequences of the conventional antisense-type ribozymes and Rz37 are shown in the lower panel. The sequence of L6 *BCR-ABL* near the junction is expanded. The *bcr* exon 2 sequence near the junction is depicted by capital letters and that of the *abl* exon 2 sequence is shown in lower-case letters. The sites of cleavage by antisense-type ribozymes (81-mer Rz, 41-mer Rz and 52-mer Rz) and the control ribozyme, Rz37, are indicated. The site of cleavage by the dimeric minizyme is identical to that of Rz37 and the 29 nt recognition site for the dimeric minizyme is also indicated by underlining.

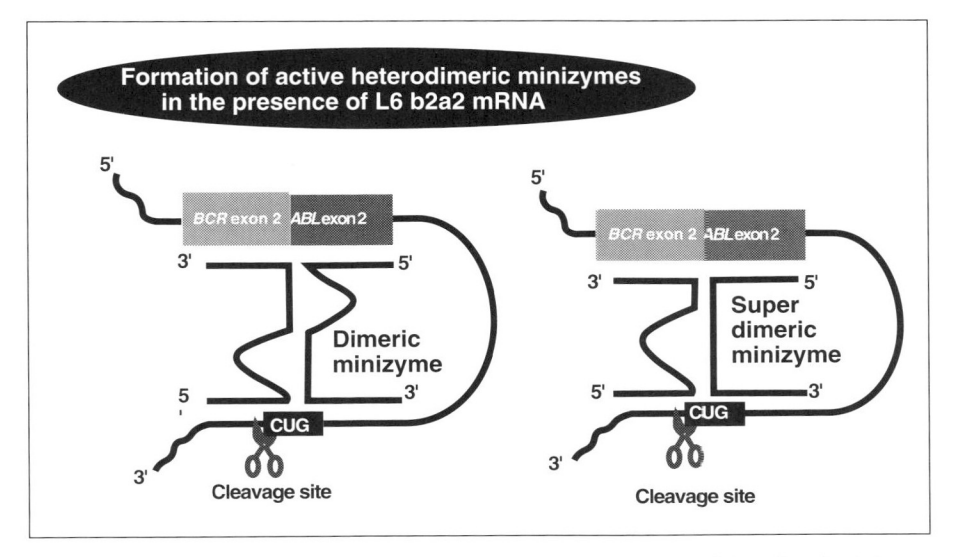

Novel RNA Motif Capable of Cleaving L6 BCR-ABL Fusion mRNA with High Specificity

Fig. 5.5. Cleavage of L6 b2a2 mRNA by dimeric minizymes. Minizyme left (MzL) and minizyme right (MzR) form a dimeric structure with a common stem II in the presence of L6 b2a2 mRNA. One unit of the substrate-recognition sequences is used to recognize the abnormal *BCR-ABL* junction. One of the catalytic cores of the heterodimeric minizyme can be deleted completely to yield a "super dimeric minizyme" (right figure).

use one of the substrate-binding regions, within an active heterodimeric minizyme, as the recognition arms for the abnormal *BCR-ABL* junction (Fig. 5.5). One of the catalytic cores of the heterodimeric minizyme can be deleted completely to yield a "super dimeric minizyme". In order to achieve high substrate-specificity, the heterodimeric minizyme should retain its active conformation only in the presence of the abnormal *BCR-ABL* junction, while its conformation should remain inactive in the presence of the normal *abl* mRNA. The novel minizyme, MzL (minizyme left) and MzR (minizyme right), shown in Figure 5.6 should enable such conformational changes depending on the presence or absence of the abnormal b2a2 mRNA. One unit of the substrate-recognition sequences is used to recognize the abnormal *BCR-ABL* junction. As a control ribozyme, Rz37, designed to target the same site as the dimeric minizyme on L6 b2a2 mRNA, was also prepared. Rz37 is expected to cleave not only the abnormal chimeric *BCR-ABL* mRNA but also the normal *abl* mRNA since the cleavage site is located far from the *BCR-ABL* junction (Fig. 5.4B).

In order to examine the specificity of cleavage reactions catalyzed by conventional ribozymes or by our novel heterodimeric minizyme, we examined three types of RNA substrate (Figs. 5.7 and 5.8), namely, the normal *abl* substrate, the chimeric *BCR-ABL* substrate, and a short *BCR-ABL* substrate with lengths, respectively, of 92, 121 and 16 nucleotides. Enzymes with high specificity should cleave the chimeric *BCR-ABL* substrate (Fig. 5.7) or the 16-mer short *abl* substrate in the presence of a pseudo-substrate that has the b2a2 junction sequence (Fig. 5.8), without cleaving the other RNAs. All kinetic measurements were made in 25 mM $MgCl_2$ and 50 mM Tris-HCl (pH 8.0), under enzyme-saturating (single-turnover) conditions at 37°C (measurements of k_{cat} or k_{obs}), namely, our standard conditions for kinetic measurements.[55]

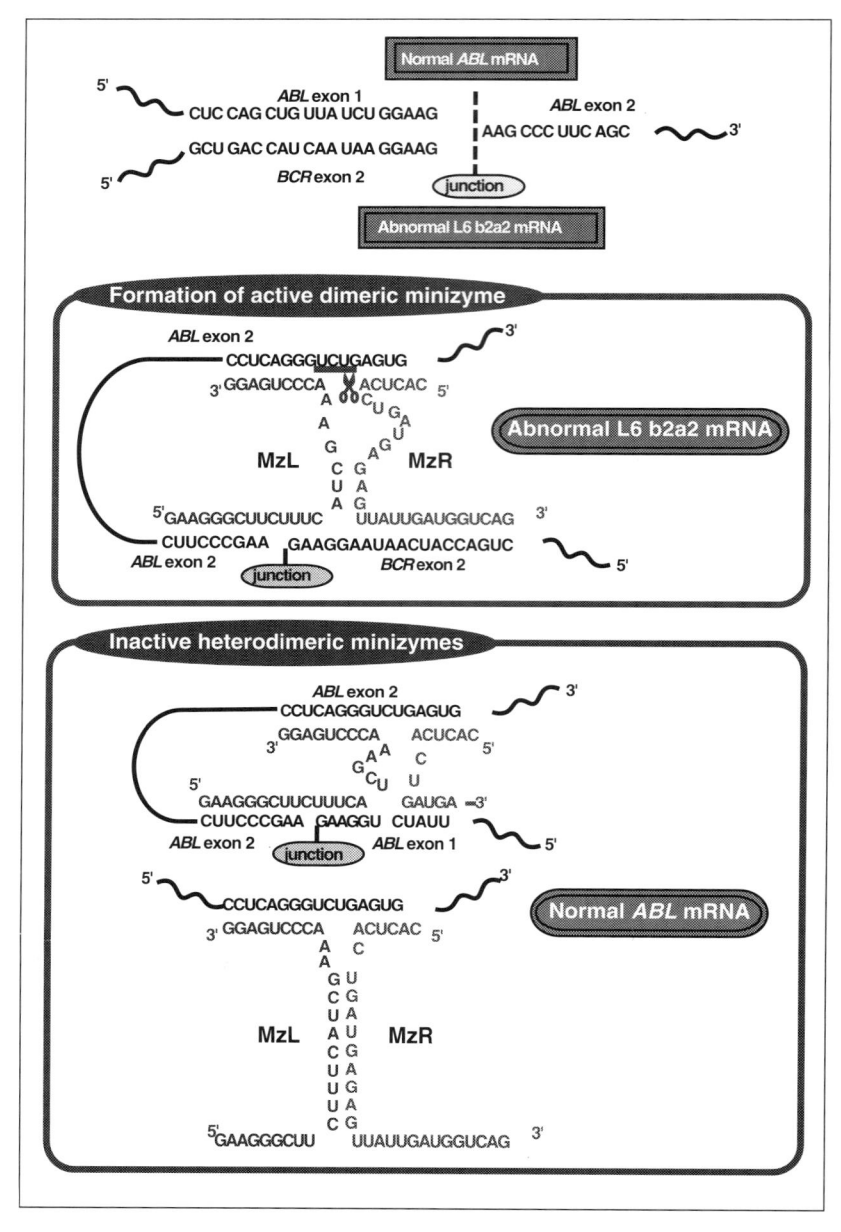

Fig. 5.6. Formation of active or inactive heterodimeric minizyme. In order to achieve high substrate-specificity, the heterodimeric minizyme components should retain their active conformation only in the presence of the abnormal *BCR-ABL* junction (middle panel), while their conformation should retain inactive in the presence or absence of the normal *abl* mRNA (bottom panel). The novel minizyme, MzL (minizyme left) and MzR (minizyme right) should enable such conformational changes depending on the presence or absence of the abnormal b2a2 mRNA.

Results of cleavage of relatively long substrates by the conventional antisense-type ribozymes and the super dimeric minizymes are shown in Figure 5.7. As expected, all the conventional ribozymes cleaved the *BCR-ABL* substrate at the anticipated sites. However, in contrast to expectations based on previous reports,[56,57] not only the control Rz37 but also the antisense-type ribozymes cleaved the normal *abl* substrate within 1 hour. Moreover, the amounts of cleavage products obtained from the normal *abl* mRNA with each ribozyme were almost the same as those obtained from the chimeric *BCR-ABL* substrate, indicating that these conventional ribozymes, with their relatively long antisense arms, recognized not only the abnormal *BCR-ABL* mRNA but also the normal *abl* mRNA as substrates. Therefore, non-specific cleavage of normal *abl* mRNA could not be avoided when we used conventionally designed ribozymes. In previous studies on these long antisense-type ribozymes,[56] one part of the target site was designed to be accessible for annealing and served to direct ribozyme nucleation, while the other part recognized the cleavage triplet in the vicinity of the *BCR-ABL* junction, where specific cleavage of the hybrid mRNA occurred. We note that, in all cases, these conventional Rzs have regions of complementary binding to the normal *abl* mRNA sequences of at least 6-8 nts. Previous studies of hammerhead ribozymes demonstrated that cleavage of the substrate could occur when one of the substrate-binding arms was three nucleotides long.[58,59] Thus, we would not expect substrate specificity from the conventionally designed ribozymes shown in Figure 5.4B.

Our novel heterodimeric minizyme was expected to show high substrate specificity for the L6 *BCR-ABL* substrate, if and only if it forms an active conformation in the presence of the abnormal b2a2 mRNA, as depicted in Figure 5.6. The specificity of the dimeric minizyme was tested by incubating the minizymes with the 5'-[^{32}P]-labeled short 16-mer substrate (S16) in the presence or absence of either a short 20-mer normal *abl* pseudo-substrate or a short 28-mer *BCR-ABL* pseudo-substrate (Fig. 5.8). In this case, one part of the target site (b2a2 mRNA junction within the *BCR-ABL* pseudo-sub) was designed to be accessible to MzL and MzR for annealing and served to direct formation of the active dimeric minizyme (Fig. 5.6), while the other part recognized the cleavage triplet in the short 16-mer *abl* substrate RNA, where specific cleavage of the latter RNA occurred (Fig. 5.8). It is to be noted that the cleavage activity of the novel heterodimeric minizyme was nearly identical to that of the control hammerhead ribozyme Rz37. In terms of substrate specificity, no products of cleavage of the substrate were detected in the absence of the *BCR-ABL* junction, demonstrating the expected high substrate-specificity of the heterodimeric minizyme. Since MzL or MzR alone, in the presence or in the absence of the pseudo-substrate, did not show any cleavage activity, the active species is clearly the heterodimeric form of the minizyme. A similar study demonstrated high substrate-specificity for the longer L6 *BCR-ABL* substrate (Fig. 5.7).

Activities and Specificities of tRNA-Embedded Minizymes

Ribozymes have been shown to be potent inhibitors of gene expression and viral function. There are two basic strategies for ribozyme delivery into cells: endogenous delivery in that a gene for the ribozyme is transcribed in cells, and exogenous delivery in that a pre-synthesized ribozyme is supplied to the cells by means of carriers. For the endogenous ribozyme expression, the gene encoding the ribozyme is inserted into a vector which can be delivered into target cells. Efficacy of ribozyme-mediated repression of a target gene in living cells depends on the level of expression and also the stability of transcribed ribozymes. For the repression of *BCR-ABL* chimeric mRNA whose products cause CML diseases, our dimeric minizyme should be particularly useful because of its high cleavage activity and specificity. For the endogenous delivery of minizymes, we chose a promoter for RNA polymerase III, which naturally drives tRNA and snRNA synthesis with high levels of expression.

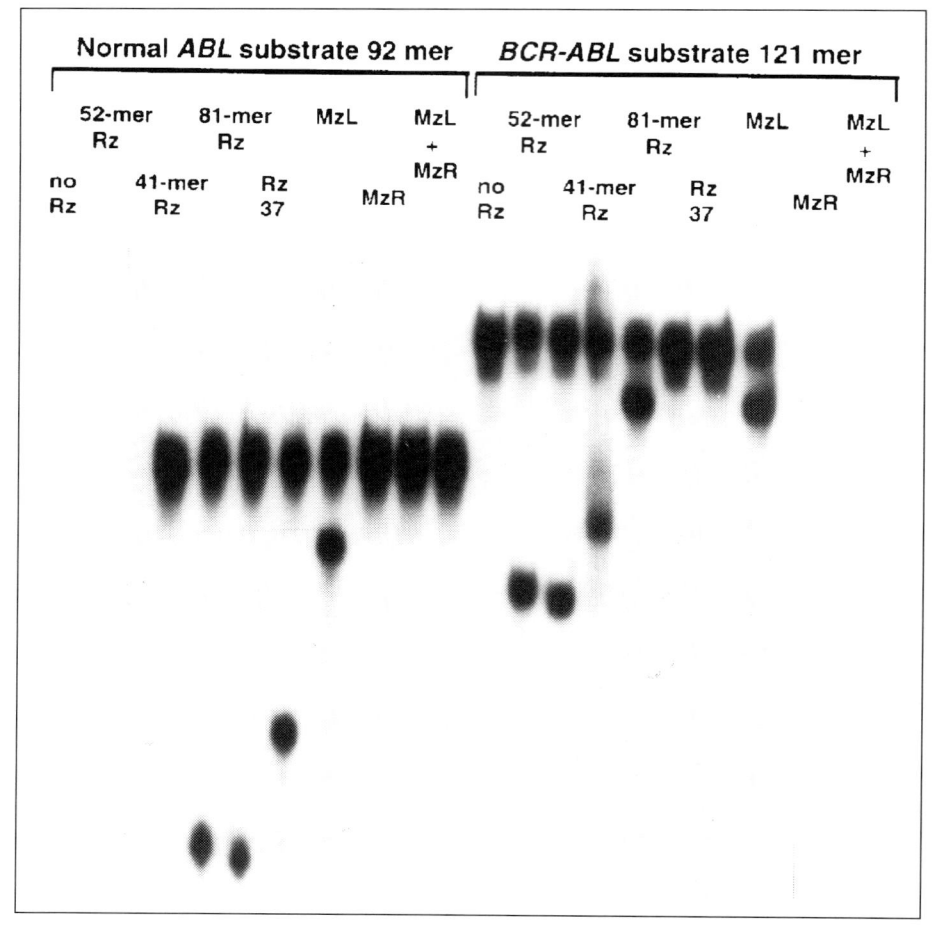

Fig. 5.7. Gel electrophoresis showing cleavage of normal and/or abnormal long substrate by conventional ribozymes and dimeric minizyme. It revealed the non-specific cleavage of chimeric BCR-ABL mRNA, as well as of normal abl mRNA, by conventional ribozymes. In contrast, the dimeric minizyme showed high cleavage specificity. Specificity was examined with the normal abl substrate (92-mer) and the chimeric BCR-ABL substrate (121-mer). Each enzyme (1 μM) and 2 nM 5'-[^{32}P]-labeled substrate were incubated at 37°C for 60 min in a solution that contained 50 mM Tris-HCl (pH 8.0) and 25 mM MgCl$_2$ and then the mixture was subjected to electrophoresis on an 8% polyacrylamide/7M urea gel.

Cleavage products from the normal *abl* substrate (92-mer) were as follows. Non-specific cleavage, at the UUC triplet located 9 nts 3' of the junction, by the 52-mer Rz generated a [^{32}P]-labeled 5'-fragment of 43 nts in length. Similarly, non-specific cleavage, at the CUU triplet located 8 nts 3' of the junction, by the 41-mer Rz generated a visible fragment of 42 nts. Non-specific cleavage, at GUA located 19 nts 3' of the junction, by the 81-mer Rz generated a fragment of 54 nts. Non-specific cleavage, at GUC located 45 nts 3' of the junction, by Rz37 generated a fragment of 79 nts.

Cleavage products from the *BCR-ABL* substrate (121-mer) were as follows. Cleavage by the 52-mer Rz generated a visible 5'-fragment of 72 nts in length. Similarly, cleavage by the 41-mer Rz generated a fragment of 71 nts. Cleavage by the 81-mer Rz generated a fragment of 83 nts. Cleavage by Rz37 and dimeric minizyme generated a fragment of 108 nts in length.

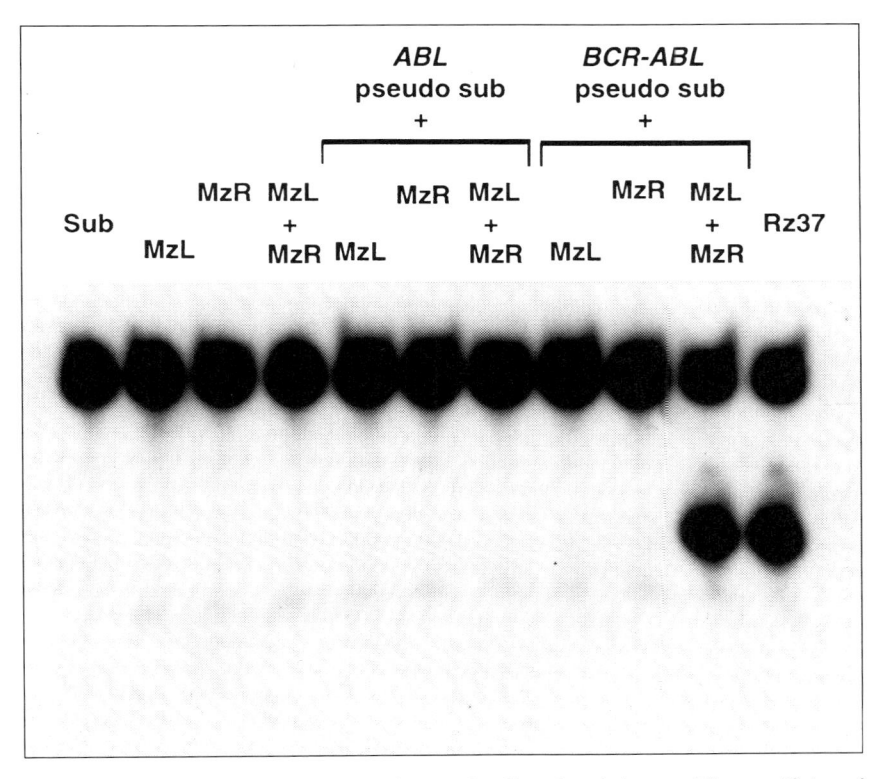

Fig. 5.8. Gel electrophoresis showing cleavage by dimeric minizymes. The specificity of dimeric minizyme-mediated cleavage was tested by incubating the minizymes with the 5'-[^{32}P]-labeled short 16-mer substrate S16 (Sub) in the presence or absence of either a short 20-mer normal *abl* pseudo-substrate (*abl* pseudo-sub) or a short 28-mer *BCR-ABL* pseudo-substrate (*BCR-ABL* pseudo-sub). Minizymes (MzL and MzR) were incubated at 0.1 µM with 2 nM 5'-[^{32}P]-labeled S16 substrate (Sub). When applicable, the concentration of pseudosubstrate, such as *abl* or *BCR-ABL*, was at 1 µM. Reactions were usually initiated by the addition of 25 mM MgCl$_2$ to a buffered solution that contained 50 mM Tris-HCl (pH 8.0) and enzyme together with the substrate, and each resultant mixture was then incubated at 37°C for 60 min. The reaction mixture was subjected to electrophoresis on an 8% polyacrylamide/7M urea gel.

In order to achieve high expression of these dimeric minizymes in vivo for future gene therapy, we embedded the dimeric minizyme portion (MzL and MzR) downstream of a tRNA^{Val} promoter sequence which could be recognized by RNA polymerase III (Fig. 5.9). For the tRNA^{Val} promoter-driven minizymes to be active, the attached tRNA^{Val} portion should not cause severe steric hindrance during the formation of dimeric minizymes. Therefore, we first examined the effect of the tRNA portion of the pol III-derived ribozyme transcripts. Results of cleavage by the tRNA-embedded dimeric minizyme are shown in Figure 5.10. In order to examine the specificity of cleavage reactions catalyzed by tRNA-embedded dimeric minizymes, we examined both chimeric *BCR-ABL* substrate (121 mer) and the normal *abl* substrate (92 mer). Template DNAs which encode the T7 promoter and tRNA-embedded dimeric minizyme sequence depicted in Figure 5.9 were prepared. In the T7 transcription reaction solution, purified [^{32}P]-labeled substrate was added. As can be seen in Figure 5.10,

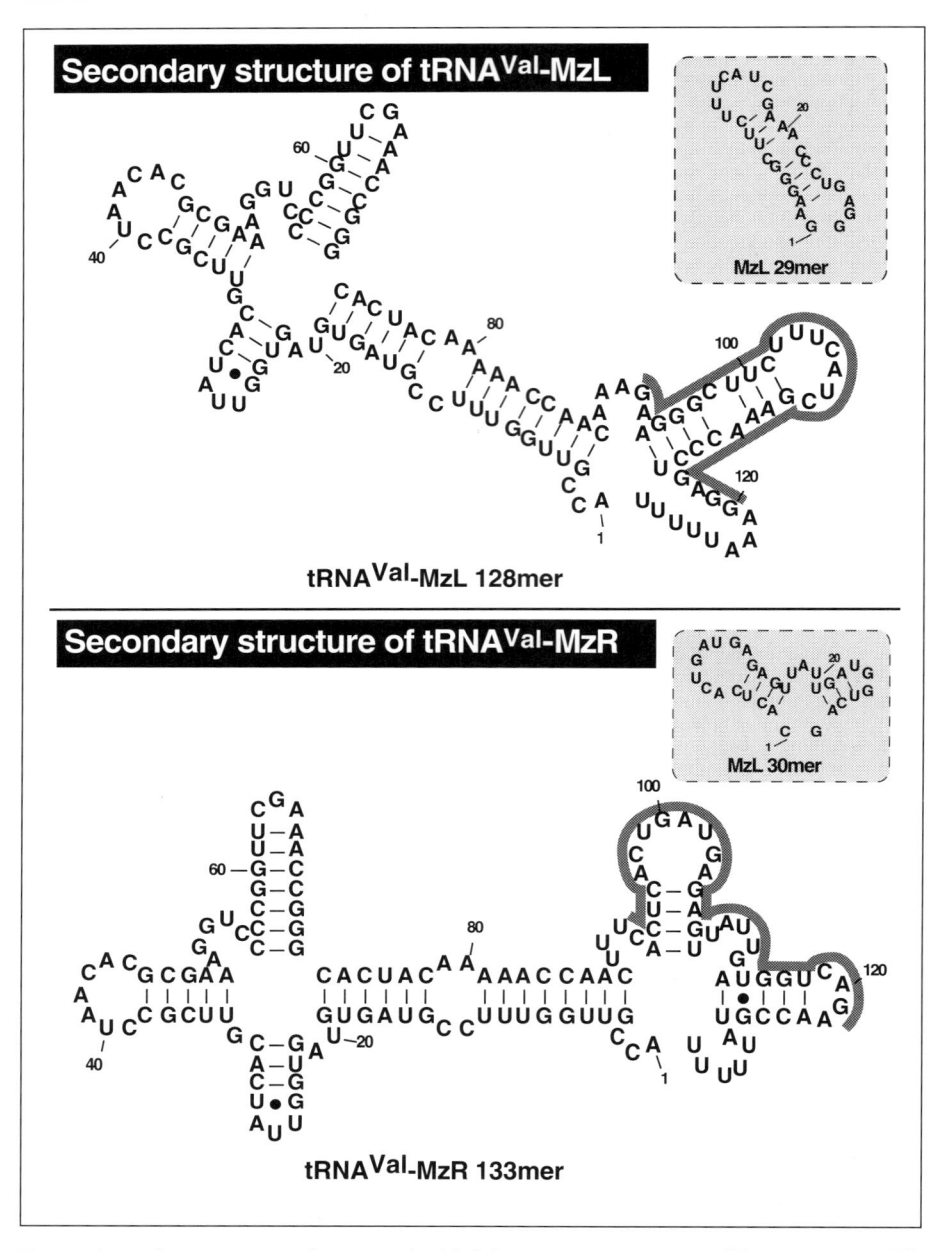

Fig. 5.9. Secondary structures of tRNA-embedded dimeric minizyme (tRNA[Val]-MzL and tRNA[Val]-MzR) and naked dimeric minizyme (MzL and MzR; upper right figure in both panels). The dimeric minizyme portion is outlined.

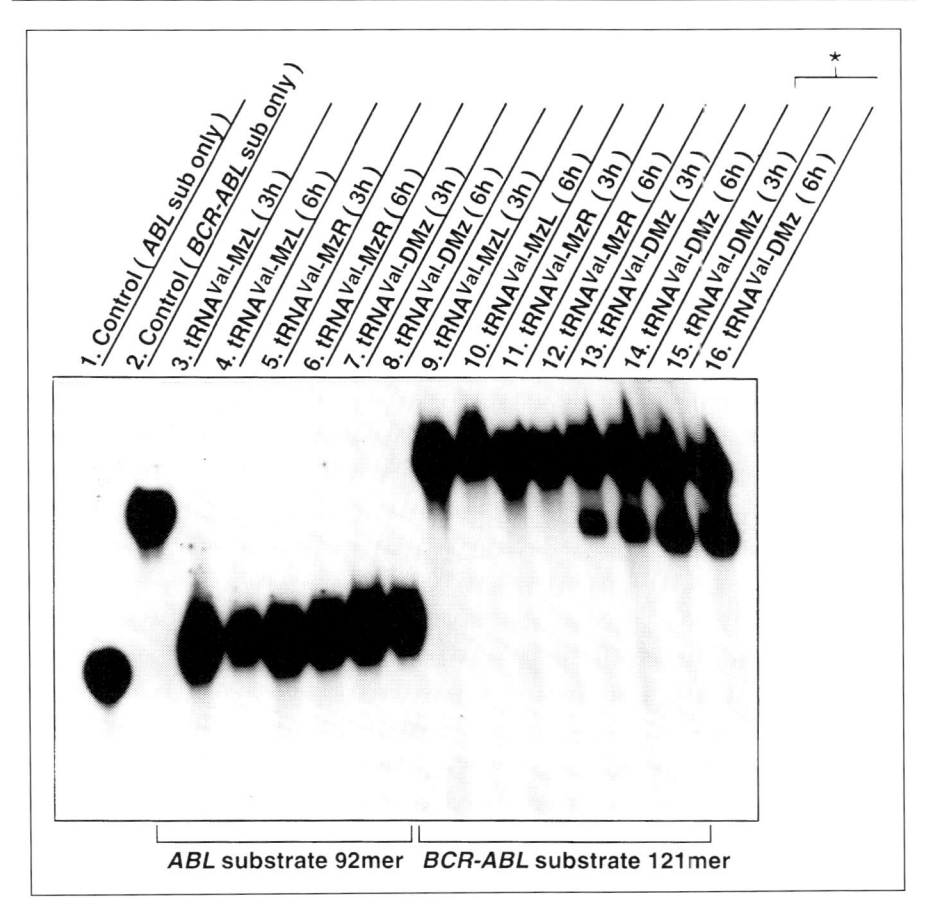

Fig. 5.10. Gel electrophoresis showing cleavage by tRNA-embedded dimeric minizyme. Minizymes (MzL and MzR) which form a dimeric structure were embedded after the tRNA^{Val} promoter sequence, namely tRNA^{Val}-MzL and tRNA^{Val}-MzR. The tRNA^{Val}-MzL and the tRNA^{Val}-MzR form an active dimer complex, namely tRNA^{Val}-DMz. The reaction solutions after 3 h and 6 h incubation for each condition was loaded on the gel (from lane 3 to lane 16). The cleavage activity and specificity was examined in the T7 transcription of tRNA-embedded dimeric minizyme with incubation of purified [^{32}P]-labeled substrate. In lanes 15 and 16 (*), the reaction solutions which contained an excess of T7 RNA polymerase were loaded.

the tRNA-embedded dimeric minizyme specifically cleaved the chimeric *BCR-ABL* substrate. No cleavage products were detected in the presence of the normal *abl* substrate. As expected, tRNA-MzL or tRNA-MzR alone did not show any cleavage. Similarly to the naked dimeric minizyme (Figs. 5.7 and 5.8), the tRNA-embedded dimeric minizyme also showed high substrate specificity. Figure 5.10 demonstrates the formation of active dimeric tRNA-minizymes, providing evidence that the attached tRNA portion did not prohibit the dimerization process.

In order to characterize in further detail the properties of tRNA-embedded dimeric minizymes, we determined kinetic parameters using a short 16-mer substrate (S16), and

Table 5.1. Kinetic parameters for the cleavage of short BCR-ABL substrate (S16)*

Enzyme	k_{cat} (min^{-1})	K_d (μM)
Dimeric minizyme	0.018	0.27
tRNA-embedded dimeric minizyme	0.013	0.21

*All reaction rates were measured, in 25 mM MgCl$_2$ and 50 mM Tris-HCl (pH 8.0) under enzyme-saturating (single-turnover) conditions at 37°C. In all cases, kinetic measurements were made under conditions where all of the substrate was expected to form a Michaelis-Menten complex, with high concentrations of enzymes. Rate constants are averages from two sets of experiments.

compared the activities between the tRNA-embedded dimeric minizyme and the naked dimeric minizyme. Kinetic analysis carried out under single-turnover conditions and the rate constants of the dimeric minizyme and tRNA-embedded dimeric minizyme determined with the S16 substrate are shown in Table 5.1. Interestingly, the cleavage activity of tRNA-embedded dimeric minizymes was almost the same as that of the naked dimeric minizymes. This result indicates that our dimeric minizyme can fully form an active dimeric structure even if the tRNA^{Val} sequence was connected at the 5' end of each minizyme (MzL and MzR). Moreover, the minizyme retains the active conformation only in the presence of the abnormal *BCR-ABL* junction (b2a2 mRNA), while the conformation remains inactive in the absence of an abnormal *BCR-ABL* junction.

Future Prospects

Potential Gene Therapy for Treatment of Chronic Myelogenous Leukemia (CML)

The specific association of nucleic acid-based drugs, such as our novel heterodimeric minizymes, with their targets via base pairing and subsequent cleavage of the RNA substrate suggests that these catalytic molecules might be useful for gene therapy. There are basically two ways to introduce ribozymes into cells. One such technique is an exogenous delivery (drug-delivery) system (DDS) in which chemically pre-synthesized ribozymes are encapsulated in liposomes or other related compounds and delivered to target cells. For this exogenous delivery, chemical modifications[60] to make nuclease-resistant heterodimeric minizymes and/or DNA enzymes[44,61] should be useful. Another way to introduce ribozymes into cells is by transcription from the corresponding DNA template (gene therapy). Current gene-therapy technology is limited primarily by the necessity for ex vivo manipulations of target tissues and the technology is practical for endogenous delivery systems.[62] Ribozymes with natural components but not chemically modified counterparts can be transcribed in vivo. In this context, our novel heterodimeric minizymes driven by a pol III promoter are superior to the other nucleic acid-based drugs, because of their extremely high substrate specificity and high cleavage activity, for the treatment of chronic myelogenous leukemia (CML), especially in the case of L6 translocations.

References

1. Symons RH. Self-cleavage of RNA in the replication of small pathogens of plants and animals. Trend Biochem Sci 1989; 14:445-450.
2. Haseloff J, Gerlach WL. Simple RNA enzymes with new and highly specific endonuclease activities. Nature 1988; 334:585-591.
3. Uhlenbeck OC. A small catalytic oligonucleotide. Nature 1987; 328:596-600.

4. Koizumi M, Iwai S, Ohtsuka E. Cleavage of specific sites of RNA by designed ribozymes. FEBS Lett 1988; 239:285-288.
5. Ruffer DE, Stormo GD, Uhlenbeck OC. Sequence requirements of the hammerhead RNA self-cleavage reaction. Biochemistry 1990; 29:10695-10702.
6. Perriman R, Delves A, Gerlach WL. Extended target-site specificity for a hammerhead ribozyme. Gene 1992; 113:157-163.
7. Shimayama T, Nishikawa S, Taira K. Generality of the NUX rule: Kinetic analysis of the results of systematic mutations in the trinucleotide at the cleavage site of hammerhead ribozymes. Biochemistry 1995; 34:3649-3654.
8. Zoumadakis M, Tabler M. Comparative analysis of cleavage rates after systematic permutation of the NUX consensus tartget motif for hammerhead ribozymes. Nucleic Acids Res 1995; 23:1192-1196.
9. Sarver N, Cantin E, Chang P et al. Ribozymes as potential anti-HIV-1 therapeutic agents. Science 1990; 247:1222-1225.
10. Homann M, Tzortzakaki S, Rittner K et al. Incorporation of the catalytic domain of a hammerhead ribozyme into antisense RNA enhances its inhibitory effect on the replication of human immunodeficiency virus type 1. Nucleic Acids Res 1993; 21:2809-2814.
11. Mulligan RC. The basic science of gene therapy. Science 1993; 260:926-932.
12. Altman S. RNA enzyme-directed gene therapy. Proc Natl Acad Sci USA 1993; 90:10898-10900.
13. Marschall P, Thomson JB, Eckstein F. Inhibition of gene expression with ribozymes. Cell Mol Neurobiol 1994; 14:523-538.
14. Sullivan SM. Development of ribozymes for gene therapy. J Invest Dermatol 1994; 103:85-89.
15. Cameron FH, Jennings PA. Multiple domains in a ribozyme construct confer increased suppressive activity in monkey cells. Antisense Res Dev 1994; 4:87-94.
16. Ohkawa J, Yuyama N, Takebe Y et al. Importance of independence in ribozyme reactions: Kinetic behavior of trimmed and of simply connected multiple ribozymes with potential activity against human immunodeficiency virus. Proc Natl Acad Sci USA 1993; 90:11302-11306.
17. Sun LQ, Pyati J, Smythe J et al. Resistance to HIV-1 infection conferred by transduction of human peripheral blood lymphocytes with ribozyme, antisense or polyTAR constructs. Proc Natl Acad Sci USA 1995; 92:7272-7276.
18. Christoffersen RE, Marr JJ. Ribozymes as human therapeutic agents. J Med Chem 1995; 38:2023-2037.
19. Ferbeyre G, Bratty J, Chen H et al. Cell cycle arrest promotes trans-hammerhead ribozyme action in yeast. J Biol Chem 1996; 271:19318-19323.
20. Kiehntopf M, Brach MA, Licht T et al. Ribozyme-mediated cleavage of the MDR-1 transcript restores chemosensitivity in previously resistant cancer cells. EMBO J 1994; 13:4645-4652.
21. Kiehntopf M, Esquivel EL, Brach MA et al. Ribozymes: Biology, biochemistry, and implications for clinical medicine. J Mol Med 1995; 73:65-71.
22. Thompson JD, Ayers DF, Malmstrom TA et al. Improved accumulation and activity of ribozymes expressed from a tRNA-based RNA polymerase III promoter. Nucleic Acids Res 1995; 23:2259-2268.
23. Thompson JD, Macejak D, Couture L et al. Ribozymes in gene therapy. Nature Med 1995; 1:277-278.
24. Tuschl T, Thomson JB, Eckstein F. RNA cleavage by small catalytic RNAs. Curr Opin Struct Biol 1995; 5:296-302.
25. Kawasaki H, Ohkawa J, Tanishige N et al. Selection of the best target site for ribozyme-mediated cleavage within a fusion gene for adenovirus E1A-associated 300kDa protein (p300) and luciferase. Nucleic Acids Res 1996; 24:3010-3016.
26. Eckstein F, Lilly DMJ eds. In: Catalytic RNA, Nucleic Acids and Molecular Biology. Vol 10. Berlin:Springer-Verlag, 1996.
27. Nowell PC, Hungerford DA. A minute chromosome in human chronic granulocytic leukemia. Science 1960; 132:1497-1499.

28. Rowley JD. A new consistent chromosomal abnormality in chronic myelogenous leukaemia identified by quinacrine fluorescence and Giemsa staining. Nature 1973; 243:290-293.
29. Bartram CR, de Klein A, Hagemeijer A et al. Translocation of c-abl oncogene correlates with the presence of a Philadelphia chromosome in chronic myelocytic leukaemia. Nature 1983; 306:277-280.
30. Heisterkamp N, Stephenson JR, Groffen J et al. Localization of the c-abl oncogene adjacent to a translocation break point in chronic myelocytic leukaemia. Nature 1983; 306:239-242.
31. Groffen J, Stephenson JR, Heisterkamp N et al. Philadelphia chromosomal breakpoints are clustered within a limited region, bcr, on chromosome 22. Cell 1984; 36:93-99.
32. Schtivelman E, Lifshitz B, Gale RP et al. Fused transcript of abl and bcr genes in chronic myelogenous leukaemia. Nature 1985; 315:550-553.
33. Shtivelman E, Lifschitz B, Gale RP et al. Ribozyme-mediated inhibition of bcr-abl gene expression in a Philadelphia chromosome-positive cell line. Cell 1986; 47:277-284.
34. Konopka JB, Watanabe SM, Witte ON. An alteration of the human c-abl protein in K562 leukemia cells unmasks associated tyrosine kinase activity. Cell 1984; 37:1035-1042.
35. Shore SK, Nabissa PM, Reddy EP. Ribozyme-mediated cleavage of the BCR-ABL oncogene transcript: in vitro cleavage of RNA and in vivo loss of P210 protein-kinase activity. Oncogene 1993; 8:3183-3188.
36. Snyder DS, Wu Y, Wang JL et al. Ribozyme-mediated inhibition of bcr-abl gene expression in a Philadelphia chromosome-positive cell line. Blood 1993; 82:600-605.
37. Lange W, Cantin EM, Finke J et al. In vitro and in vivo effects of synthetic ribozymes targeted against BCR/ABL mRNA. Leukemia 1993; 7:1786-1794.
38. Wright L, Wilson SB, Milliken S et al. Ribozyme-mediated cleavage of the bcr/abl transcript expressed in chronic myeloid leukemia. Exp Hematol 1993; 21:1714-1718.
39. Lange W, Daskalakis M, Finke J et al. Comparison of different ribozymes for efficient and specific cleavage of BCR/ABL related mRNAs. FEBS Lett 1994; 338:175-178.
40. Kearney P, Wright LA, Milliken S et al. Improved specificity of ribozyme-mediated cleavage of bcr-abl mRMA. Exp Hematol 1995; 23:986-989.
41. Leopold LH, Shore SK, Newkirk TA et al. Multi-unit ribozyme-mediated cleavage of bcr-abl mRNA in myeloid leukemias. Blood 1995; 85:2162-2170.
42. Kronenwett R, Haas R, Sczakiel G. Kinetic selectivity of complementary nucleic acids: bcr-abl-directed antisense RNA and ribozyme. J Mol Biol 1996; 259:632-644.
43. Leopold LH, Shore SK, Reddy EP. Multi-unit anti-BCR-ABL ribozyme therapy in chronic myelogenous leukemia. Leuk Lymphoma 1996; 22:365-373.
44. Kuwabara T, Warashina M, Tanabe T et al. Comparison of the specificities and catalytic activities if hammerhead ribozymes and DNA enzymes with respect to the cleavage of BCR-ABL chimeric L6 (b2a2) mRNA. Nucleic Acids Res 1997; 25:3074-3082.
45. Amontov S, Taira K. Hammerhead minizymes with high cleavage activity: A dimeric structure as the active conformation of minizymes. J Am Chem Soc 1996; 118:1624-1628.
46. Goodchild J, Kohli V. Ribozymes that cleave an RNA sequence from human immunodeficiency virus: The effect of flanking sequence on rate. Arch Biochem Biophys 1991; 284:386-391.
47. McCall MJ, Hendry P, Jennings PA. Minimal sequence requirements for ribozyme activity. Proc Natl Acad Sci USA 1992; 89:5710-5714.
48. Tuschl T, Eckstein F. Hammerhead ribozymes: Importance of stem-loop II activity. Proc Natl Acad Sci USA 1993; 90:6991-6994.
49. Thomson JB, Tuschl T, Eckstein F. Activity of hammerhead ribozymes containing non-nucleotidic linkers. Nucleic Acids Res 1993; 21:5600-5603.
50. Fu DJ, Benseler F, Mclaughlin LW. Hammerhead ribozymes containing non-nucleoside linkers are active RNA catalysts. J Am Chem Soc 1994; 116:4591-4598.
51. Long DM, Uhlenbeck OC. Kinetic characterization of intramolecular and intermolecular hammerhead RNAs with stem II deletions. Proc Natl Acad Sci USA 1994; 91:6977-6981.
52. Hendry P, McCall MJ, Santiago FS et al. In vitro activity of minimised hammerhead ribozymes. Nucleic Acids Res 1995; 23:3922-3927.

53. Amontov S, Nishikawa S, Taira K. Dependence on Mg^{2+} ions of the activities of dimeric hammerhead minizymes. FEBS Lett 1996; 386:99-102.
54. Sugiyama H, Hatano K, Saito I et al. Catalytic activities of hammerhead ribozymes with a triterpenoid linker instead of stem/loop II. FEBS Lett 1996; 392:215-219.
55. Kuwabara T, Amontov S, Warashina M et al. Characterization of several kinds of dimer minizyme: Simultaneous cleavage at two sites in HIV-1 tat mRNA by dimer minizymes. Nucleic Acids Res 1996; 24:2302-2310.
56. Pachuk CJ, Yoon K, Moelling K et al. Selective cleavage of bcr-abl chimeric RNAs by a ribozyme targeted to non-contiguous sequence. Nucleic Acids Res 1994; 22:301-307.
57. James H, Mills K, Gibson I. Investigating and improving the specificity of ribozymes directed against the bcr-abl translocation. Leukemia 1996; 10:1054-1064.
58. Hertel KJ, Herschlag D, Uhlenbeck OC. Specificity of hammerhead ribozyme cleavage. EMBO J 1996; 15:3751-3757.
59. Birikh KR, Heaton PA, Eckstein F. The hammerhead ribozyme—structure, function and application. Eur J Biochem 1997; 245:1-16.
60. Jarvis TC, Wincott FE, Alby LJ et al. Optimizing the cell efficacy of synthetic ribozymes. Site selection and chemical modifications of ribozymes targeting the proto-oncogene c-myb. J Biol Chem 1996; 271:29107-29112.
61. Santoro SW, Joyce GF. A general purpose RNA-cleaving DNA enzyme. Proc Natl Acad Sci USA 1997; 94:4292-4266.
62. Morgan RA, Anderson WF. Human gene therapy. Annu Rev Biochem 1993; 62:191-217.

CHAPTER 6

Using Ribozymes to Attenuate Gene Expression in Transgenic Mice

Shimon Efrat

Introduction

The development of efficient methods for downregulation of cell-specific gene expression in vivo is of great value for gaining new insights into complex biological systems, and for advancing gene therapy for human diseases. Recent progress in gene targeting approaches in transgenic mice utilizing the Cre-loxP DNA recombination system opened the way for disrupting gene function in a cell-specific and time-specific manner.[1] By placing the Cre recombinase under control of an inducible regulatory system, such as that of the bacterial tetracycline operon,[2] one can control the timing of elimination of a certain gene function from a particular cell type in vivo.

Many applications, however, require partial attenuation of gene expression, rather than the all-or-none effect of gene disruption. For such purposes the transcript-specific downregulation of RNA levels and activity using antisense RNA techniques represents a promising approach. The use of antisense RNA in vivo has met with some success in a number of transgenic experiments (reviewed in ref. 3), while in many other cases it failed to affect a significant change in gene expression. One major obstacle has been the need to maintain relatively high intracellular levels of the antisense RNA, which interacts stoichiometrically with the target transcript.

The discovery of ribozymes opened the way for incorporating catalytic RNA elements into antisense RNA. This allows one antisense RNA molecule to interact with and inactivate multiple target RNA molecules, thus reducing the constraint to overexpress a vast excess of the antisense RNA in the target cells. In principle this advantage appears very attractive. It is, therefore, surprising that only a handful of publications have reported the successful application of ribozymes in transgenic animals.

The choice of target may be an important factor. Ribozymes, and antisense RNA approaches in general, may be effective against constitutively expressed genes that are not regulated at the transcriptional level. In contrast, a gene with a capacity to sense the ribozyme-induced downregulation of expression by some feedback mechanism, and respond by upregulating its transcription, may be much harder to downregulate with this approach.

Examples of Ribozyme Applications in Transgenic Mice

Our laboratory has chosen to apply ribozymes to downregulate the expression of the enzyme glucokinase (GK) in pancreatic β cells in transgenic mice.[4] GK is a high-K_m member of the hexokinase family of enzymes. It is expressed specifically in β cells and hepatocytes,

Ribozymes in the Gene Therapy of Cancer, edited by Kevin J. Scanlon and Mohammed Kashani-Sabet.
©1998 R.G. Landes Company.

where it represents the major activity responsible for phosphorylation of glucose to glucose-6-phosphate.[5] This is the first and rate-limiting step in glycolysis, which in β cells generates signals for insulin secretion.[6] Thus GK has been denoted the "glucose sensor" of β cells, in charge of coupling extracellular glucose levels to the correct amounts of secreted insulin.[5] Reduced glucokinase activity may result in decreased sensitivity of β cells to glucose, leading to abnormal insulin secretion and diabetes. DNA polymorphism studies have established a linkage between the GK locus and diabetes in patients with a non insulin-dependent diabetes (type II) form termed MODY (maturity-onset diabetes of the young).[7,8] This disease is characterized by an early age of onset and an autosomal dominant inheritance. Sequencing of the GK gene from MODY patients has detected a number of nonsense and missense mutations which are associated with regions of the enzyme molecule involved in glucose and ATP binding.[7,8] The molecular mechanism which makes these mutations dominant remains unknown, but a gene dosage effect has been suggested. The inheritance pattern of the disease suggests that the patients' β cells contain normal enzyme molecules encoded by the wild type allele. The mutant proteins manifest drastically reduced enzymatic activities.[9,10] Since GK expression in β cells is not transcriptionally regulated,[11,12] the wild type allele can not compensate for this reduction. The decreased GK activity may be sufficient to shift the threshold for glucose sensing, thereby resulting in impaired insulin secretion at physiological glucose levels. However, it remains unclear whether abnormal glucose metabolism in the liver contributes to the disease. Glucose uptake into the liver, where it is stored as glycogen, is an important component in maintaining normal blood glucose levels. This function depends on normal glucokinase activity. The GK gene is transcribed in hepatocytes through a specialized promoter that was shown to be upregulated by insulin.[11,13] Thus, it is possible that the hepatocytes of MODY patients can correct the reduced GK activity by increased transcription of the wild type allele. Yet, as this regulation depends on insulin, it may not be effective when insulin secretion is impaired, as is the case in MODY patients.

Understanding of the human disease can benefit from an animal model, which will allow detailed biochemical and physiological studies. We aimed at generating transgenic mice in which GK activity is specifically impaired in β cells, leaving the liver activity intact, to dissect the relative contribution of these two cell types to the MODY phenotype. To this end a GK-specific ribozyme was expressed in β cells in transgenic mice under control of the insulin promoter.[4]

A synthetic DNA fragment was generated consisting of two 12 bp fragments of mouse GK gene exon 3 sequence in antisense orientation that flank a hammerhead ribozyme catalytic element[14,15] (Fig. 6.1a). The length of the regions complementary to the target represents a compromise between the need to provide target specificity on one hand and catalytic turnover on the other hand. The region of the transcript chosen as target should be unique to assure target specificity. The only target RNA sequence requirements for cleavage by the ribozyme is a GUX element (X = A, C or U). The ribozyme cleaves the target RNA immediately 3' to the X (Fig. 6.1a). A number of ribozymes directed against different regions of the transcript may need to be tested for each target in cultured cells, in order to choose the most efficient one for in vivo expression.

The hybrid DNA fragment was placed downstream of the rat insulin II promoter and an intron element, and upstream of the SV40 late polyadenylation site (Fig. 6.1b). Stable transfection of this construct, denoted RIP-GKRZ, into a murine β cell line (βTC6) resulted in a 45% reduction in GK mRNA levels; however no cleavage products could be detected (Fig. 6.2b). This likely results from the fact that the two cleavage products lack either a cap site or a poly-A tail, both of which are needed for RNA stability. In their absence the RNA is rapidly degraded. In the absence of demonstrable degradation products it is hard to prove

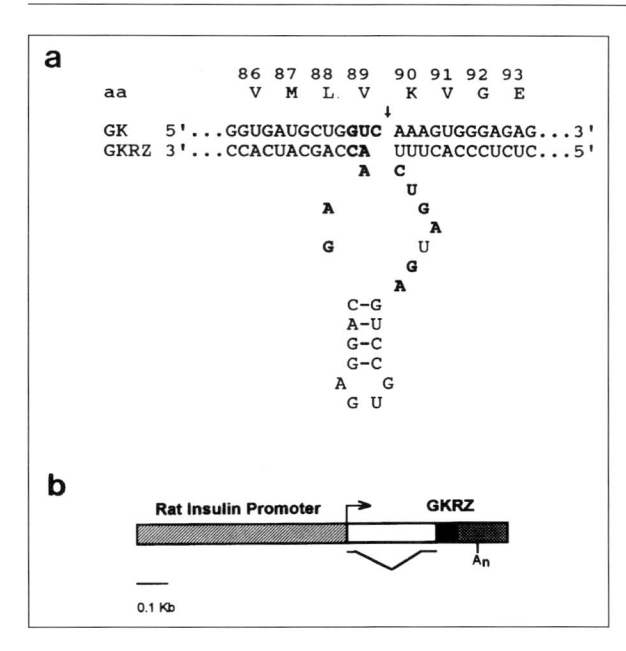

Fig. 6.1. Design of the RIP-GKRZ construct. (a) The GKRZ transcript hybridized with the target GK mRNA. The conserved ribozyme nucleotides are shown in bold letters. The arrow marks the putative cleavage site. (b) The RIP-GKRZ hybrid gene consists of a synthetic DNA fragment encoding the ribozyme flanked by GK antisense sequences (GKRZ), an upstream intron element and a downstream polyadenylation site. Reproduced with permission from Efrat S et al, Proc Natl Acad Sci USA 1994; 91: 2051-2055.

that the reduction in mRNA levels occurs as a result of ribozyme activity, as opposed to a simple antisense effect, which could lead to degradation of the target GK transcript through the formation of a duplex RNA. It is not known whether the ribozyme cleavage activity and the subsequent RNA degradation take place in the nucleus or in the cytoplasm. Immunoblotting analysis of the transfected cells revealed a 2- to 3-fold reduction in GK protein levels, compared to untransfected cells (Fig. 6.2c). This suggests that in addition to RNA degradation, attenuation may be achieved through reduced translational activity of the GK mRNA, presumably by the formation of double-stranded RNA hybrids with the GKRZ transcripts, as has been observed in other antisense RNA experiments.[16]

The RIP-GKRZ construct was microinjected into mouse embryos, and two independent transgenic lines were shown to express the transgene by RT-PCR analysis of islet RNA. Immunohistochemical analysis of pancreas sections with a GK antiserum revealed a reduced staining intensity in transgenic islets, compared with normal controls (Fig. 6.3).

Glucose phosphorylation activity at various glucose concentrations was assayed in islets isolated from the transgenic mice. GK activity in RIP-GKRZ islets was reduced by 70%, compared to normal islets, while the activity of the related low-K_m hexokinases remained essentially unaffected (Fig. 6.4). This finding demonstrates the sequence specificity of the approach. The incomplete inhibition of expression obtained with the antisense approach may represent an advantage for studying its consequences in vivo, since it mimics the situation in MODY. In addition, total shutoff of GK expression in β cells is lethal, as demonstrated by gene disruption experiments.[17-19]

Although no data on islet GK activity is available from MODY patients, it is assumed that the wild type GK allele produces half of the normal activity. Therefore islet GK activity in the RIP-GKRZ mice is likely to be as low or lower than that of MODY patients. Nevertheless, the RIP-GKRZ mice maintained normal fasting plasma glucose and insulin levels and manifested normal glucose tolerance. In contrast, analysis of glucose-induced insulin secretion from in situ-perfused pancreas (Fig. 6.5) revealed a markedly reduced response, for the

Fig. 6.2. Analysis of pRIP-GKRZ effect on GK expression in transfected β cells. (a) RT-PCR analysis of GKRZ expression in the transfected (+) vs. untransfected (-) cells. Expression is manifested by the 200 bp band that results from spliced transcripts. P represents the size of an unspliced fragment amplified from pRIP-GKRZ DNA. (b) Northern blotting analysis of GK mRNA. Ribosomal RNA bands serve as size markers. An α-tubulin probe was used to correct for loading. (c) Immunoblotting analysis of GK protein. Size markers are in kilodaltons. Reproduced with permission from Efrat S et al, Proc Natl Acad Sci USA 1994; 91:2051-2055.

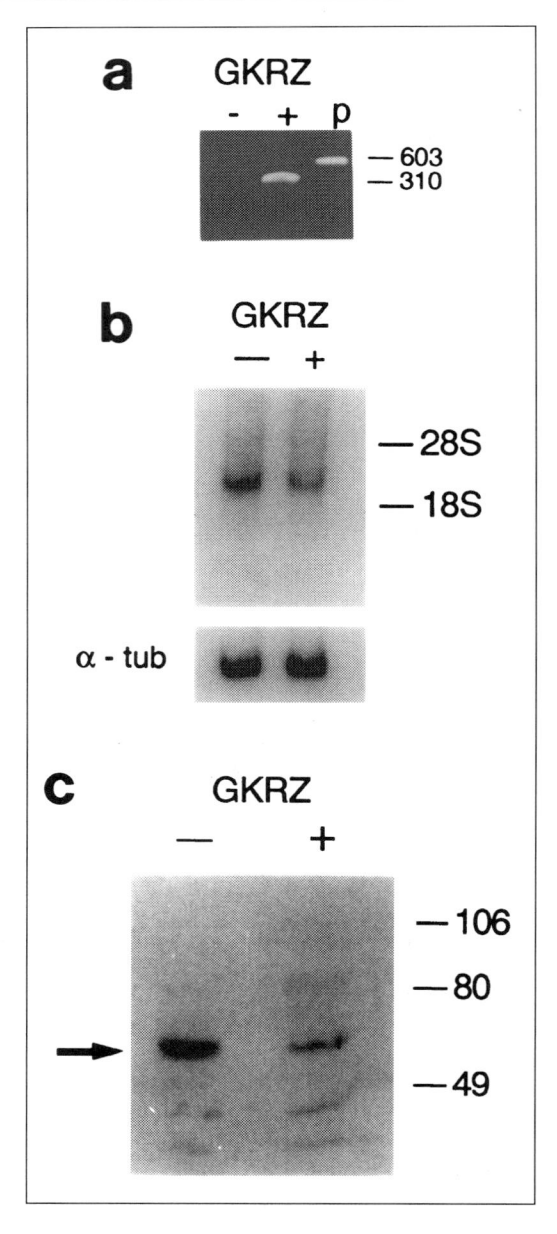

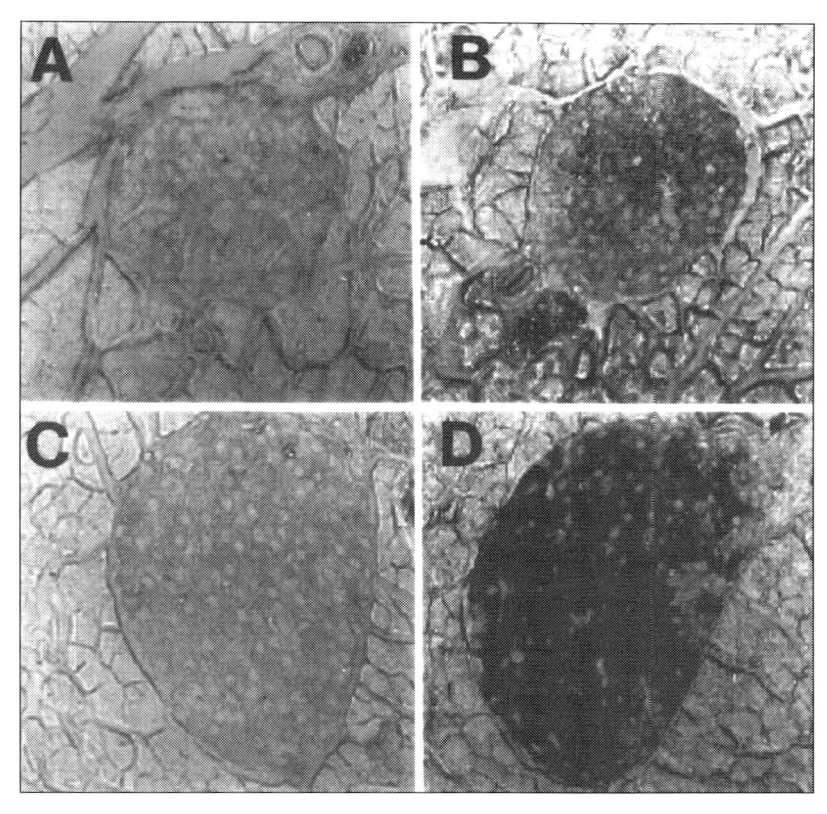

Fig. 6.3. Immunohistochemical analysis of RIP-GKRZ pancreas. Tissue sections were incubated with a sheep-anti-GK serum followed by a biotinylated second antibody, and visualized with horseradish peroxidase-conjugated avidin. (A) transgenic islet stained with pre-immune sheep serum; (B) transgenic islet stained with anti-GK serum; (C) normal islet stained with pre-immune serum; (D) normal islet stained with anti-GK serum. Magnification is x200. Reproduced with permission from Efrat S et al, Proc Natl Acad Sci USA 1994; 91:2051-2055.

Fig. 6.4. Glucose phosphorylation activity in RIP-GKRZ islets. The great difference in K_m, 0.05 and 8 mM for hexokinase and glucokinase, respectively, allows distinction between the two enzymatic activities. Solid bar, normal islets; dotted bar, RIP-GKRZ islets, lineage 2; hatched bar, RIP-GKRZ islets, lineage 4. Values are expressed in units per gram of islet protein. 1 U = 1 µmol product per minute. Values are mean ± SEM (n = 3). Transgenic and normal GK activity differences are statistically significant (p <0.0001 by t test). Reproduced with permission from Efrat S et al, Proc Natl Acad Sci USA 1994; 91:2051-2055.

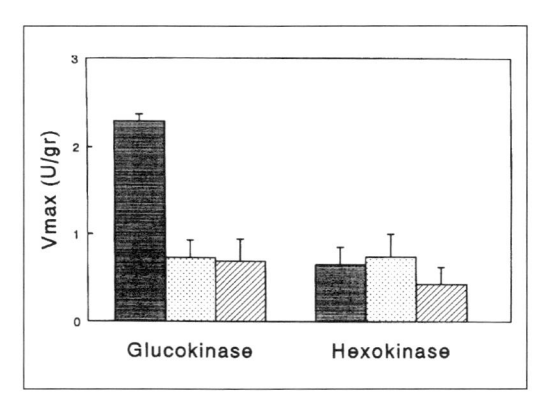

Fig. 6.5. Insulin secretion from in situ-perfused control (open circle) and transgenic (closed circle) mouse pancreas. Values are mean ± SEM (n = 5). Reproduced with permission from Efrat S et al, Proc Natl Acad Sci USA 1994; 91:2051-2055.

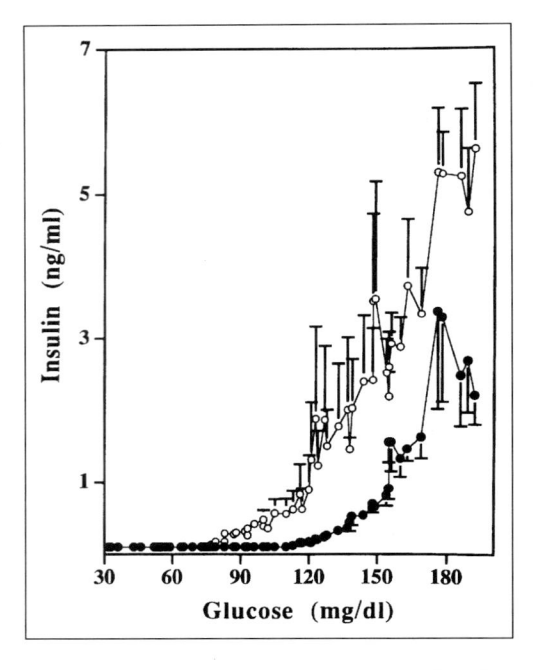

glucose concentration range of 75-200 mg/dl, in the transgenic pancreas compared to that of normal controls.

Thus, in spite of the considerable reduction in β cell GK activity, below the level that gives rise to diabetes in MODY patients, and the reduced insulin secretory response to glucose, in a manner similar to that observed in MODY patients,[20] the RIP-GKRZ mice did not develop overt diabetes. It is possible that in the mouse other insulin secretagogues can compensate for the reduction in glucose-induced secretion. Alternatively, these results indicate that an impaired liver function, in addition to that of β cells, is required for the induction of overt diabetes by GK deficiency, as suggested by the gene disruption experiments.[17-19] Such liver impairments have been documented in MODY patients.[21] The finding that partial attenuation of expression of the normal GK protein is sufficient to impair the sensitivity of β cells to glucose supports the interpretation of the dominance of the GK mutations in MODY as a gene dosage effect, rather than a gain-of-function negative dominant effect of the mutant protein.

The reduced β cell GK activity in the RIP-GKRZ mice may cause a predisposition to diabetes. This may develop into overt disease in certain physiological conditions, such as those caused by age, sex, weight, diet, and genetic background differences. Thus, these mice provide an experimental system for studying the effect of such factors on the development of type II diabetes.

A second example of an effective ribozyme application in transgenic mice is the targeting of $β_2$-microglobulin ($β_2$M) mRNA.[22] This protein is required for antigen peptide presentation by class I major histocompatibility molecules on the surface of most mammalian cells. A hammerhead ribozyme directed to exon 2 was expressed in transgenic mice under the cytomegalovirus promoter. Expression was detected in lung, kidney and spleen, with the greatest reduction (>90%) in $β_2$M mRNA levels observed in the lungs, although considerable variation was noted among individual mice in the same lineage. Unfortunately, the phenotype of these mice has not been described.

Recently, mice were generated carrying a transgene that encodes a hammerhead ribozyme directed against bovine α-lactalbumin (α-lac) under control of the mouse mammary tumor virus long terminal repeat.[23] The ribozyme was targeted to the 3' untranslated region of the transcript and was flanked by 12-nucleotide segments of complementary sequence. The mice were crossed to a transgenic line over-expressing a bovine α-lac transgene in the mammary gland. Expression of the ribozyme resulted in up to 78% reduction in target mRNA and protein. The endogenous murine transcript and protein levels were not affected, demonstrating the specificity of the approach.

Future Directions

These successful studies demonstrate the feasibility of employing ribozymes in the attenuation of gene expression in vivo. Although they represent an encouraging beginning, much work remains to be done to render this approach more efficient and widely applicable. Better understanding of the ribozyme mechanism of action and the subcellular site of action is needed to design improved targeting constructs. Ways to improve ribozyme synthesis in the cells and increase ribozyme stability will result in enhanced function. The parameters guiding the choice of the optimal cleavage site within the target transcript need to be established. Improved in vitro assays, in which the cleavage products can be preserved, may assist in some of these tasks. In addition, a rigorous comparison of antisense and ribozyme approaches is needed to establish their relative efficiency in individual systems.

In spite of the seemingly slow progress, this methodology continues to hold a great promise for research and therapy alike. In combination with conditional gene expression approaches, it should be possible to effectively utilize ribozymes for cell-specific and time-specific downregulation of gene expression in vivo.

Acknowledgments

The research in my laboratory has been supported by the Juvenile Diabetes Foundation International, by a Career Scientist Award from the Irma T. Hirschl Foundation and by an NIDDK James A. Shannon Director's Award.

References

1. Gu H, Marth JD, Orban PC et al. Deletion of a DNA polymerase beta gene segment in T cells using cell type-specific gene targeting. Science 1994; 265:103-106.
2. Gossen M, Bujard H. Tight control of gene expression in mammalian cells by tetracycline-responsive promoters. Proc Natl Acad Sci USA 1992; 89:5547-5551.
3. Sokol DL, Murray JD. Antisense and ribozyme constructs in transgenic animals. Transgen Res 1996; 5:363-371.
4. Efrat S, Leiser M, Wu Y-J et al. Ribozyme-mediated attenuation of pancreatic β-cell glucokinase expression in transgenic mice results in impaired glucose-induced insulin secretion. Proc Natl Acad Sci USA 1994; 91:2051-2055.
5. Meglasson MD, Matschinsky FM. Pancreatic islet glucose metabolism and regulation of insulin secretion. Diabetes Metab Rev 1986; 2:163-214.
6. Meglasson MD, Matschinsky FM. New perspectives in pancreatic islet glucokinase. Am J Physiol 1984; 246:E1-13.
7. Vionnet N, Stoffel M, Takeda J et al. Nonsense mutation in the glucokinase gene causes early-onset non-insulin-dependent diabetes mellitus. Nature 1992; 356:721-722.
8. Stoffel M, Froguel P, Takeda J et al. Human glucokinase gene: Isolation, characterization, and identification of two missense mutations linked to early-onset non-insulin-dependent (type 2) diabetes mellitus. Proc Natl Acad Sci USA 1992; 89:7698-7702.
9. Gidh-Jain M, Takeda J, Xu LZ at al. Glucokinase mutations associated with non-insulin-dependent (type 2) diabetes mellitus have decreased enzymatic activity: Implications for structure/function relationships. Proc Natl Acad Sci USA 1993; 90:1932-19336.

10. Takeda J, Gidh-Jain M, Xu LZ et al. Structure/function studies of human β-cell glucokinase. J Biol Chem 1993; 268:15200-15204.
11. Iynedjian PB, Pilot PR, Nouspikel T et al. Differential expression and regulation of the glucokinase gene in liver and islets of Langerhans. Proc Natl Acad Sci USA 1989; 86:7838-7842.
12. Liang Y, Najafi H, Matschinsky FM. Glucose regulates glucokinase activity in cultured islets from rat pancreas. J Biol Chem 1990; 265:16863-16866.
13. Magnuson MA, Shelton KD. An alternate promoter in the glucokinase gene is active in the pancreatic beta cell. J Biol Chem 1989; 264:15936-15942.
14. Forster AC, Symons RH. Self-cleavage of plus and minus RNAs of a virusoid and a structural model for the active sites. Cell 1987; 49:211-220.
15. Hasellof J, Gerlach WL. Simple RNA enzymes with new and highly specific endoribonuclease activities. Nature 1988; 334:585-591.
16. Strickland S, Huarte J, Belin D et al. Antisense RNA directed against the 3' noncoding region prevents dormant RNA inactivation in mouse oocytes. Science 1988; 241:680-684.
17. Bali D, Svetlanov A, Lee H-W et al. Animal model for maturity-onset diabetes of the young generated by disruption of the mouse glucokinase gene. J Biol Chem 1995; 270:21464-21467.
18. Grupe A, Hultgren B, Ryan A et al. Transgenic knockouts reveal a critical requirement for pancreatic beta cell glucokinase in maintaining glucose homeostasis. Cell 1995; 83:69-78.
19. Terauchi Y, Sakura H, Yasuda K et al. Pancreatic beta-cell-specific targeted disruption of glucokinase gene. Diabetes mellitus due to defective insulin secretion to glucose. J Biol Chem 1995; 270:30253-30256.
20. Byrne M, Sturis J, Clement K et al. Insulin secretory abnormalities in subjects with hyperglycemia due to glucokinase mutations. J Clin Invest 1994; 93:1120-1130.
21. Sakura H, Kawamori R, Kubota M et al. Glucokinase gene mutations and impaired glucose uptake by liver. Lancet 1993; 341:1532-1533.
22. Larsson S, Hotchkiss G, Andang M et al. Reduced beta 2-microglobulin mRNA levels in transgenic mice expressing a designed hammerhead ribozyme. Nuc Acids Res 1994; 22:2242-2248.
23. L'Huillier PJ, Soulier S, Stinnakre MG et al. Efficient and specific ribozyme-mediated reduction of bovine alpha-lactalbumin expression in double transgenic mice. Proc Natl Acad SCi USA 1996; 93:6698-6703.

CHAPTER 7

Retroviral Delivery of Ribozymes

Lun-Quan Sun and Geoff Symonds

Retroviral Properties and Life cycle

Retroviruses (RNA tumor viruses) have been used as vectors for gene transfer since the early 1980s. They possess structural and enzymatic properties that make them suitable vectors. These properties are summarized in Table 7.1. The long terminal repeats (LTRs) are involved in integration of the provirus and contain promoter/enhancer elements to drive proviral transcription. The viral enzymes reverse transcriptase, polymerase and integrase are present within the virions and are essential to the retroviral life cycle. The structural genes *gag* and *env* encode internal (Gag) and external (Env) viral proteins. Retroviruses infect cells via the relevant receptors. While there is some degree of cellular specificity, their ability to infect cells is quite broad. The retroviral life cycle is shown in Figure 7.1 and reviewed by Miller in ref. 1.

Retroviral Vectors and Their Design

It was shown in the late 1970s/early 1980s that internal portions of the retroviral genome could be deleted and cDNAs for a variety of genes (oncogenes, marker genes, potentially therapeutic genes) could be inserted into the viral DNA. The use of packaging cell lines (mouse and human) which supplied the missing vector functions in trans allowed the generation of virions from the cDNA, following transfection of the recombinant DNA into the packaging cell line.[1] The retroviruses that were thereby produced were termed recombinant retroviruses and, more recently, retroviral vectors (the latter term is now utilized to describe the viral backbone plus the specific insert). The mode of production of retroviral particles from engineered cDNA is shown in Figure 7.2. The variety of inserts utilized experimentally is summarized in Table 7.2.

A number of different retroviral vectors have been developed for gene transfer into human cells, generally based on the Moloney murine leukemia virus (MoMLV) backbone.[1] A wide variety of vector constructs from the original vectors, such as N2 and LNL6, have been described. These vectors include those with the long terminal repeats (LTRs) as the promoter of gene transcription,[2] those with internal promoters,[3] those with the gene of interest expressed in the reverse orientation,[4] those with self-inactivating (SIN) LTRs,[5] those with pol III and pol I promoters,[6,7] those with the expression cassette inserted in the LTRs (double-copy vectors)[8] and those with modified LTRs.[9] However, it has gradually become apparent that as the complexity of design increases, the corresponding vector titers usually decrease and there is an increasing propensity for retroviral rearrangement. This has tended to lead the field back to simple one-gene vector designs. In our laboratory, a simple design of a retroviral vector based on LNL6 has been consistently found to be very efficient in the

Ribozymes in the Gene Therapy of Cancer, edited by Kevin J. Scanlon and Mohammed Kashani-Sabet.
©1998 R.G. Landes Company.

Fig. 7.1. Retroviral life cycle. The retroviral virion binds to the cell surface generally, through an appropriate receptor. It is then uncoated and the viral genomic RNA, in association with the viral enzymes reverse transcriptase, polymerase and integrase, enters the cell. The RNA is reverse transcribed to a cDNA copy which becomes double stranded and integrates into the host genome. This proviral DNA is transcribed as for other cellular genes into RNA. The RNA is either mRNA to produce viral proteins following translation, or genomic RNA which is packaged into virions that bud from the cell surface. This is generally (except in the case of HIV and certain other lentiviruses) non-pathogenic to the host cell. The resultant virions can then infect further target cells to reinitiate the process. In the case of replication-incompetent recombinant retroviruses, there is a requirement for so-called "helper" or replication-competent retrovirus to supply those functions missing from the vector in trans. This can be accomplished to produce single-hit retroviruses by the use of appropriate packaging cell lines (see text and Fig. 7.2).

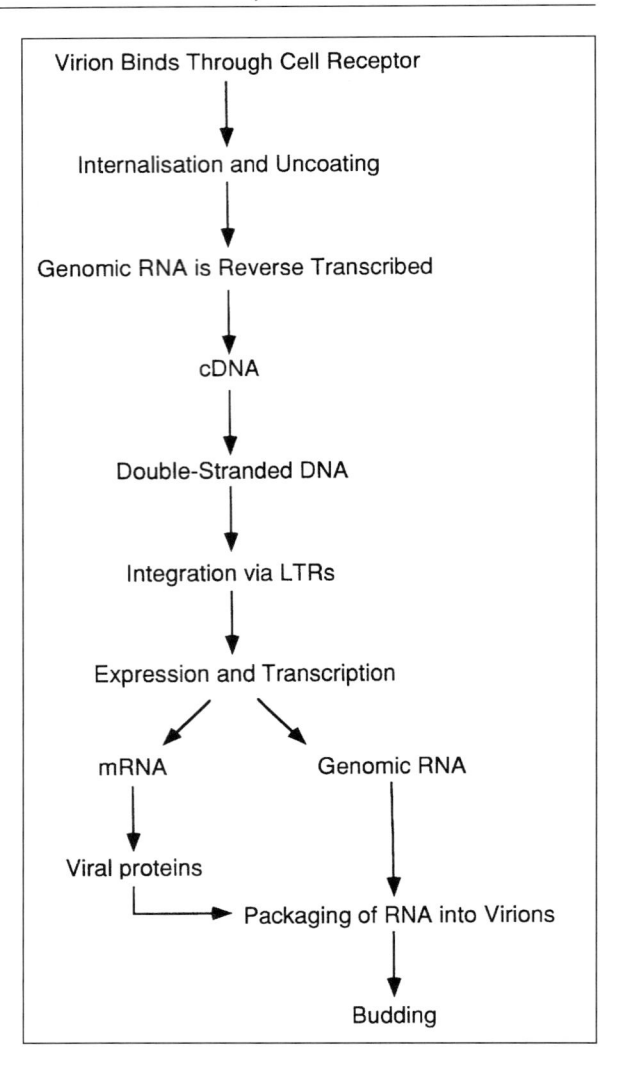

```
Virion Binds Through Cell Receptor
              ↓
   Internalisation and Uncoating
              ↓
   Genomic RNA is Reverse Transcribed
              ↓
            cDNA
              ↓
      Double-Stranded DNA
              ↓
       Integration via LTRs
              ↓
     Expression and Transcription
          ↙           ↘
       mRNA         Genomic RNA
         ↓                ↓
   Viral proteins         |
         └──────→ Packaging of RNA into Virions
                          ↓
                       Budding
```

Table 7.1. Properties of retroviruses

1. Ability to accommodate cDNA inserts through genetic engineering in the cDNA form.
2. Virions containing modified genomic RNA can be produced through the transfection/infection of relevant packaging cell lines.
3. Following infection, proviruses integrate at single to several copies into the target cell genome and hence carried to progeny cells.
4. Insert cDNA is expressed from viral long terminal repeat or from internal promoters via cellular transcriptional machinery.
5. Envelope can be modified to be cell targeted.
6. Non-toxic and can be modified to reduce the risk of replication competent retroviruses (RCR) generation.

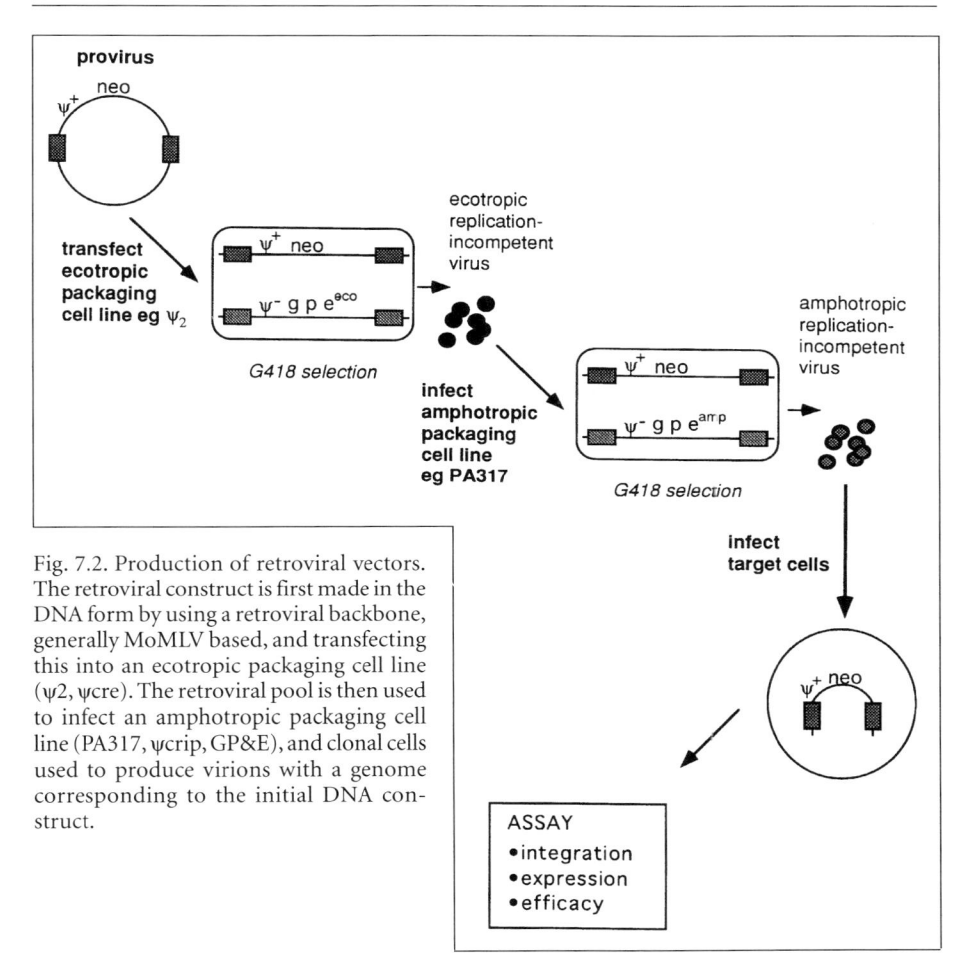

Fig. 7.2. Production of retroviral vectors. The retroviral construct is first made in the DNA form by using a retroviral backbone, generally MoMLV based, and transfecting this into an ecotropic packaging cell line ($\psi 2$, ψcre). The retroviral pool is then used to infect an amphotropic packaging cell line (PA317, ψcrip, GP&E), and clonal cells used to produce virions with a genome corresponding to the initial DNA construct.

Table 7.2. Retroviral cDNA inserts

1. Marker genes, e.g., *neo*, hygromycin to select cells and follow cell fate.
2. Potentially therapeutic genes, e.g., adenosine deaminase, β-globin, to impact on cell phenotype.
3. Oncogenes, e.g., *myc*, *erbB*, to induce cell transformation/oncogenesis.
4. Tumor suppressor genes, e.g., *p53, p21, Rb*, to reverse transformation.
5. Ribozymes, antisense, decoys and transdominant protein genes to suppress gene expression.
6. Suicide genes, e.g., HSV-tk, to kill cancer cells

transduction of T lymphocyte cell lines and human peripheral blood lymphocytes (PBLs) in terms of vector titers, transduction efficiency as measured by G418 resistance, duration of transgene expression and stability of transgene transcripts.

Cell Type Specific Promoters

Retroviral vectors are widely used vehicles for the effective delivery of ribozyme genes constructs into mammalian cells. The lack of regulation of these expression vectors represents an obstacle for appropriate and controlled expression of foreign genes. The large number of well-characterized regulatory elements controlling cell specific gene expression and the identification of responsive/inducible elements within promoter sequences has laid the foundation for utilizing these elements in the construction of retroviral vectors (Table 7.3). Second and third generation retroviral vectors which harbor cell specific promoters or elements responding to regulatory signals represent an important component for safe, selective, and controlled expression of therapeutic genes. Furthermore, exploitation of cell type specific promoter sequences for gene expression in the appropriate cell type could augment the efficacy and stability of gene expression.

Packaging Cell Lines

Recent generation packaging cell lines have been designed to reduce the chance of generation of replication competent retrovirus (RCR). RCR have the potential to develop following extensive passaging in packaging cell lines. Such RCR, also termed "helper viruses", are generated through recombination events. To reduce the possibility of recombination, the PA317 packaging cell line was designed with deletion not only of the ψ packaging signal but also of two other regions in the 5' and 3' LTR.[10] Also, a modified version N2 vector, LNL6,[11] was designed. The start codon of the *gag* gene in the previous vector N2 was replaced by a stop codon; some of the MoMLV sequences of LTR in N2 vector were replaced by Moloney murine sarcoma virus (MSV) to decrease the homology between the vector and helper virus genome. This combination (LNL6 and PA317) has been used in most of the clinical studies to date. Other alterations of packaging cell lines (Ψ-cre and Ψ-crip) include deletion of the packaging signal (as previously) as well as expression of the *gag-pol* and *env* genes on two separate plasmids to decrease the possibility of recombination.[12] More recently, transient packaging cell line systems have been developed, including the PHOENIX system.[13]

Targeting of Retroviruses

Research has been conducted into cell-specific retroviral targeting by modifications in viral envelope protein sequences, using antibodies as specific mediators in viral infection, and modified ligands or receptors. The strategies for modification of the target cell specificity of retroviral vectors are summarized as follows. Generally this involves re-engineering the *env* gene by replacing segments with epitopes that recognize receptors other than those normally used by the virus. This is achieved by manipulation of the *env* gene in the proviral construct of the packaging cell line.[14]

Antibody-Mediated Binding

Retroviral vector particles can be engineered that contain an antigen binding site of an Ab molecule (single chain antigen binding proteins, scFv) in place of the natural retroviral receptor binding peptide.[15] This single chain antibody can be targeted to specific cellular membrane proteins. An antibody (Ab) bridge can thus be engineered between a retroviral vector and the designated target cell that does not contain a receptor for the virus. In addition, antibodies directed against a specific known protein that is located on the target cell

Table 7.3. Cell-specific promoters and their target cells.

Promoters	Target cells
β-Globin promoter/LCR	Erythroid cells
Immunoglobin promoters	B lymphoma
CD11a, b promoters	Leucocytes
Albumin promoter	Hepatocytes
HIV-LTR	HIV-infected T cells
Tat/Rev responsive elements	CD4+ T cells
CEA promoter	Colon and lung carcinomas
AFP promoter	Hepatocellular carcinomas
Tyrosinase promoter	Melanomas
MMTV-LTR	Mammary carcinoma
Egr-1 promoter	Irradiated tumors
HSP70 promoter	Tumor treated with hyperthermy

surface can be linked by streptavidin to antibodies against viral Env proteins. The Ab-streptavidin complex functions as a bridge to link the virus to its target cells via the novel, specific receptor.

Asialoglycosylation

The retroviral Env proteins can be chemically modified so that they are recognized by receptors expressed on the surface of the target cell. One such example is to asialate the Env proteins by the coupling of lactose. By this means, the hepatocyte-specific asialoglycoprotein receptors can be targeted using modified retroviral vectors.[16]

Pseudotyped Vectors

This is based on the concept that cell tropism is determined by the source of the viral Env protein present on the vector virions. One such example is the recently developed packaging cell line, PG13.[17] This packaging cell line can pseudotype the MoMLV vector with the gibbon ape leukemia virus (GALV) envelope, and these pseudotyped retrovirus vectors appear able to infect a larger number of human cells more efficiently than comparable MoMLV-based amphotropic retroviruses.

Ribozyme Action

As noted in the previous chapters, ribozymes are RNA molecules with catalytic properties enabling them to cleave target RNA substrates.[18-25] The two main types of ribozymes are hairpin and hammerhead.[21,22] They differ in their structure, but each has been shown to be amenable to modifications in which the substrate and catalytic components are separated to enable cleavage in trans.[21,22] Several features of ribozymes make them attractive as potential therapeutic agents—in particular, their specificity of cleavage and their potential ability to cleave multiple substrate molecules. Having shown their ability to cleave in vitro-derived substrates, ribozyme DNA constructs can then be incorporated into a variety of vectors. Such vectors include relatively simple expression vectors in which the ribozyme is incorporated downstream of a mammalian promoter, generally as a chimeric gene construct, or in more complicated vectors which are based on the genome of retroviruses or other viruses.

The ribozyme is engineered in the DNA form by complementarity to the target sequence, which in the case of hammerhead ribozymes possesses a GUX or, in certain cases, NUX (where N represents any nucleotide and X represents A, C or U) motif. The cDNA is incorporated into the retroviral cDNA and the new genomic material is produced following transfection into the packaging cell line. We, and others, have used this approach to introduce a variety of ribozymes into retroviruses. We have previously detailed the production of anti-HIV retroviruses.[26]

As to stability of the ribozyme within cells, it is likely that many factors contribute. These include structure of the RNA transcript, the cellular compartment in which ribozyme transcripts are produced and transported, and whether the ribozyme is embedded within another gene. To date, tRNA, U1 or U6 snRNA have been used as expression cassettes for ribozymes. We consistently found that the insertion of a ribozyme sequence into the 3' untranslated region of the neomycin resistance gene within an expression vector led to a high level expression of the neo/ribozyme chimeric RNA transcript.[27,28]

Ribozymes have been shown to affect the expression of a number of genes in tissue culture systems. Various read-outs can be utilized to monitor the effectiveness of ribozyme action. Such read-outs include modulation of gene expression (structural genes, cytokines) monitored by Northern or Western blots, modification of cellular phenotype as measured by microscopy or FACS, and inhibition of viral replication determined by ELISA or viral RNA dot-blots. Once introduced into cell lines or primary cells, ribozyme-mediated inhibition can be assayed in appropriate test systems. Two major systems where ribozymes have shown efficacy in tissue culture are:

1. the reversion of the transformed cellular phenotype; and
2. the inhibition of HIV replication.

The overall construction and testing procedure used by this group for such studies is outlined in Figure 7.3. Reversion of the transformed cellular phenotype is based on ribozyme mediated downregulation of oncogene expression. In inhibiting HIV replication, the ribozymes act to cleave genomic or sub-genomic mRNA molecules of HIV. Ribozymes that have been utilized for these two purposes are detailed at length in other chapters of this book. The following focuses on one example of retroviral delivery of ribozymes—the one that has been used most extensively to date—the use of ribozymes targeted to inhibition of retroviral replication, in particular, that of HIV.

Murine Model Systems for Retroviral-Ribozyme Delivery and Inhibition of Gene Expression

By using a Moloney murine leukemia virus (MoMLV) model system, we have shown that the ψ packaging site, the site essential for packaging of viral genomic RNA, is an effective ribozyme target site and can be used to effectively inhibit MoMLV replication.[27] The efficiency of substrate cleavage by these ψ packaging site-targeted ribozymes correlated with the ability of the corresponding ribozyme expression constructs to inhibit MoMLV replication.[27] We have used retroviral vectors containing ribozymes to this site to demonstrate the utility of retroviral vectors (and the specificity of the packaging site as a target) by demonstrating that ribozymes could be designed to specifically cleave a MoMLV ψ packaging site target, though not the MoMSV variant sequence, within the retroviral vector itself. This was despite the high degree of homology between the two ψ packaging site sequences. Virus could be produced from the recombinant ribozyme containing provirus (without an apparent inhibition of vector titer) and cells transduced with this ribozyme-containing virus were shown to inhibit target MoMLV replication.[29] This shows the utility of retroviral-ribozyme constructs.

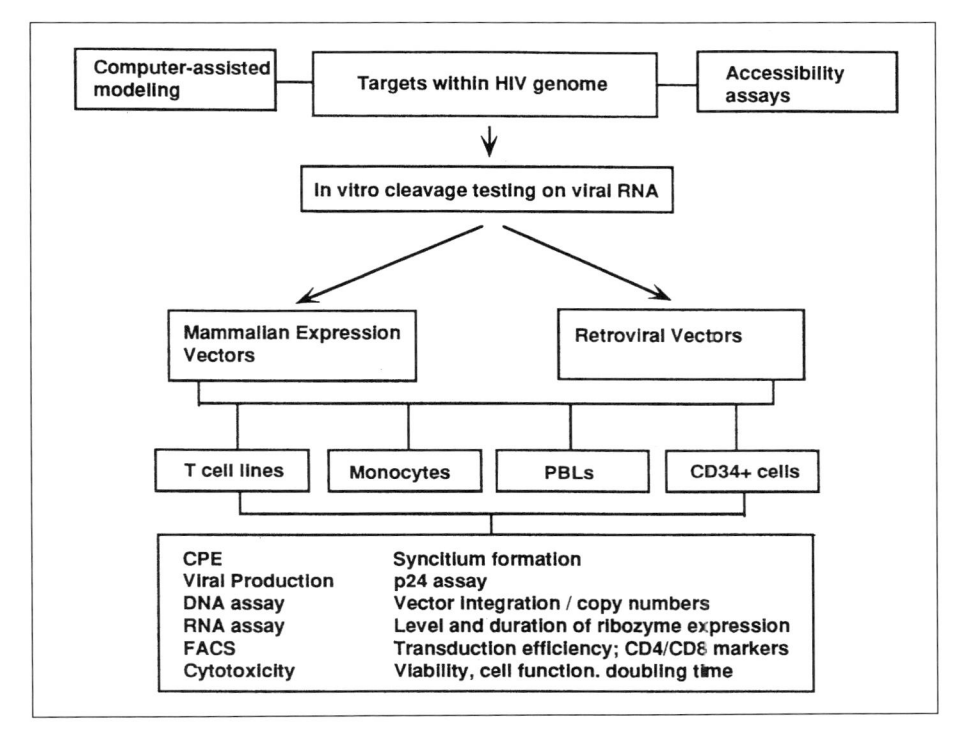

Fig. 7.3. Strategy of construction and testing of anti-viral ribozyme constructs. Ribozymes are designed based on the accessibility of their corresponding target RNA. This can be assessed by computer modeling and/or in vitro assays such as RNAase mapping. After testing for in vitro cleavage, the ribozymes are cloned into expression or retroviral vectors. They can then be tested in different cell systems using the various read-outs as shown.

Anti-HIV Retroviral Ribozyme Constructs

A number of studies have employed ribozymes to show effective inhibition of HIV replication. These studies have been previously summarized both by ourselves and other groups and are briefly outlined here.

Sarver and colleagues used a ribozyme construct targeted to the HIV-1 *gag* sequence and showed inhibition of HIV replication.[30] The retroviral (MoMLV) transfer of HIV-1 (5' leader sequence) targeted ribozymes into a stable T cell line (MT4) resulted in resistance to HIV-1 infection.[31] Other investigators used a ribozyme construct engineered to specifically cleave the HIV-1 *tat* gene.[32] Retrovirally transduced cells showed a delay in measurable HIV p24 levels—15 days compared to 7 days in control cells. In addition, a hairpin ribozyme expressed from a tRNA^{Val} transcriptional cassette within various expression vectors, including retroviruses, was shown to confer resistance to several HIV-1 isolates.[33-38]

In our own experiments we used ribozyme constructs in which the ribozyme was:
1. cloned into the 3' region of the *neo* gene and driven by the SV40 promoter in an expression vector; or
2. inserted into a MoMLV-based retroviral vector.

Using ribozymes which were targeted against either the HIV *tat* gene or the ψ packaging site of HIV-1,[27,28,39] we observed protection of transfected or retrovirally transduced T lymphocyte (SupT1) cells from HIV-1 infection—both in terms of delay of HIV-1 replication and absolute virus levels (assayed by syncytia and p24 ELISA antigen assay). Replication of the virus was inhibited by 70-95% for the laboratory adapted HIV-1 isolates (SF2, IIIB) and by 2-4 logs for primary clinical isolates. The most effective ribozyme in both expression systems was one directed to the first coding exon of *tat*, termed Rz2; within the MoMLV vector LNL6 this is termed RRz2.[27,28,39] These results were borne out in a second T lymphocyte cell line, a pooled CEM T4 cell line system, in which the most effective construct was RRz2. This construct elicited an anti-viral effect, reducing p24 antigen levels by 70-80% compared to vector/marker- alone (LNL6) controls. An antisense retroviral construct termed RASH-5 with sequences complementary to a 550 base 5' region of the HIV-1 genome exhibited a similar level of inhibition (Smythe, Sun, Pyati, Gerlach, Symonds, unpublished results).

These results using retroviral-ribozyme constructs were confirmed in non-HIV infected, normal peripheral blood lymphocytes (PBLs)—both total and CD4+ enriched. The RRz2 retroviral construct, shown to be effective in the pooled T lymphocyte assay, was also effective (70-90% inhibition) in this assay. Other ribozyme-containing constructs were somewhat less effective. For the retroviral assay systems, another recombinant retrovirus, engineered to contain polyTAR—a construct similar to that shown by others to be effective in T cell lines,[40] was used as a positive control. In the PBL assay, this polyTAR retrovirus was found to be somewhat less efficient than the Rz2 and antisense viruses.[28] In addition, RRz2 and LNL6 vectors were also used to transduce PBLs from HIV-1 infected patients. Paired analysis showed that cell viability in the ribozyme-transduced HIV-1 infected PBLs was significantly higher than that in the vector-transduced cells. This difference in viability (between RRz2 and LNL6 transduced cells) was not observed in PBLs from non-infected donors.[40a] This observation is the first evidence that a ribozyme can impact on the survival of HIV-1 infected patient-derived PBLs in cell culture, and implies that the ribozyme-expressing cells may have a growth viability advantage over non-transduced cells within HIV-1-infected patients.

Recent work from this group has confirmed the specificity of ribozyme action. In a study addressing this issue, a different ribozyme, Rz1, targeted to the 5' splicing region of the *tat* gene was designed to cleave GUC N, in which N is G in HIV-1 IIIB and N is A in HIV-1 SF2. The data from both in vitro and in vivo studies showed that the ribozyme could protect cells from challenge by only those HIV isolates whose genomic sequence was cleavable in vitro, and demonstrated the importance of the first base pair distal to the NUX within helix I of the hammerhead structure for both in vitro and in vivo ribozyme activities.[39]

To address issues of the impact of ribozyme expression on the viral population, including virus sequence integrity, a multiple-passage assay was developed in our group to analyze HIV-1 sequence variation and viral replication dynamics in ribozyme-expressing cells. The results demonstrated that Rz2 ribozyme expression in transduced human T cells yields:
1. no mutations within the ribozyme targeting region over five sequential viral passages; and
2. rapid disappearance of certain quasi-species of HIV-1.[40a] This further indicates the potential for clinical use of an anti-HIV ribozyme.

Taken together, these results show that retroviral-ribozyme constructs effectively inhibit HIV-1 replication.

General Aspects of Retroviral and Other Delivery Systems

Probably the major hurdle to be overcome in gene therapy is the efficient delivery of the therapeutic gene(s) into relevant cell populations within patients. At present, retroviral vectors are generally the delivery system of choice due to their relative efficiency, observed safety, stable integration and persistent expression.[1,41,42] Well over 150 gene therapy clinical trials have been approved in the USA to date and, of these, a large majority rely on a retroviral vector to carry marker or therapeutic genes into the target cell genome. Most of these viral vectors are derived from MoMLV.[1] However, retroviral vectors also have some limitations. Their host range may be restricted (to date amphotropic retroviruses have generally been used) and, probably more importantly, they require cell division for integration of their genomic material.

Recently, advances have been made by investigators[17,43,44] who described the construction and use of gibbon ape leukemia virus (GaLV) components or vesicular somatitis virus (VSV) G-glycoprotein pseudotyped retroviral vectors. These vectors appear able to somewhat more efficiently infect a larger number of human cells than amphotropic virus, thereby potentially yielding higher transduction efficiencies compared to MoMLV-based amphotropic retroviruses.[45] However, to a certain extent, lowering the viral harvest temperature to 32°C and using concentrated virus (both increasing the effective MOI) to initially infect the cells, can mitigate this apparent advantage by acting to increase amphotropic viral transduction efficiency.

As previously discussed, both the retroviral cDNA vector backbone and the "helper" provirus within the various packaging cell lines have been manipulated to minimize the risk of generating replication competent retrovirus (RCR). This has been accomplished by deleting portions of the two retroviral genomes (backbone and "helper") to minimize the chance of recombination.[1,41,42] As RCR can cause insertional mutagenesis, the use of retroviruses for gene therapy in humans is dependent on demonstration of lack of RCR. Assays have been developed to show whether or not RCR exist within retroviral pools.

Other potential delivery systems for ribozymes include adeno-associated virus (AAV), which has been shown to be capable of stable and efficient insertion of other anti-HIV-1 genes into hematopoietic cells.[46] Chatterjee and colleagues have reported the use of AAV to transduce an HIV-1 antisense construct into human T cells, resulting in a significant reduction of HIV-1 levels following challenge of the transduced cells.[47] There are several potential advantages of AAV vectors that are relevant for HIV-1 gene therapy.[48] They appear to have no potential for homologous recombination, and have high transduction efficiency for hematopoietic cells, including progenitor cells. In addition, AAV is non-pathogenic and replication-incompetent, and non-dividing cells can be transduced. However, for practical application, there are still three main problems:

1. a limit of approximately 4.7 kb for insertion of therapeutic genes (though similar to retroviruses);
2. potential adenovirus contamination; and
3. the possible excision or instability of the integrated gene.

Another approach being investigated is the use of another retroviral system,[49] namely HIV-1 based vectors, in which the positive aspects:

1. HIV-1 target cell specific expression;
2. ability to infect non-dividing cells; and
3. possibility of tat inducible expression,

need to be balanced by potential negatives:

1. possibility of recombination with HIV-1; and
2. a present lack of robust producer cell lines.

Adenoviruses have also been used as gene delivery vectors; adenoviral delivery of ribozymes is dealt with in other chapters.

Clinical Application of Retroviral Delivery of Ribozymes

Ex Vivo *Transduction of Peripheral Blood Lymphocytes in Gene Therapy*

The concepts for a genetic type of therapy were developed almost 20 years ago and have recently been transformed (albeit with limited success) into clinical reality.[1] In 1990 the first gene therapy study for the treatment of ADA deficiency began, followed by a rapidly growing number of clinical gene therapy trials, which covered diseases caused by genetic disorders, viral infections, and malignancies.[1]

For the clinical application of gene therapy for AIDS, a simple approach to treating HIV-infected patients is the infusion of transduced and "protected" CD4$^+$ PBLs. Recent findings about how the AIDS virus population behaves in the body suggest that the battle between the immune system and the virus is so evenly matched that any approaches which weaken the virus replication and give the immune system a slight but maintained edge might be enough to show a significant effect.[50,51] Therefore, if ribozyme constructs can protect CD4$^+$ T cells from HIV-1 infection and its sequelae in patients, the decline in the numbers of CD4$^+$ T cells could be halted or even potentially reversed and HIV-infected individuals could benefit clinically. It is relevant that the half life of an HIV infected and producing CD4$^+$ T lymphocyte is of the order of only two days.[50,51] Recently, we and others proposed and are conducting clinical trials of HIV-1 gene therapy. Although it is only Phase I studies that are underway for ribozymes, overall these clinical trials will address such issues as safety, efficacy and the issue of potential emergence of escape mutants in HIV-1 infected patients.

A scheme for gene transfer into PBLs in a clinical application is outlined in Figure 7.4. Patient PBLs are collected by apheresis. After separation on a Ficoll/Hypaque gradient, cells are depleted of the CD8$^+$ subpopulation of T cells by binding to antibody-coated plates. Enriched PBLs are then stimulated with OKT-3 antibody. Following stimulation, PBLs are transduced with retroviral vectors in the presence of interleukin-2. This is the scheme that we have employed for a ribozyme-based clinical trial in AIDS.

Currently, there are several procedures being used in the transduction and expansion of PBLs. The simplest is to use tissue culture flasks for both transduction and expansion, such as the Lifecell Tissue Culture Flask of Baxter.[52] This method is easy to use, and relatively inexpensive, but is very labor intensive. Furthermore, since this system is not a closed one, there is a potential risk of contamination.

The second protocol is to transduce and expand PBLs in tissue culture bags (Wong-Staal et al, Clinical protocol (Ribozyme), NIH RAC). This is very similar to that using tissue culture flasks except that a large volume of media is used (normally about 0.5 to 1 liter) to produce the requisite number of cells. Recently, closed Artificial Capillary Systems have been developed for transduction of PBLs and for large scale cell manipulation for clinical therapy.[53] These systems, such as the CELLMAX system of Cellco, consist of an electronically controlled pump that perfuses culture medium through a capillary cartridge designed for the growth of a particular cell type. The culture cartridge used for PBLs is the 'Peripheral Blood Lymphocyte-Moderate Pore Size' which has been specifically designed to support the growth of OKT-3 stimulated human mononuclear lymphocytes. Up to 5 x 10^9 lymphoid cells can be obtained from each cartridge. The advantages of this system over conventional methods are:

1. it permits optimum expansion of PBLs with minimal operator manipulation and interference, thus having less chance of potential contamination and cell stress; and

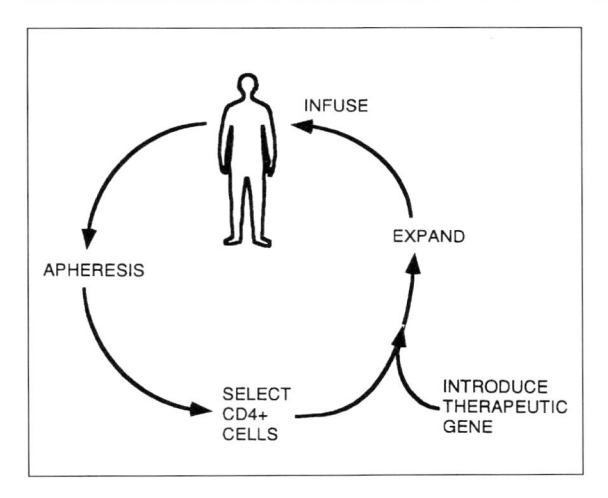

Fig. 7.4. Retrovirus-mediated gene transfer of CD4+ cells in a clinical setting. Peripheral blood mononuclear cells are isolated from the patient's or donor's blood by apheresis followed by Ficoll-Hypaque. Following a purification step to deplete CD8+ T lymphocytes, they are stimulated with an agent such as OKT-3 and expanded with the T cell cytokine interleukin-2. They are then transduced with the retrovirus, expanded further and infused into the recipient.

2. it allows for the concentration of retroviral vectors in the closed system, that is, a greater effective multiplicity of infection (MOI)

The latter appears to be an important issue for PBL transduction.

Ex Vivo *Transduction of Human CD34+ Cells*

Gene therapy protocols targeting human stem cells (HSC) have primarily used recombinant retroviruses as delivery vehicles. HSC-based therapies require long-term expression of the transgene, limiting the choice of vector to those which allow stable integration into the host genome. The success of gene transfer in the murine system has led to in vitro and in vivo studies with HSCs and the initiation of clinical trials. High levels of gene transfer routinely reported for murine progenitors were achieved by co-cultivation of target cells with the retroviral producer cells. While transduction by co-cultivation has been shown to be superior to cell-free viral supernatant,[54] co-cultivation is generally not suitable for clinical protocols due to the potential risk of contamination of cellular infusions with the producer cells.[55] Strategies to overcome this problem have included a high MOI and multiple rounds of infection with viral supernatant, which is now standard in most clinical gene therapy protocols. Fibronectin fragments are also under trial.

The challenge in this area is to identify culture conditions which will induce cell cycling, thus rendering the cells susceptible to infection, while maintaining pluripotentiality. Most clinical protocols include overnight pre-culture in media supplemented with the growth factors interleukin-3, interleukin-6 and stem cell factor (SCF) to induce cell cycling, followed by addition of retroviral supernatant daily for 2-4 days. The primary concern has been to minimize the time in ex vivo culture to limit the degree of differentiation induced by the recombinant cytokines. Recent studies have shown that FLT-3/FLK-2 ligand and KIT ligand, as well as megakaryocyte growth and development factor (MGDF) are capable of expanding progenitor cell numbers while maintaining the reconstituting ability of the cells.[56,57]

Concluding Remarks

Ribozymes cleave oncogenes to suppress cell transformation and cleave genomic and subgenomic HIV to suppress the latter's replication. This has been shown in cell culture systems. The key question is: Can ribozymes affect the disease course of cancer and AIDS?

In the case of AIDS, can they impact on the two surrogate markers of advancing disease, viral load and CD4+ T cell counts? Initial approaches have been made to address these questions in Phase I safety clinical trials presently being conducted, or about to be conducted, by a number of groups including our own.

Ribozymes are but one of several possible gene therapeutic approaches. It can be expected that continued improvement in the design of antigenes such as ribozymes will augment the potential for gene therapeutic approaches to AIDS, cancer or some genetic diseases. Concomitantly, improvements in delivery systems, the use of combinations of different strategies (multi-targeted gene therapy, drugs, immune modulation), as well as specific means for the introduction into appropriate target tissue or cells, will result in realization of the potential clinical applications of ribozyme-based gene therapy.

Acknowledgments

We thank Halley Hanlen for assistance with preparation of this manuscript and Janet Macpherson for preparation of the figures. Much of the work described herein from the authors' laboratories was funded by contract with Gene Shears Pty Ltd, Australia.

References

1. Miller AD. Human gene therapy comes of age. Nature 1992; 357:455-459.
2. Hock RA, Miller AD, Osborne WRA. Expression of human adenosine deaminase from various strong promoters after gene transfer into human haematopoietic cell lines. Blood 1989; 74:876-881.
3. Overell RW, Wesser KE, Cosman D. Stably transmitted triple-promoter retroviral vectors and their use in transformation of primary mammalian cells. Mol Cell Biol 1988; 8:1803-1808.
4. Dzierzak EA, Papayannopoulou T, Mulligan RC. Lineage-specific expression of a human β-globin gene in murine bone marrow transplant recipients reconstituted with retrovirus-transduced stem cells. Nature 1988; 331:35-41.
5. Yee JK, Moores JC, Jolly DJ et al. Gene expression from transcriptionally disabled retroviral vectors. Proc Natl Acad Sci USA 1987; 84:5179-5201.
6. Sullenger BA, Lee TC, Smith CA et al. Expression of chimeric tRNA-driven antisense transcripts renders NIH 3T3 cells highly resistant to Moloney murine leukemia virus replication. Mol Cell Biol 1990; 10:6512-6523.
7. Palmer TD, Miller AD, Reeder RH et al. Efficient expression of a protein coding gene under the control of an RNA polymerase I promoter. Nucleic Acids Res 1993; 21:3451-3457.
8. Hantzopoulos PA, Sullenger BA, Ungers G et al. Improved gene expression upon transfer of the adenosine deaminase minigene outside the transcriptional unit of a retroviral vector. Proc Natl Acad Sci USA 1989; 86:3519-3523.
9. Hawley RG, Sabourin LA, Hawley TS. An improved retroviral vector for gene transfer into undifferentiated cells. Nucleic Acids Res 1989; 17:4001.
10. Miller AD, Buttimore C. Design of retrovirus packaging cells to avoid recombination leading to helper virus production. Mol Cell Biol 1986; 6:2895-2902.
11. Bender MA, Palmer TD, Gelinas RE et al. Evidence that the packaging signal of Moloney leukemia virus extends into the gag region. J Virol 1987; 61:1639-1646.
12. Danos O, Mulligan RC. Safe and efficient generation of recombinant retroviruses with amphotropic and ecotropic host ranges. Proc Natl Acad Sci USA 1988; 85:6460-6464.
13. Pear WS, Nolan GP, Scott ML et al. Production of high-titer retroviruses by transient transfection. Proc Natl Acad Sci USA 1993; 90:8392-8396.
14. Bushman F. Targeting retroviral integration. Science 1995; 267:1443-1444.
15. Etienne-Julan M, Roux P, Carillo S et al. The efficiency of cell targeting by recombinant retroviruses depends on the nature of the receptor and the composition of the artificial cell-virus linker. J Gen Virol 1992; 73:3251-3255.

16. Neda H, Wu CH, Wu GY. Chemical modification of an ecotropic murine leukemia virus results in redirection of its target cell specificity. J Biol Chem 1991; 266:14143-14146.
17. Miller AD, Garcia JV, von Suhr N et al. Construction and properties of retrovirus packaging cells based on gibbon ape leukemia virus. J Virol 1991; 65:2220-2224.
18. Cech T. The chemistry of self-splicing RNA and RNA enzymes. Science 1987; 236:1532-1539.
19. Uhlenbeck OC. A small catalytic oligoribonucleotide. Nature (London) 1987; 328:596-600.
20. Forster A, Symons R. Self-cleavage of plus and minus RNAs of a virusoid and a structural model for the active sites. Cell 1987; 49:211-220.
21. Hampel A, Nesbitt S, Tritz R et al. The hairpin ribozyme. Meth Enzymol 1987; 5:37-42.
22. Haseloff J, Gerlach WL. Simple enzymes with new and highly specific endoribonuclease activity. Nature (London) 1988; 334:585-591.
23. Hertel KJ, Herschlag D, Uhlenbeck OC. Specificity of hammerhead ribozyme cleavage. EMBO J 1996; 14:3751-3757.
24. Rossi JJ. Ribozymes. Curr Opin Biotech 1992; 3:3-7.
25. James W, Al-Shamkhani A. RNA enzymes as tools for gene ablation. Curr Opin Biotec 1995; 6:44-49.
26. Sun LQ, Gerlach WL, Symonds G. The design, production and validation of an anti-HIV type 1 ribozyme. Methods in Molecular Medicine 1998; 4:51-64.
27. Sun LQ, Warrilow D, Wang L et al. Ribozyme-mediated suppression of Moloney murine leukemia virus and human immunodeficiency virus type 1 replication in permissive cell lines. Proc Natl Acad Sci USA 1994; 91:9715-9719.
28. Sun LQ, Pyati J, Wang L et al. Resistance to HIV-1 infection conferred by transduction of human peripheral blood lymphocytes with ribozyme, antisense or polyTAR constructs. Proc Natl Acad Sci USA 1995; 92:7272-7276.
29. Lowenstein P, Symonds G. Inhibition of Moloney murine leukemia virus (MoMLV) by a retroviral vector LNL6, carrying ribozymes, targeted to the 5' non-coding sequence. J Gen Virol 1997; 78:2587-2590.
30. Sarver N, Cantin EM, Chang PS et al. Ribozymes as potential anti-HIV-1 therapeutic agents. Science 1990; 247:1222-1225.
31. Weerasinghe M, Liem SE, Asad S et al. Resistance to human immunodeficiency virus type 1 (HIV-1) infection in human CD4+ lymphocyte-derived cell lines conferred by using retroviral vectors expressing an HIV-1 RNA-specific ribozyme. J Viol 1991; 65:5531-5534.
32. Lo KMS, Biasolo MA, Dehni G et al. Inhibition of replication of HIV-1 by retroviral vectors expressing *tat*-antisense and anti-*tat* ribozyme RNA. Virology 1992; 190:176-183.
33. Leavitt MC, Yu M, Yamad O et al. Transfer of an anti-HIV-1 ribozyme gene into primary human lymphocytes. Human Gene Ther 1994; 5:1115-1120.
34. Yu M, Ojwang JO, Yamada O et al. A hairpin ribozyme inhibits expression of diverse strains of human immunodeficiency virus type 1. Proc Natl Acad Sci USA 1993; 90:6340-6344.
35. Ojwang JO, Hampel A, Looney DJ et al. Inhibition of human immunodeficiency virus type 1 expression by a hairpin ribozyme. Proc Natl Acad Sci USA 1992; 89:10802-10806.
36. Yu M, Leavitt MC, Maruyama M et al. Intracellular immunization of human fetal cord blood stem/progenitor cells with a ribozyme against human immunodeficiency virus type 1. Proc Natl Acad Sci USA 1995; 92:699-703.
37. Yu M, Poeschla E, Yamada O et al. In vitro and in vivo characterization of a second functional hairpin ribozyme against HIV-1. Virology 1995; 206:381-386.
38. Yamada O, Kraus G, Leavitt MC et al. Activity and cleavage site specificity of an anti-HIV-1 hairpin ribozyme in human T cells. Virology 1994; 205:121-26.
39. Sun LQ, Wang L, Gerlach WL et al. Target sequence-specific inhibition of HIV-1 replication by ribozymes directed to tat RNA. Nucleic Acids Res 1995; 23:2909-2913.
40. Lisziewicz J, Sun D, Smythe J et al. Inhibition of human immunodeficiency virus type 1 replication by regulated expression of a polymeric Tat activation response RNA decoy as a strategy for gene therapy in AIDS. Proc Natl Acad Sci USA 1993; 90: 8000-8004.

40a. Wang L, Witherington C, King A, Gerlach W, Carr A, Penny R, Cooper D, Symonds C, Sun L-Q. Preclinical characterization of an anti-tat ribozyme for therapeutic application. Human Gene Therapy 1998; 9:1283-1291.
41. Miller AD, Rosman GJ. Improved vectors for gene transfer and expression. BioTechniques 1989; 7:980-986.
42. Jolly D. (1994) Viral vector systems for gene therapy. Cancer Gene Ther 1994; 1:51-64.
42. Kavanaugh MP, Miller DG, Zhang W et al. Cell-surface receptors for gibbon ape leukemia virus and amphotropic retrovirus are inducible sodium-dependent phosphate symporters. Proc Natl Acad Sci USA 1994; 91:7071-7075.
44. Bums JC, Friedmann T, Driever W et al. Vesicular stomatititis virus G glycoprotein pseudotyped retroviral vectors: Concentration to very high titer and efficient gene transfer into nonmammalian cells. Proc Natl Acad Sci USA 1993; 90:8033-8037.
45. Von kalle C, Kiem HP, Goehle SO et al. Increased gene transfer into human haematopoietic progenitor cells by extended in vitro exposure to pseudotyped retroviral vector. Blood 1994; 84:2890-2897.
46. Kuzczyka N. Use of adeno-associated virus as a general transduction vector in mammalian cells. Curr Top Microbiol Imuunol 1992; 158:97-129.
47. Chatterjee S, Johnson PR,Wong KK Jr. Dual-target inhibition of HIV-1 in vitro by means of an adeno-associated virus antisense vector. Science 1992; 258:1485-1488.
48. Carter DJ. Adeno-associated virus vectors. Curr Opin Biotechnol 1992; 3:533-539.
49. Lever AML. HIV and other lentivirus-based vectors. Gene Therapy 1996; 3:470-471.
50. Ho DD, Neumann AU, Perelson AS et al. Rapid turnover of plasma virions and CD4 lymphocytes in HIV-1 infection. Nature (London) 1995; 373:123-126.
51. Wei X, Ghosh SK, Taylor ME et al. Viral dynamics in human immunodeficiency virus type 1 infection. Nature (London) 1995; 373:117-122.
52. Woffendin C, Ranga U, Yang Z-Y et al. Expression of a protective gene prolongs survival of T cells in human immunodeficiency virus-infected patients. Proc Natl Acad Sci USA 1996; 93:2889-2894.
53. Packard BS. Mitogenic stimulation of human tumor-filtrating lymphocytes by secreted factors from human tumor cell lines. Proc Natl Acad Sci USA 1990; 87:4058-4062.
54. Havenga M, Hoogerbrugge P, Valerio D et al. Retroviral stem cell gene therapy. Stem Cell 1997; 15:162-179.
55. Gordon MY. Adhesive properties of haemopoietic stem cells. Br J Haematol 1988; 68:149.
56. Yonemura Y, Ku H, Ltman SD et al. In vitro expression of hematopoietic progenitors and maintenance of stem cells: Comparison between FLT-3/FLK-2 ligand and KIT ligand. Blood 1997; 89:1915-1921.
57. Rasko JE, O'Flaherty E, Begley CG. Mpl ligand (MGDF) alone in combination with stem cell factor (SCF) promotes proliferation and survival of human megakaryocyte, erythroid and granulocyte/macrophage progenitors. Stem Cells 1997; 15:33-42.
58. Amado RG, Symonds G, Jamieson BD, Zhao G, Rosenblatt JD, Zack JA. Effects of megakaryocyte growth and development factor on survival and retroviral transduction of T-lymphoid progenitor cells. Human Gene Therapy 1998; 9:173-183.

CHAPTER 8

Adeno-Associated Virus (AAV) Mediated Ribozyme Expression in Mammalian Cells

Piruz Nahreini and Beth Roberts

Introduction

Gene therapy has increasingly become an ideal method for the treatment of many hereditary and acquired human diseases.[1] Efficient delivery, regulated expression, low toxicity, lack of adverse immune responses, and in most cases long-term stable expression of a therapeutic gene in target cells are desired features for a successful gene therapy. Several viral and nonviral methods of gene delivery into cells have been developed, but none has a universal application for diseases amenable to genetic treatment.[2] Each method, however, has its unique set of advantages for a given human disorder.

For example, adenoviral vectors are very efficient in gene delivery.[3] However, the expression of a therapeutic gene is sustained for only several weeks because these vectors do not integrate stably into the chromosomal DNA of target cells. Therefore, adenovirus is a suitable vector if transient expression of a therapeutic gene is sufficient to ameliorate a disease state, provided that the associated immunogenicity of these vectors does not interfere with the treatment process. On the other hand, retrovirus and adeno-associated virus (AAV), by virtue of integrating into chromosomal DNA, are suitable vectors when stable, long-term expression of a therapeutic gene is preferred.[4-6] Retroviral vectors are dependent on cell mitosis for efficient integration into chromosomal DNA, and this explains the inefficient expression of a gene of interest in non-dividing cells.[7] A new generation of retroviral vectors, the lentiviruses, have recently been reported to efficiently express a transgene in non-dividing cells.[8] The strong enhancer and promoter of retroviral long terminal repeats (LTR) can potentially be a problem when a regulated expression of a therapeutic gene is warranted. When regulated, long-term expression in non-dividing, as well as dividing cells, is desired, AAV may be the ideal vector.

In this chapter, we focus on the utility of AAV as a vector for gene expression, and emphasize certain issues which have direct impact on the feasibility of its broader use in human gene therapy. We report here some of our own observations with regard to vector production and transgene expression, particularly hammerhead ribozyme expression. These small, catalytic RNA molecules are potentially attractive for gene therapy for a variety of human disorders. The expression of a ribozyme using retroviral and adenoviral vectors has

Ribozymes in the Gene Therapy of Cancer, edited by Kevin J. Scanlon and Mohammed Kashani-Sabet. ©1998 R.G. Landes Company.

been reported in several studies;[9-13] however the utility of AAV for ribozyme expression has not been investigated extensively.

AAV Life Cycle and Genetics

Adeno-associated virus (AAV) is a small non-pathogenic human parvovirus which infects a variety of mammalian cells with a broad host range.[4-5] The AAV genome (4681 bases) is a single-stranded DNA (ss-DNA) of either polarity flanked by inverted terminal repeats (ITRs). Plus and minus viral strands are encapsidated into mature virions at the same frequency. AAV can establish a lytic or latent infection in mammalian cells in the presence or absence of a helper virus, respectively. The ITRs, which are 145 bases in length, are the sole cis-acting elements essential for chromosomal excision (rescue), integration, replication, and encapsidation of nascent viral DNA.[4-5] The viral genome consists of two major open reading frames (ORF). The left ORF encodes the overlapping AAV replication proteins, Rep68 and Rep78 from the p5 promoter and Rep40 and Rep52 from the p19 promoter. The right ORF encodes AAV capsid proteins (VP1, VP2, and VP3) driven by the p40 promoter.[4-5]

A schematic representation of the AAV life cycle and recombinant AAV (rAAV) production is shown in Figure 8.1. Productive AAV infection is dependent on a helper virus, usually adenovirus; however herpesvirus and vaccinia virus can also perform this function.[4] The helper virus may primarily optimize the host milieu for productive AAV infection. In support of this, several stress-inducing agents (ultraviolet light, gamma-irradiation, chemical carcinogens, metabolic inhibitors, and heat shock) that alter the intracellular milieu, support productive AAV infection in the absence of a helper virus, albeit less efficiently (~ two logs lower).[14-18] In the absence of a helper virus, the AAV genome preferentially integrates into a defined region of human chromosome 19 (q13.3-qter), and establishes a stable latent infection.[19-21] The frequency of the site-specific integration of AAV is estimated to be up to 70% in established human cell lines such as HeLa and Detroit-60.[19] The presence of viral Rep proteins (Rep68 or Rep78) in trans and ITRs in cis are essential for the site-specific integration of the viral genome on chromosome 19.[22] Efficient rescue and replication of the integrated viral genome from chromosomal DNA ensues when latently AAV infected cells are superinfected with a helper virus.[4-5]

Positive and Negative Features of AAV Vectors

Attractive features of AAV for use in human gene therapy include:

1. non-pathogenicity—AAV has not been linked directly to the cause of any human disease and has not been associated with tumorigenicity, although it is frequently isolated from certain tissues (in fact, current data indicate that AAV may function as an anti-oncogenic virus);[23-24]
2. broad host range—AAV infects a broad host range including dividing and non-dividing cells. However, transduction of the former is more efficient;[25]
3. stable integration—AAV stably integrates into chromosomal DNA, allowing long-term transgene expression;[4-5]
4. stable virions—AAV virions are very stable and tolerate conditions which readily inactivate enveloped viruses, such as retroviruses;[4]
5. stem cell infection—AAV infects human (CD34[+]) and mouse (Lin[-]Sca-1[+]) hematopoietic progenitor cells;[26-31]
6. absence of promoter interference—unlike the retrovirus LTR, the AAV-ITR is devoid of enhancer and TATA box-containing promoter elements, and it is less likely to interfere with the transgene expression.[32] However, it has an initiator sequence characteristic of a TATA-less promoter and binding sites for the SP1 transcription factor;[33] and

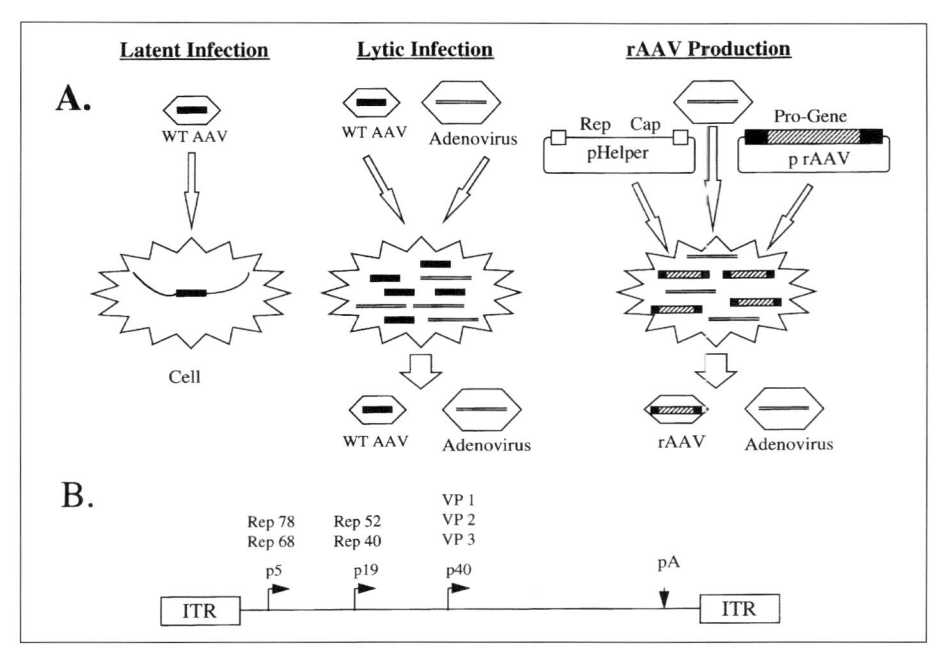

Fig. 8.1. Schematic representation of AAV life cycle, rAAV production, and wild type (wt) AAV genome. (A) In the absence of a helper virus, the wt AAV integrates into the chromosomal DNA site-specifically (latent infection). In the presence of a helper virus, the wt AAV undergoes a productive infection (lytic infection). Helper plasmid (pHelper), recombinant AAV plasmid (prAAV), and adenovirus are required for generating recombinant AAV (rAAV production). Open squares in pHelper depict the adenovirus ITRs, and filled rectangles in prAAV depict AAV-ITRs which flank the expression cassette for the gene of interest (Pro-Gene) (B) The wt AAV genomic map. Inverted terminal repeats (ITRs), promoters (p5, p19, p40) with the associated gene products (replication {Rep} and capsid {VP} proteins), and the polyadenylation site (pA) are indicated. See text for detail.

7. low immunogenicity—AAV, in contrast to adenovirus, has no observed significant adverse immune responses to rAAV vectors.[34-36] This is probably due to the absence of AAV ORFs in most rAAV vectors.

There are, however, certain undesirable features of rAAV for use as a vector for gene therapy, such as:

1. There is no simple method for large scale rAAV generation, as currently is possible for recombinant adenovirus and retrovirus production;
2. AAV-mediated gene expression is dependent on the efficient conversion of its ss-DNA genome into double-stranded form in most cells.[37-40] This rate limiting step is dependent on cell type, and can be dramatically enhanced by certain factors and conditions, such as helper virus infection, genotoxic treatments (e.g., gamma radiation), and tyrosine phosphorylation;[37-40]
3. Integration efficiency varies depending on cell type, and in some instances the viral genome remains episomal in the host cell nuclei, conferring transgene expression up to several weeks;[41-42]

4. The packaging capacity for foreign DNA into rAAV is limited to 4.5 kb, which exceeds the size of many human therapeutic cDNA genes;[43-45] and
  5. 80-90% of the human population is seropositive for AAV,[46] which may pose a problem for in vivo transduction of human cells.

Generation of Recombinant AAV

Background

The molecular cloning of an intact double-stranded form of the AAV genome into a bacterial plasmid facilitated the study of AAV genetics and paved the way for the production of rAAV.[47-48] Rescue and replication of the AAV genome from a plasmid was demonstrated in adenovirus infected cells.[47-48] Nascent viral DNAs were shown to be packaged into biologically infectious virions.[47-48] Genetic studies using the cloned AAV revealed that foreign DNA, substituted for the entire AAV Rep and Cap coding region and flanked by AAV-ITRs, can undergo rescue/replication in host cells in the presence of AAV Rep proteins and helper adenovirus (see Fig. 8.1).[49] Furthermore, replicated DNA fragments between ~2-5 kb can be packaged into mature AAV virions, provided that AAV Cap proteins are provided in trans.[43,49] Recombinant viral genomes ranging in size between 4-5 kb are efficiently packaged into virions, whereas smaller recombinant genomes are packaged inefficiently.[43-45]

Methods for rAAV Production

Early work on developing a method for generating rAAV made use of a two-plasmid system. The "helper plasmid" contained an intact cloned AAV genome with a 1 kb lambda DNA insertion just upstream of the right ITR.[43] Upon rescue and replication in adenovirus infected cells, this modified AAV genome is too large to be packaged into mature virions, but provides AAV Rep and Cap expression. The "recombinant plasmid" (prAAV) contains a gene of interest flanked by AAV ITRs. The rescue, replication, and packaging of the recombinant genome occurs in the presence of the Rep and Cap proteins provided in trans by the helper plasmid. The major problem with this method of generating the rAAV is the production of contaminating wild type AAV (wt AAV), which can range from 10%-50% of the total virus produced.[43] This is primarily due to the homologous AAV sequences in the helper and recombinant plasmids.

Samulski et al constructed new helper and recombinant backbone plasmids which resulted in a significant increase in rAAV titer and dramatically reduced wt AAV contamination.[50-51] The new helper plasmid (pAAV/Ad) consists of the entire AAV coding region (Rep and Cap ORFs) flanked by the first 107 bp of adenovirus type 5 terminal repeats (Ad-ITR).[51] The insertion of adenovirus termini was originally intended to amplify the helper plasmid in cells; however helper plasmid amplification was not detected. Instead, the strong enhancer within the Ad-ITR significantly augments AAV Rep and Cap expression. For construction of the recombinant AAV plasmids, the cloned AAV backbone vector was modified for easy replacement of the entire AAV coding region with a gene of interest. The resulting absence of homologous AAV sequences in the helper and recombinant plasmids has resulted in a dramatic reduction in the generation of wt AAV.[51]

Vector Constructions

We have constructed several rAAV backbone plasmids which were tailor-made for the insertion of ribozyme expression cassettes driven from either pol II or pol III promoters (Fig. 8.2). To allow for selection in the target cell, either the bacterial neomycin phosphotransferase (NPT II) gene driven by the herpes simplex thymidine kinase promoter, or a modified nerve growth factor receptor (NGFR) gene, driven by cytomegalovirus early

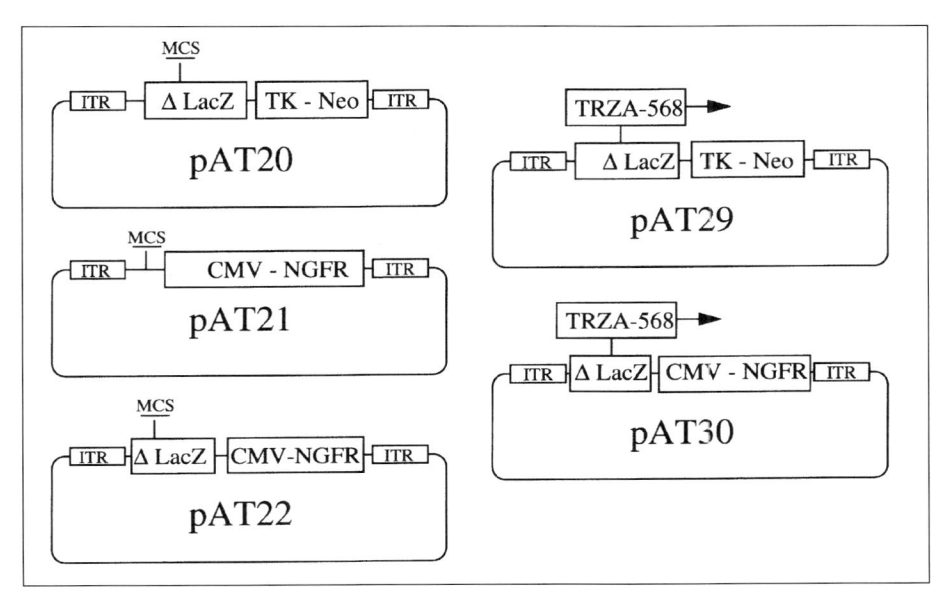

Fig. 8.2. Schematic drawing of recombinant AAV plasmids. Recombinant AAV plasmids pAT29 and pAT30 contain the "TRZA568" transcription unit, a hammerhead ribozyme targeted against a site in the HIV-LTR, driven by a modified tRNA promoter.[52] See text for additional detail.

promoter, was cloned into these rAAV constructs. The NGFR expressed from these constructs is biologically nonfunctional because of a deletion in the C terminus of the cDNA. However, the expression of this truncated NGFR can be readily detected on the membrane of transduced cells by fluorescence activated cell sorting (FACS). In contrast, the NPT II selection requires the neomycin analog G418, which is toxic to uninfected cells. Due to its rapid selection and lack of toxicity, NGFR expression is a preferred method of selection in our laboratory. A 1.6 kb stuffer fragment originating from the bacterial LacZ gene, and containing a multiple cloning site (MCS), was inserted in two of the constructs to increase the size of the recombinant genome for efficient packaging. The pol II and III promoters used for driving hammerhead ribozyme (Rz) expression are modified versions of mammalian tRNA, U1, and U6, and viral (CMV) promoters. The molecular design and details of the construction of these modified promoters are described elsewhere (Unpublished data for U1, U6, and CMV).[52]

Rescue and Replication

Rescue and replication of these rAAV, with or without ribozyme transcription units, was examined in 293 cells (Fig. 8.3). The characteristic viral replicative intermediates (monomer, dimer, tetramer, etc.) were detected, similar to the rescue/replication pattern of cloned AAV.[49-50] Rescue and replication of pAT20 appears to be more efficient as compared to the other recombinant AAV plasmids, as shown in Figure 8.3. The reproducibility of this observation has not been investigated. Rolling and Samulski examined the stability in rAAV of exogenous sequences with secondary structures, such as the adenovirus polymerase III VA RNA promoter, the internal ribosomal entry site (IRES) of encephalomyocarditis virus (EMCV), and the 3' untranslated region of Factor IX (FIX).[53] With the exception of the 3'

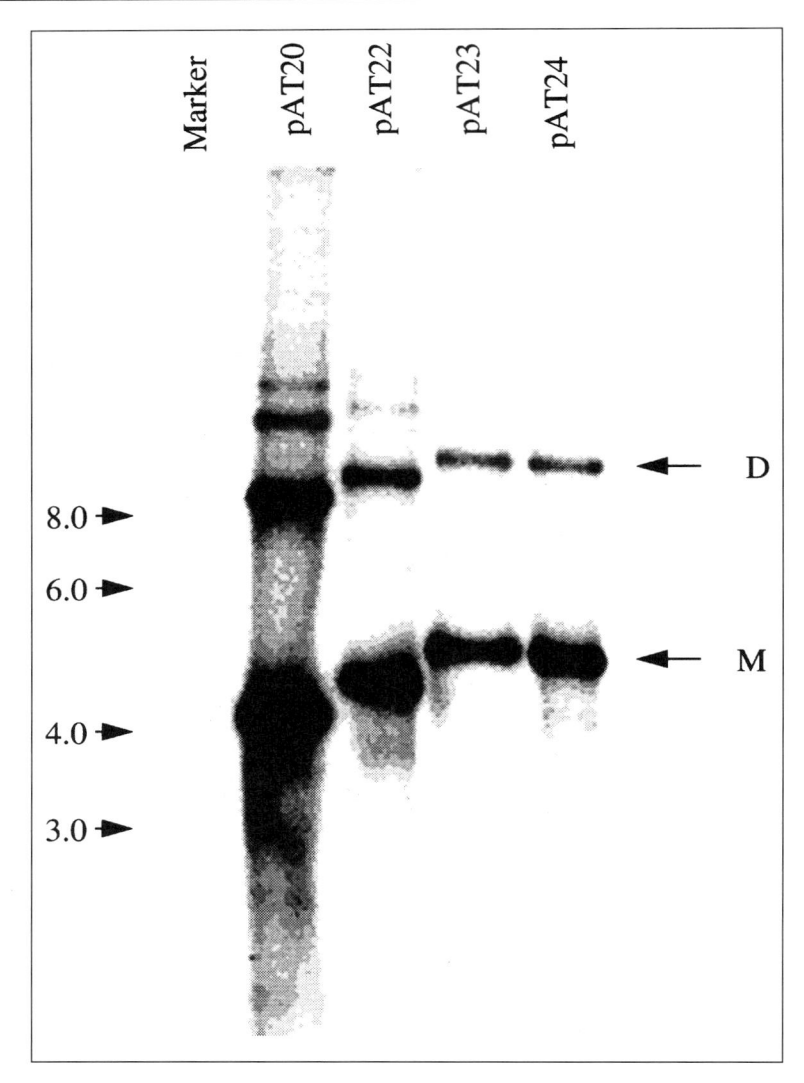

Fig. 8.3. Rescue and replication of rAAV plasmids. Adenovirus-infected 293 cells were cotransfected with the helper plasmid (pAAV/Ad) and with pAT20, pAT22, pAT23, or pAT24 using a calcium phosphate transfection method (Promega). Recombinant AAV plasmids pAT23 and pAT24 contain a hammerhead ribozyme expression cassette targeted against a metalloproteinase mRNA driven by a U1 promoter. The expression cassettes were cloned into the MCS of the pAT22 in either the forward or reverse orientation, (pAT23 and pAT24, respectively). Low molecular weight (LMW) DNAs were isolated 48 h post-transfection/infection using the protocol described by Hirt.[75] LMW DNAs (~20 µg) were digested with the restriction enzyme *Dpn*I (digests unreplicated, methyated DNA), resolved by electrophoresis on a 1% agarose gel, transferred to a nitrocellulose membrane (Genescreen plus), and probed with [^{32}P]-labeled LacZ DNA. M and D denote the monomeric and dimeric forms of the rAAV DNA replicative intermediates, respectively.

untranslated region (UTR) of FIX, these sequences did not interfere with rescue/replication or virus production. The 3' UTR of FIX in rAAV vectors resulted in significant reduction of viral yield due to progressive deletion of recombinant sequence during replication.[53] To date, none of our hammerhead Rz transcription units have caused aberrant replication in the context of rAAV plasmids. rAAV titers, with or without Rz-transcription units, are approximately the same, ranging between 7.5-8.5 x 10^8 total IU/ml obtained from large scale preparations as described below.

Viral Production and Titer Determination

For large scale preparation of rAAV, 293 cells were cotransfected with pAAV/Ad and prAAV (100 µg of each plasmid per 500 cm^2 plate) using a calcium phosphate transfection method. Transfection is carried out for 12-16 h, followed by adenovirus infection (MOI:5-10). Cells are processed for rAAV purification when adenovirus cytopathic effect (CPE) is visible microscopically (65-72 h p.i.). The cell pellet is frozen and thawed 3-4 times at -70°C and 37°C, respectively, and the cell lysate is centrifuged to collect the supernatant (also referred to as the "crude rAAV" preparation). The rAAV particles in this crude preparation are further purified by CsCl equilibrium gradient centrifugations. The rAAV with a genomic size similar to that of AAV has a density of 1.42-1.45 g/cm^3 as compared to the 1.33 g/cm^3 density of adenovirus in CsCl solution. We further purified the crude viral preparations by two CsCl step gradient centrifugations (1.33/1.55 g/cm^3 densities). The rAAV band is located at the junction between 1.33 and 1.5 CsCl densities, just below the visible band of adenovirus. The portion of the gradient containing rAAV is collected and dialyzed against PBS containing 1% sucrose. The dialyzed rAAV preparation is concentrated by centrifugation through an Amicon Centriplus membrane system.

The titer of dialyzed rAAV preparations is routinely determined by two different methods. The copy number of rAAV genomes is determined using a previously described slot-blot hybridization method.[54] The number of infectious units per ml are determined by FACS analysis of cell surface NGFR expression. In our experience, the use of slot-blot hybridization for particle number determination results in a 1-2 log higher rAAV titer than the phenotypic assay. This discrepancy is most likely due to defective interfering particles giving rise to artificially high apparent titers. A typical rAAV titer determination is shown in Figure 8.4.

An Update on New Strategies for rAAV Production

One of the major obstacles for rAAV application in human gene therapy has been the lack of an efficient system to generate high titer recombinant virus, free of AAV and adenovirus. A complete packaging cell line that inducibly expresses AAV Rep and Cap proteins and adenovirus VA I and II RNAs, and constitutively expresses the remaining helper functions of adenovirus (E1A, E1B, E2A, and E4), would be an ideal cell line for generating rAAV. Progress on developing alternative methods for the production of rAAV is briefly discussed below.

To date, at least two different cell lines that inducibly express AAV Rep have been established.[55-56] In one line, the mouse metallothionein-inducible promoter was used to drive the expression of the entire Rep ORF in 293 cells.[55] Clonal isolates showed variable levels of Rep expression which influenced cell growth rate. Interestingly, Rep78 could be induced in one subclone of the primary isolate to 50-70% of the level present in 293 cells coinfected with AAV and adenovirus. Rep52 was constitutively expressed in these cell lines. No expression of Rep40 was detected in any of the isolated clones. In the second cell line, the glucocorticoid-responsive promoter of mouse mammary virus was used to drive the expression of the entire Rep ORF in HeLa cells.[56] Two promising clonal isolates have been found to

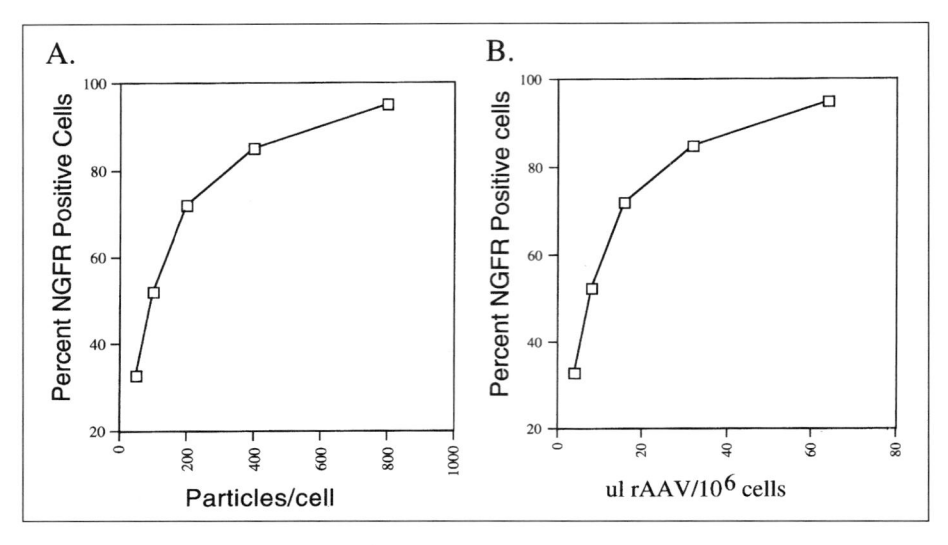

Fig. 8.4. rAAV titer determination. The recombinant AAV plasmid pAT30 contains a hammerhead ribozyme expression cassette, targeted against a site in the HIV LTR, driven by a modified tRNA promoter cloned into the MCS of pAT22. The plasmid pAT30 was used to generate a large scale preparation of rAAV-AT30 in 293 cells as described in the text. HeLa cells were infected with dilutions of the CsCl gradient purified rAAV-AT30. (A) The particle concentration was determined by measuring viral genome copy number using slot blot hybridization as previously described.[54] (B) The percentage of cells expressing cell surface NGFR was determined by FACS analysis at 48 h p.i.

express Rep78 in the presence of dexamethasone, and have been shown to complement the replication of a Rep mutant rAAV.[56] In contrast to Rep-expressing 293 cells, no growth inhibitory effect was noted. Even though these two HeLa clones efficiently express all three AAV capsid proteins upon trans-activation by Rep in the presence of adenovirus, neither clone supported the packaging of a Rep-deficient rAAV. Interestingly, transient expression of any one of the AAV Rep proteins (Rep78, 68, 52 or 40) in these clones was sufficient to obviate the packaging problem.[57] Thus, lack of packaging in these HeLa cell lines was explained to be due to low level of Rep proteins. Furthermore, high levels of Rep78 expression can compensate for the absence of Rep52, which is critical for the accumulation of ss-DNA and subsequent packaging.[57] This suggests redundancy of some function(s) among Rep proteins. It appears that development of a cell line which expresses all four Rep proteins to a similar level as that in 293 cells coinfected with AAV and adenovirus is a challenging task; however, ongoing progress is directed toward achieving this goal.

The utility of an EBV-based vector to maintain an AAV Rep and Cap expression cassette, a gene of interest flanked with AAV-ITR, or a combination of both on the same episomal vector, was investigated in 293 and HeLa cell lines.[58-59] Results indicate that continuous Rep expression is either toxic (e.g., 293 cells) or insufficient (e.g., HeLa cells) for efficient rAAV production. Since the rAAV-EBV-based vectors, without an AAV Rep ORF, were shown to be stable episomally in clonal isolates of 293 or HeLa cells, the incorporation of AAV Rep genes driven by an inducible promoter in this system might be warranted.

Several alternative methods for the production of rAAV were presented at the VII International Parvovirus Workshop, held in Heidelberg, Germany in September, 1997. First, a recombinant herpesvirus containing AAV Rep and Cap expression cassettes was constructed and tested for its use in generating rAAV.[60] This recombinant herpesvirus can effectively substitute for helper plasmid and adenovirus, and gives rise to rAAV titers equivalent to the two-plasmid method of rAAV production.[60] Second, a plasmid containing the helper functions of adenovirus and AAV Rep and Cap expression cassette was constructed, which can substitute for the helper plasmid and adenovirus in the current method of rAAV production.[61] The titers of rAAV using the latter plasmid were reported to be comparable to the standard two-plasmid method. Third, a packaging deficient adenoviral plasmid was tested as a substitute for adenovirus for the rAAV production.[62] The major advantage here is that the viral preparations are free of adenovirus. rAAV titers are comparable to the two-plasmid production method.[62-63] Lastly, the Cre-Lox P recombination system was used to establish cell lines with Rep and Cap expression cassettes.[64] Expression from these cassettes occurred only in the presence of Cre, which was provided by a helper recombinant adenovirus.

In view of the ease of generating high titers (10^{11}-10^{12} IU/ml) of AAV from cells coinfected with AAV and adenovirus, why is the development of an efficient large scale method for the production of high titer rAAV free of adenovirus still lacking? The foregoing studies underscore the need to better understand AAV transcriptional regulation in the presence of adenovirus. It is clear that the level of expression of AAV Rep proteins (78, 68, 54, 40) and Cap (VP1, 2, 3) is essential for optimal rAAV production,[65-66] as this is tightly regulated in cells coinfected with AAV and adenovirus. The activity of the AAV promoters, p5, p19, and p40, are tightly coordinated and significantly influenced by AAV-ITRs, AAV Rep proteins, adenovirus, and cellular transcription factors.[67-68] The design of an efficient method for the production of rAAV has to utilize a transcriptional regulation system similar to one existing in cells coinfected with AAV and adenovirus.

rAAV Infection and Transgene Expression

Role of Helper Virus and Host in AAV-Mediated Expression

The conversion of AAV ss-DNA genome into ds-DNA form is essential for initiation of AAV replication, gene expression, and presumably for integration. Although adenovirus helper functions are required for productive AAV infection, none of the adenovirus gene products have been demonstrated to be directly involved in supporting AAV replication, expression, and integration.[4-5] The adenovirus E1 and E4 gene products are indirectly implicated in efficient conversion of single-stranded AAV genomes to the transcriptionally active double-stranded form, presumably via enhancing host DNA polymerase(s) activity.[37-38] In support of this, helper virus-independent AAV production was demonstrated in some hamster and human cells pretreated with hydroxyurea, ultraviolet (UV) light, or cyclohexamide.[14-15] These observations signify that the helper virus primarily induces some host functions which support the initiation of AAV replication and expression. Consistent with this, rAAV devoid of Rep and Cap genes and containing either NPT II or alkaline phosphatase (ALP) genes transduces human diploid fibroblasts primarily during S-phase of the cell cycle.[25] Interestingly, factors that influence host cell DNA metabolism, such as DNA synthesis inhibitors (e.g., aphidicolin, hydroxyurea) or topoisomerase inhibitors (e.g., etoposide, ectoposide, and camptothecin) significantly augment rAAV transduction (expression and/or integration) in normal human diploid fibroblasts.[14-18] It appears that the viral or non-viral factors which support AAV replication and expression induce some host cell functions which are normally turned on in the S-phase of the cell cycle.

In an elegant report, Qing et al identified a cellular protein, named "double stranded D-sequence-binding protein" (dsD-BP), which specifically interacts with the D sequence at the 3' end of the AAV genome.[39] Tyrosine phosphoration and dephosphorylation of dsD-BP is hypothesized to block, or permit, second strand AAV DNA synthesis, respectively. Interestingly, some of the aforementioned factors (adenovirus E4 ORF6, hydroxyurea), which are implicated in enhancing second strand DNA synthesis, promote the dephosphorylation of dsD-BP bound to the AAV genome.[39,40] Furthermore, a specific inhibitor of tyrosine kinases, genistein, is shown to completely substitute for adenovirus in augmenting rAAV expression.[39] The discovery of dsD-BP not only paves the way for improvising new strategies to realize the utility of rAAV for gene therapy, it underscores a plausible role of dsD-BP in the regulation of leading-strand DNA synthesis in human cells. It is reasonable to speculate that in the S-phase of the cell cycle tyrosine dephosphorylation of the dsD-BP triggers initiation of leading strand DNA synthesis. In view of this, AAV replication and expression is intimately linked to host DNA and RNA synthesis.

We were interested in testing whether adenovirus is the sole factor required for optimal rAAV transgene expression in cells coinfected with rAAV and adenovirus. To address this, the titer of a crude rAAV-LacZ preparation was determined on 293 cells. The preparation was either titered directly, titered after heat treatment to inactivate the adenovirus, or titered after heating followed by the addition of increasing amounts of exogenous adenovirus (Fig. 8.5B). Heat treatment of the rAAV-LacZ decreased the titer from 8×10^7 to 10^5, a reduction of ~2-3 logs in LacZ expression. We tested whether addition of exogenous adenovirus to the heat-treated rAAV-LacZ preparation would fully reconstitute LacZ expression. The titer of heat-treated rAAV-LacZ increased as the MOI of adenovirus increased. However, only ~ 5% reconstitution of LacZ expression was achieved following maximum addition of adenovirus. In a separate experiment, rAAV-LacZ and adenovirus titers were determined in a preparation which was partially purified by polyethylene glycol precipitation and further purified by CsCl gradient centrifugation (no heat treatment), to remove contaminating adenovirus. The rAAV-LacZ titer was determined prior to CsCl gradient centrifugation, in rAAV-containing CsCl gradient fractions, and following addition of exogenous adenovirus to the rAAV-containing fractions (Fig. 8.5A). The addition of exogenous adenovirus to the purified rAAV preparation reconstituted LacZ expression to near that of the original titer. Lack of complete reconstitution of rAAV titer can be explained by loss of rAAV particles during the CsCl purification step.

Our data suggest that, besides adenovirus, one or more heat-labile element(s) might be critical for rAAV expression in 293 cells. It is possible that rAAV may package heat-labile factors (rAAV Rep, dsD-BP, etc.) which may play crucial roles in vector-mediated gene expression following viral uncoating in the cells. Interestingly, AAV Rep has been detected in the mature AAV virions, and is implicated in the growth inhibitory effect of rAAV, devoid of Rep gene, on primary human cells.[69] Whether encapsidated AAV Rep plays a role, alone or by interacting with cellular factors such as dsD-BP, in the early stage of viral replication remains to be investigated. In view of the critical role of dsD-BP in either inhibiting or stimulating second strand DNA synthesis, it would be interesting to investigate whether dsD-BP is encapsidated in mature AAV virions.

To address the possibility that the aforementioned observations might be related to a specific transcription unit (e.g., the CMV promoter driving the LacZ gene), we tested rAAV containing other transcription units. The "TRZ" transcription unit, containing an anti-HIV ribozyme driven by a modified tRNA promoter,[52] was cloned into two of our rAAV backbone plasmids as shown in Figures 8.2 and 8.6. Ribozyme expression was detected at low levels in 293 cells infected with rAAV-AT29 and -AT30, which were heat-treated to inactivate contaminating adenovirus. In contrast, the addition of exogenous adenovirus to the heat-treated rAAV sample dramatically augmented TRZ expression. Our data is in agreement with the results of other investigators who reported the effect of adenovirus on enhancing rAAV-mediated gene expression, independent of the nature of the transgene pro-

A. Effect of Adding Exogenous Adenovirus to rAAV-LacZ Partially Purified by CsCl Step Gradient

B. Effect of Heat-Inactivation and Addition of Exogenous Adenovirus on rAAV-LacZ Titer

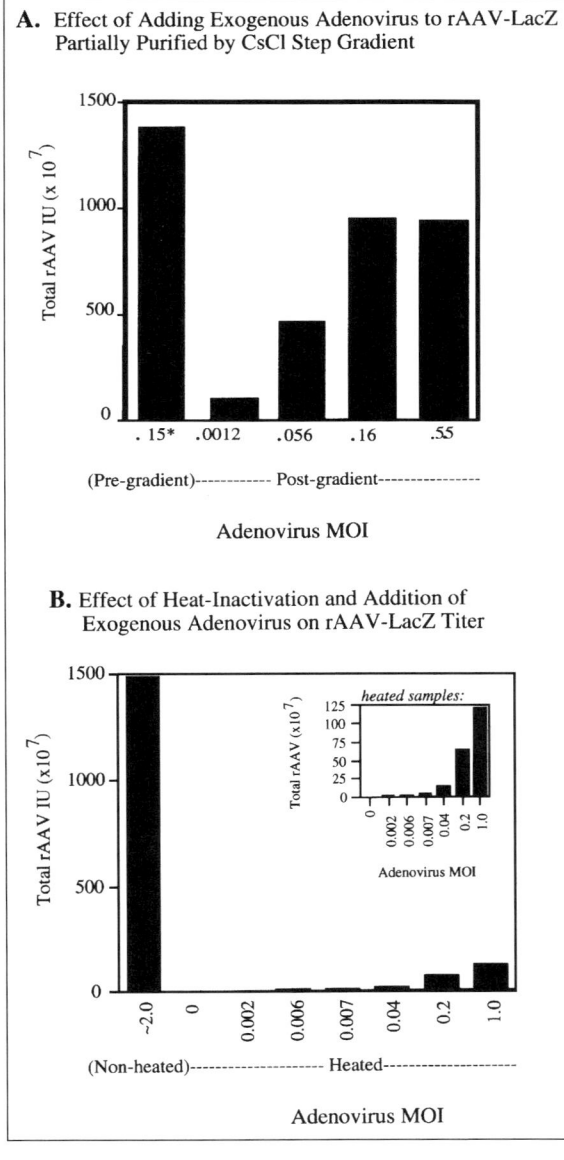

Fig. 8.5. Adenovirus enhancement of rAAV-LacZ expression. (A) The total IU of a rAAV-LacZ preparation, which was partially purified by polyethylene precipitation, was determined before CsCl gradient centrifugation (*), to remove adenovirus, and after purification, with the addition of the indicated MOIs of exogenous adenovirus (dl312). (B) Effect of heat-treatment and addition of exogenous adenovirus on rAAV-LacZ titer. The total infectious unit (IU) of a crude rAAV-LacZ preparation was determined on 293 cells using the nonheat-treated sample or the heat-treated (56°C, to inactivate adenovirus) sample with or without the addition of the indicated MOIs of exogenous adenovirus (dl312).

moter and its coding region.[37-39] In our system, adenovirus enhancement of ribozyme expression can be explained by considering the following possibilities:
1. adenovirus augments the second-strand synthesis of rAAV genomic DNA, which is indispensable for transcription initiation;
2. contaminating wt AAV, generated during the production of rAAV preparations, can increase the copy number of rAAV genomic templates, leading to higher expression; and
3. adenovirus activates the tRNA promoter driving the ribozyme expression.

These possibilities are being addressed in our laboratory.

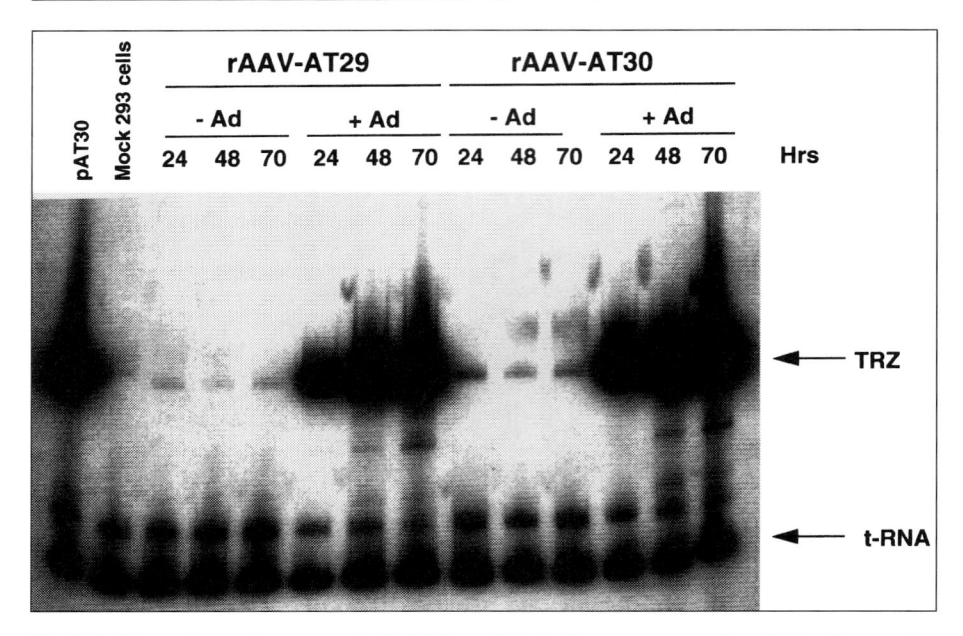

Fig. 8.6. Adenovirus enhancement of rAAV-mediated ribozyme expression. 293 cells were infected with heat-treated rAAV-AT30 or rAAV-AT29 with or without the addition of exogenous adenovirus (MOI:2). Cells were harvested at the indicated time points p.i., and RNA purification and Northern blot analysis were carried out as described previously.[52] As a positive control, 293 cells were transfected with pAT30 using a calcium phosphate transfection protocol (Promega), and total RNA was analyzed 48 h post-transfection (labeled as pAT30). This blot was hybridized with a [^{32}P]-labeled T7 transcript containing the ribozyme and modified tRNA promoter sequences which also hybridizes to the endogenous species of tRNAs.

Host Range, Transduction, and Gene Expression

An attractive feature of rAAV as a vector for human gene therapy is its ability to infect a broad range of mammalian cell types, such as human, mouse, and rat. In addition, rAAV-mediated transgene expression appears to be stable for a long period of time without any deleterious immune response. These features facilitate the testing of safety and efficacy of rAAV in vivo, in animal models of human disease.

The transduction efficiency of rAAV varies significantly among different cell types within a species. Several recent studies have shown that muscle, brain, and liver are among the best tissues for rAAV-mediated transgene expression.[34-36,70-73] When rAAV-LacZ was injected intravenously in mice, LacZ expression was predominately detected in liver hepatocytes, (cells which are non-dividing); however moderate expression of LacZ was shown in lung and kidney tissues.[72] This finding paves the way for target-specific therapeutic application of rAAV. Efficient transduction of non-dividing liver cells with rAAV containing the expression cassette for the human factor IX (hFIX) was recently reported with a single administration of rAAV to mice.[71] This study demonstrated stable, persistent, and therapeutic levels of factor IX expression in mice, without any significant immune response.

Efficient expression of LacZ and hFIX was demonstrated in mouse muscle cells.[34] High levels and stable LacZ expression was detected in mice following intramuscular injection of rAAV, which integrated into chromosomal DNA of differentiated muscle fibers.[34] In this study, no humoral or cellular immune responses were elicited against the E. coli β-galactosidase. Furthermore, neutralizing antibody against AAV capsid proteins did not prevent readministration of rAAV vector. In the case of rAAV-mediated hFIX expression in mouse muscle, the level of plasma factor IX reached therapeutic levels, and was sustained for 6 months.[34] The efficient expression of LacZ or factor IX mediated by rAAV in muscle did not induce any detectable cytotoxic T lymphocyte response; however, immune competent mice developed circulating antibodies to hFIX.[34] This is in stark contrast to adenovirus-mediated expression of LacZ or Factor IX, which induces a massive immune response leading to complete abrogation of transgene expression.[3,34]

These observations underscore the potential of rAAV-mediated gene therapy in muscle tissues for the treatment of inherited and acquired human diseases. Muscle tissues are also a good reservoir for the systemic delivery of therapeutic molecules like blood clotting factors, growth factors, or hormones.

Several reports have demonstrated the efficient expression of transgenes in neuronal cells.[70,73] LacZ expression was detected in caudate nucleus, amygdala, striatum, and hippocampus of the adult rat brain 3 days following stereotactic microinjection of rAAV-LacZ.[70] Transduction efficiency into various regions of the rat brain was estimated to be about 10%, which closely matches that of transgene delivery with HSV or adenovirus. Neuronal expression of LacZ was detected in caudate nucleus for up to 3 months. Kaplitt et al investigated the therapeutic benefits of expressing tyrosine hydroxylase (AAVth) in a rat model for Parkinson's disease.[70] Tyrosine hydroxylase expression was detected in striatal neurons and glia for up to 4 months following vector injection into the denervated striatum of unilateral 6-hydroxydopamine-lesioned rats. Significant behavioral recovery in lesioned rats was noted with rAAVth versus AAVLacZ treated animals.

The ability of rAAV to infect primary mouse (Lin$^-$Sca-1$^+$) and human (CD34$^+$) hematopoietic progenitor cells, capable of multilineage differentiation, has also been documented in several studies.[26-31] For example, murine hematopoietic cells transduced ex vivo with an rAAV containing a human β-globin expression cassette followed by transplantation into lethally irradiated congenic mice resulted in long-term expression of β-globin in bone marrow cells for up to 6 months.[29] When bone marrow cells from these primary mice were transplanted into secondary animals, the expression of human β-globin was detected in bone marrow cells for up to 3 months.[29] Although rAAV-mediated LacZ expression in human hematopoietic progenitor cells (CD34$^+$) has been reported in vitro, transgene expression varies in CD34$^+$ cells from different donors, ranging between 0% to 80%.[28] When bone marrow cells that are refractory to rAAV infection are induced with growth factors to undergo differentiation, they become permissive to rAAV transduction and transgene expression.[28] The stable expression of the transgene was detected in the differentiated lineages of the primary infected hematopoietic cells, such as myeloid, during the course of experiments. The observed variability of rAAV transduction of human hematopoietic cells is linked to the differential expression of a putative AAV receptor on CD34$^+$ cells.[28]

Flotte et al reported in several studies the utility of rAAV-mediated expression of the cystic fibrosis transmembrane regulator (CFTR) gene in respiratory epithelial cells, which are a suitable target for the treatment of cystic fibrosis (CF).[33,41] Efficient expression of the human CFTR gene has been demonstrated in an immortalized human bronchial epithelial cell line in vitro and subsequently in rabbit and rhesus monkey respiratory epithelium in vivo. Fiberoptic bronchoscopy was used to deliver the rAAV-CFTR to a lobe of the lung in the aforementioned animals.[41] This resulted in efficient and stable expression of the CFTR gene in lung epithelium, with minimal toxicity and no deleterious immune responses. These promising observations set the stage for testing the utility of CFTR-expressing rAAV in the ongoing clinical trial in CF patients.

Table 8.1. Summary of rAAV transduction

Cell Line	Species	Cell Type	vAT30 (μl)	MOI	% NGFR+	Heat Inact. Ad
HeLa	Human	Cervical Carcinoma	64	10	95	
H4[a]	Human	Neuroglioma	32	5	99	
SK-N-SH	Human	Neuroblastoma	64	20	80	Yes[b]
MVEC[c]	Human	Endothelium	50	20	93	
LNCap.FGC	Human	Prostate Carcinoma	64	20	85	Yes[b]
MDA-MB-435S	Human	Breast Carcinoma	64	20	80	
T-47D	Human	Breast Carcinoma	64	20	8	Yes[b]
HT-29	Human	Colon Carcinoma	64	20	35	
HS-27[c]	Human	Foreskin fibroblast	100	25	98	
RSF[c]	Rabbit	Synoviocyte	100	25	95	
B16	Mouse	Melanoma	100	25	78	
HL60	Human	Promelocytic Leukemia	60	90	0	

An approximately equivalent number of cells for each cell line (~5 x 10[5]) were infected with the indicated volume of rAAV-AT30. The percentage of cells expressing NGFR was determined by FACS analysis 3 days post-infection. [a]Transduction (percentage of NGFR-expressing cells) was approximately the same with or without heat-treatment of rAAV-AT30. [b]rAAV-AT30 was heat-treated (56°C for 30 min) to inactivate adenovirus, as the non-heated viral inoculum was toxic to these cell lines 3 days p.i., presumably due to lytic infection by adenovirus. [c]Primary cell lines.

We were interested in comparing and evaluating the transduction efficiency of rAAV containing a ribozyme expression cassette in a variety of mammalian cell lines. In pursuit of this, rAAV-AT30 was used to infect a variety of mammalian cell lines. The titer of rAAV-AT30 vector was determined on HeLa cells as shown in Figure 8.4. Table 8.1 is a summary of our transduction data based on measuring cell surface NGFR expression by FACS.

In contrast to 293 cells, approximately equivalent transduction of the neuroglioma (H4) cell line was achieved with either the nonheat-treated or the heat-treated rAAV-AT30. One likely explanation might be the efficient synthesis of second strand rAAV DNA in the H4 neuroglioma cells, independent of the adenovirus E4 ORF helper function. This observation is in agreement with others who reported that the conversion of ss-DNA of the rAAV genome to transcriptionally active ds-DNA may vary significantly in different cell types and tissues.[40] This may explain the reason for efficient expression of rAAV transgene in liver, muscle, and neuronal cells, and poor expression in other cell types, in vivo. In our experience, the rAAV transduction of human monolayer cell lines generally were more efficient than suspension cell lines.

The levels of NGFR expression from three cell lines in Table 8.1 is shown in Figure 8.7. The H4 neuroglioma cell line is highly susceptible to rAAV transduction as compared to other cell lines tested in our laboratory so far. We also noted that, although some cell lines, such as HeLa and H4, show very similar transduction efficiencies as measured by NGFR expression, the level of transgene expression can vary. Differences in gene expression might be due to several factors:
1. AAV receptor density may vary in different cell lines;
2. The conversion of rAAV ss-DNA into ds-form might be more efficient in some cell lines as compared to others; and
3. The activity of a promoter driving the transgene expression is influenced by the cell type.

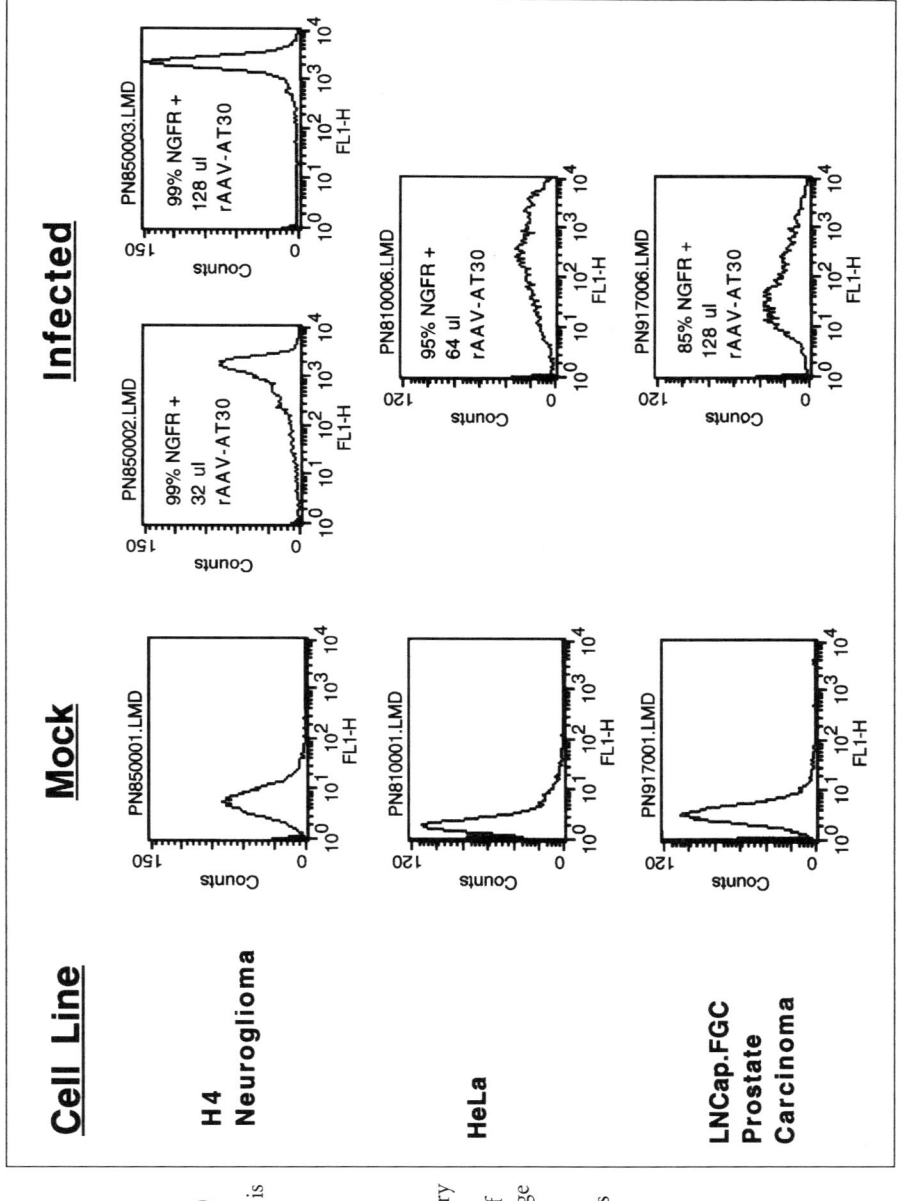

Fig. 8.7. FACS profile of the rAAV-AT30-mediated NGFR expressing cells. The pattern of NGFR expression for three human cell lines (H4, HeLa, and LNCap.FGC) transduced with the rAAV-AT30 (Table 8.1) is shown. Cells were infected at an MOI (based on particle concentration) of 5 (H4), 10 (HeLa), or 40 (LNCap.FCG). The particle:IU ratio can vary with cell line, but is typically in the range of 50–500:1. The percentage of cells expressing NGFR, in mock- and rAAV-infected cells, was determined by FACS analysis.

The expression of an anti-HIV ribozyme from an rAAV vector (TRZA568) was readily detected in several of these cell lines (Fig. 8.8). The modified tRNA promoter is highly active in most of the cell lines tested in our laboratory. Since rAAV-mediated TRZ expression is very efficient in the H4 neuroglioma cell line, it would be interesting to examine the inhibitory effect of this on HIV infection, similarly to what has been attempted using retroviruses. Retroviral vectors have been used to transduce either the hairpin or the hammerhead ribozyme expression cassette into a variety of cell lines.[10-13,74] The majority of these studies focused on targeting HIV transcripts, including Tat, Tat/Rev, and Gag mRNAs. For instance, retroviral mediated expression of a hammerhead ribozyme specific for Tat or Tat/Rev in CD4$^+$ cell lines (CEM, SupT) showed significant levels of resistance against HIV infection as demonstrated by the reduction of p24 antigen.[12-13] In the latter studies, the hammerhead ribozyme was embedded in the body of a NPT II transcript driven by Molony LTR, or it was inserted in the 3' LTR driven by a modified tRNA in a LN retroviral vector. In a separate study, macrophage-like cells differentiated from the CD34$^+$ cells, which were transduced with a retrovirus containing a hammerhead ribozyme expression cassette specific for the HIV genome, were significantly resistant to a macrophage tropic HIV-1 infection.[74]

The efficacy of vector-mediated ribozyme expression in cells is dependent on several factors, including the levels of ribozyme and target RNA expression, the half-life of the ribozyme and target RNA transcripts, absence of inhibitory secondary structure, and colocalization of ribozyme with its target RNA transcript. Bertrand et al addressed some of the aforementioned issues by constructing ribozyme expression cassettes specific for the TAR region of the simian immunodeficiency virus (SIV) driven by modified RSV, human U1, U6, and tRNA promoters cloned into retroviral or AAV backbone plasmids.[32] The transcripts of U1, U6, and tRNA were primarily localized in the nucleus, and were not effective in reducing heterologous mRNA containing the TAR region of SIV. However, RSV-LTR driven transcripts containing the SIV-TAR specific ribozyme were primarily localized in the cytoplasm, and significantly reduced the SIV LTR driven heterologous transcript. In the aforementioned study, the U6 and tRNA driven ribozyme expression were active in the context of an AAV plasmid; however, these cassettes were inactive in a retroviral plasmid, presumably due to transcriptional interference by Molony LTR.

Concluding Remarks

Progress in the basic biology of AAV has answered several key questions regarding the potential of this vector for broad use as an efficient delivery vehicle for laboratory experimentations, and ultimately for applications in human gene therapy. We would like to highlight some of the salient features of AAV as a vector, and emphasize existing knowledge gaps pertinent to its use for gene therapy.

First, a better understanding of AAV transcriptional regulation is essential for optimizing rAAV production or establishing an "ideal packaging cell line". Second, we now know that AAV infection is receptor mediated. It may be useful to further characterize this putative receptor, to facilitate an understanding of the molecular mechanisms of viral entry into cells. It might be feasible in the near future to augment rAAV transgene delivery via a transient induction of AAV receptors on target tissues prior to viral transduction. Third, in light of the importance of second strand DNA synthesis for AAV-mediated transgene expression, it would be prudent to characterize associated viral and host cell factors, and formulate strategies to enhance this in tissues in which this step is rate limiting. Fourth, stable viral integration is indispensable for long-term therapeutic gene expression. The lack of integration reported in certain systems should be investigated, to define the underlying mechanism which dictates the efficiency of viral integration. Fifth, site specific integration on chromosome 19 is one of the hallmarks of wt AAV infection, and it would be desirable to

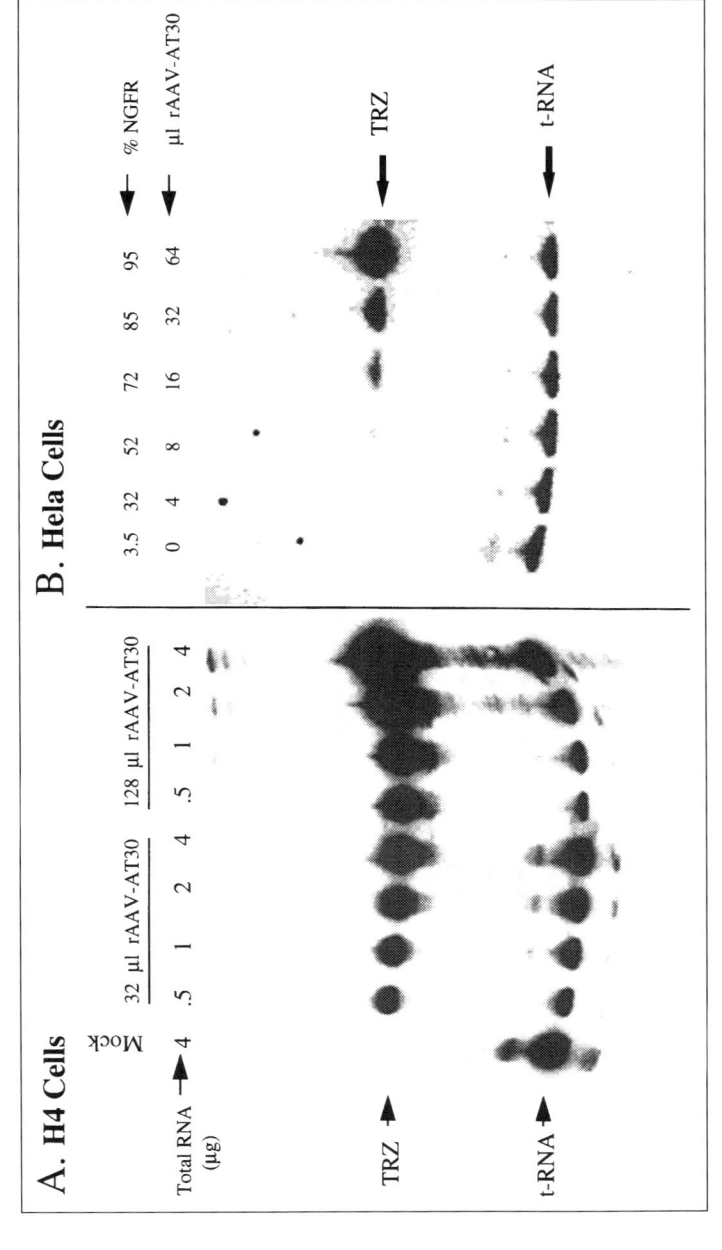

Fig. 8.8. Ribozyme expression profile of rAAV-AT30 transduced cells. The levels of TRZ expression in H4 (A) and HeLa (B) cell lines transduced with rAAV-AT30 (same infections as shown in Table 8.1 and Fig. 8.7). Cells were harvested 3 days p.i. for FACS and RNA analysis. RNA purification and Northern blot analysis were carried out as described previously.[52] Blots were hybridized with the same [^{32}P]-labeled probe as in Fig. 8.3.

impart this feature to rAAV vectors. This unique feature could reduce the risk of insertional mutagenesis associated with randomly integrating vectors, such as retroviral and current rAAV vectors. Sixth, although the overall in vivo safety and lack of deleterious immunogenicity are attractive features of rAAV vectors, the reproducibility of these features in human gene therapy awaits comprehensive clinical testing.

To end this review with a humorous note, AAV is no longer an acronym for "Almost A Virus"; instead it stands for "All Activity Vehicle" for gene delivery, which was, ironically, coined by the automobile industry rather than by parvovirologists.

Acknowledgments

We are grateful to Drs. Dennis Macejak, Jude Samulski, Arun Srivastava, and Jim Thompson for the generous gifts of plasmids and ribozyme expression cassettes. We are indebted to Dr. Larry Couture for his help and guidance through the course of this study. We also thank Drs. Larry Couture and Dennis Macejak for critical reading of this manuscript. We thank Kristi Jensen and Tim McKenzie for excellent technical assistance. We are grateful to Dr. A. Srivastava for communicating his unpublished data to us.

References

1. Anderson WF. Gene therapy. Sci Amer 1995; 273:124-128.
2. Mulligan RC. The basic science of gene therapy. Science 1993; 260:926-932.
3. Hitt MM, Addison CL, Graham FL. Human adenovirus vectors for gene transfer into mammalian cells. Adv Pharmacol 1997; 40:137-206.
4. Muzyczka N. Use of adeno-associated virus as a general transduction vector for mammalian cells. Curr Top Microbiol and Immunol 1992; 158:97-129.
5. Berns KI, Giraud C. Biology of adeno-associated virus. Curr Top Microbiol Immunol 1996; 218:1-23.
6. Miller AD, Miller DG, Garcia JV et al. Methods Enzymol 217:581-599.
7. Roe T, Reynolds TC, Yu G et al. Integration of murine leukemia virus DNA depends on mitosis. EMBO J 1993; 12: 2099-2108.
8. Naldini L, Blomer U, Gallay P et al. In vivo gene delivery and stable transduction of nondividing cells by a lentiviral vector. Science 1996; 272:263-266.
9. Huang S, Stupack D, Mathias P et al. Growth arrest of Epstein-Barr virus immortalized B lymphocytes by adenovirus-delivered ribozymes. Proc Natl Acad Sci USA 1997; 94:8156-8161
10. Couture LA, Stinchcomb DT. Anti-gene therapy: Use of ribozymes to inhibit gene function. Trends in Genetics 1996; 12:510-515.
11. Sarver N, Cantin EM, Chang PS et al. Ribozymes as potential anti-HIV-1 therapuetic agents. Science 1990; 247:1222-1225.
12. Zhou I, Bahner C, Larson GP et al. Inhibition of HIV-1 in human T-lymphocytes by retrovirally transduced anti-tat and rev hammerhead ribozymes. Gene1994; 149:33-39.
13. Zhou C. I. Bahner, Rossi JJ et al. Expression of hammerhead ribozymes by retroviral vectors to inhibit HIV-1 replication: Comparison of RNA levels and viral inhibition. Antisense and nucleic acid drug development 1996; 6:17-24.
14. Yakobson B, Koch T, Winocour E. Replication of adeno-associated virus in synchronized cells without the addition of a helper virus. J Virol 1987; 972-981.
15. Yakobson B, Hrynko TA, Peak MJ, Winocour E. Replication of adeno-associated virus in cells irradiated with UV light at 254 nm. J Virol 1989; 63:1023-1030.
16. Alexander IA, Russell DW, Miller AD. DNA-damaging agents greatly increase the transduction of nondividing cells by adeno-associated virus vectors. J Virol 1994; 68:8282-8287.
17. Alexander IA, Russell DW, Spence AM et al. Effects of gamma irradiation on the transduction of dividing and nondividing cells in brain and muscle of rats by adeno-associated virus vectors. Hum Gene Therap 1996; 7:841-850.
18. Russell DW, Alexander IE, Miller AD. DNA synthesis and topoisomerase inhibitors increase transduction by adeno-associated virus vectors. Proc Natl Acad Sci USA 1995; 92: 5719-5723.

19. Kotin RM, Siniscalco M, Samulski RJ et al. Site-specific integration by adeno-associated virus. Proc Natl Acad Sci USA 1990; 87:2211-2215.
20. Kotin RM, Linden RM, Berns KI. Characterization of a preferred site on human chromosome 19q for integration of adeno-associated virus DNA by non-homologous recombination. EMBO J 1992; 11:5071-5078.
21. Samulski RJ, Zhu X, Xiao X et al. Targeted integration of adeno-associated virus (AAV) into human chromosome 19. EMBO J 1991; 10:3941-3950.
22. Weitzman, MD, Kÿostio SRM, Kotin RM et al. Adeno-associated virus (AAV) rep proteins mediate complex formation between AAV DNA and its integration site in human DNA. Proc Natl Acad Sci USA 1994; 91:5805-5812.
23. Tobiasch E, Rabreau M, Geletneky K, Larue-Charlus S et al. Detection of adeno-associated virus DNA in human genital tissue and in material from spontaneous abortion. J Med Virol 1994; 44(2):215-222.
24. Hermonat PL, Plott RT, Santin AD, Parham GP et al. Adeno-associated virus Rep78 inhibits oncogenic transformation of primary human keratinocytes by a human papillomavirus type 16-ras chimeric. Gynecol Oncol 1997; 66:487-494.
25. Russell DW, Miller AD, Alexander IE. Adeno-associated virus vectors preferentially transduce cells in S phase. Proc Natl Acad Sci USA 1994; 91:8915-8919.
26. Zhou SZ, Broxmeyer HE, Cooper S et al. Adeno-associated virus 2-mediated gene transfer in murine hematopoietic progenitor cells. Exp Hematol 1993; 21:928-933.
27. Chatterjee S, Lu D, Podsakoff G et al. Strategies for efficient gene transfer into hematopoietic cells: The use of adeno-associated virus vectors in gene therapy. Ann NY Acad Sci 1995; 770:79-90.
28. Ponnazhagan S, Mukherjee P, Wang X-S et al. Adeno-associated virus Type 2-Mediated transduction in primary human bone marrow-derived CD34+ hematopoietic progenitor cells: Donor variation and correlation of transgene expression with cellular differentiation. J Virol 1997; 71:8286-8267.
29. Ponnazhagan S, Yoder MC, Srivastava A. Adeno-associated virus type 2-mediated transduction of murine hematopoietic cells with long-term repopulating ability and sustained expression of a human globin gene in vivo. J Virol 1997; 71:3098-3104.
30. Einerhand MPW, Antoniou M, Zolotukhin S et al. Regulated high-level human beta-globin gene expression in erythroid cells following recombinant adeno-associated virus-mediated gene transfer. Gene Ther 1995; 2:336-343.
31. Goodman S, Xiao X, Donahue RE et al. Recombinant adeno-associated virus mediated gene transfer into hematopoietic progenitor cells. Blood 1994; 84:1492-1500.
32. Bertrand E, Castanotto D, Zhou C et al. The expression cassette determines the functional activity of ribozymes in mammalian cells by controlling their intracellular localization. RNA 1997; 3:75-88.
33. Flotte TR, Afione SA, Solow R et al. Expression of the cystic fibrosis transmembrane conductance regulator from a novel adeno-associated virus promoter. J Biol Chem 1993; 268:3781-3790.
34. Fisher KJ, Jooss K, Alston J et al. Recombinant adeno-associated virus for muscle directed gene therapy. Nat Med 1997; 3(3):306-312.
35. Herzog RW, Hagstrom JN, Kung SH et al. Stable gene transfer and expression of human blood coagulation factor IX after intramuscular injection of recombinant adeno-associated virus. Proc Natl Acad Sci USA 1997; 94(11):5804-5809.
36. Snyder RO, Miao CH, Patijn GA et al. Persistent and therapeutic concentrations of human factor IX in mice after hepatic gene transfer of recombinant AAV vectors. Nat Genet 1997; 16(3):270-276.
37. Fisher KJ, Gao G-P, Weitzman MD et al. Transduction with recombinant adeno-associated virus for gene therapy is limited by leading-strand synthesis. J Virol 1996; 70(1):520-532.
38. Ferrari FK, Samulski T, Shenk T et al. Second-strand synthesis is a rate-limiting step for efficient transduction by recombinant adeno-associated virus vectors. J Virol 1996; 70:3227-3234.

39. Qing K, Wang X-S, Kube DM et al. Role of tyrosine phosphorylation of a cellular protein in adeno-associated virus 2-mediated transgene expression. Proc Natl Acad Sci USA 1997; 94(20):10879-10884.
40. Qing K, Khuntirat B, Mah C et al. Adeno-associated virus type 2-mediated gene transfer: Correlation of tyrosine phosphorylation of the cellular single-stranded D sequence-binding protein with transgene expression in human cells in vitro and murine tissue in vivo. J Virol 1998; 72(2):1593-1599.
41. Carter BJ, Flotte TR. Development of adeno-associated virus vectors for gene therapy of cystic fibrosis. Curr Top Microbiol Immunol 1996; 218:119-144.
42. Malik P, McQuiston SA, Yu XJ et al. Recombinant adeno-associated virus mediates a high level of gene transfer but less efficient integration in the K562 human hematopoietic cell line. J Virol 1997; 71(3):1776-1783.
43. McLaughlin SK, Collis P, Hermonat PL, Muzyczka N. Adeno-associated virus general transduction vectors: Analysis of proviral structures. J Virol 1988; 62:1963-1973.
44. Hermonat PL, Quirk JG, Bishop BM, Han L. The packaging capacity of adeno-associated virus (AAV) and the potential for wild-type-plus AAV gene therapy vectors. FEBS Lett 1997; 407:78-84.
45. Dong JY, Fan PD, Frizzell RA. Quantitative analysis of the packaging capacity of recombinant adeno-associated virus. Hum Gene Ther 1996; 7(17):2101-2112.
46. Blacklow NR, Hoggan MD, Rowe WP. Serologic evidence for human infection with adenovirus-associated viruses. J Natl Cancer Inst 1968; 40:319-327.
47. Samulski RJ, Berns KI, Tan M et al. Cloning of adeno-associated virus into pBR322: Rescue of intact virus from the recombinant plasmid in human cells. Proc Natl Acad Sci USA 1982; 79:2077-2081.
48. Laughlin CA, Tratschin JD, Coon H, Carter BJ. Cloning of infectious adeno-associated virus genomes in bacterial plasmids. Gene 1983; 23:65-73.
49. Nahreini P, Woody MJ, Zhou SZ et al. Versatile adeno-associated virus 2-based vectors for constructing recombinant virions. Gene 1993; 124:257-262.
50. Samulski, RJ., Chang L-S, Shank T. A recombinant plasmid from which an infectious adeno-associated virus genome can be excised in vitro and its use to study viral replication. J Vriol 1987; 61:3096-3101.
51. Samulski, RJ, Chang L-S, Shenk T. Helper-free stocks of recombinant adeno-associated viruses: Normal integration does not require viral gene expression. J Virol 1989; 63:3822-3828.
52. Thompson J, Ayers D, Malmstrom T et al. Improved accumulation and activity of ribozymes expressed from a tRNA-based polymerase III promoter. Nucleic Acids Res 1995; 23:2259-2268.
53. Rolling F, Samulski RJ. Stability of sequence cassettes containing secondary structure in AAV vectors. VIth Parvovirus Workshop, Montpellier, France, 1995, 16.
54. Kube DM, Srivastava A. Quantitative DNA slot blot analysis: Inhibition of DNA binding to membranes by magnesium ions. Nucleic Acids Research 1997; 25:3375-3376.
55. Yang Q, Chen F, Trempe JP. Characterization of cell lines that inducibly express the adenoassociated virus Rep proteins. J Virol 1994; 68:4847-4856.
56. Holscher C, Horker M, Kleinschmidt JA et al. Cell lines inducibly expressing the adenoassociated virus (AAV) rep gene: Requirements for productive replication of rep-negative AAV mutants. J Virol 1994; 68:7169-7177.
57. Holscher C, Kleinschmidt JA, Burkle A. High-level expression of adeno-associated virus (AAV) Rep 78 protein is sufficient for infectious-particle formation by a rep-negative AAV mutant. J Virol 1995; 69: 6880-6885
58. Lebkowski J, Okarma TB, Philip R. The challenges of recombinant adeno-associated virus manufacturing: Alternative use of adeno-associated virus plasmid/liposome complexes for gene therapy applications. Curr Top Microbiol Immunol 1996; 218:51-59.
59. Neyns B, Rijcke MD, Teugels, Hermonat P et al. Establishment of recombinant adenoassociated virus producer cell lines that provide the rep and cap complementor functions

from an episomal plasmid. VIIth International Parvovirus Workshop, Heidelberg, Germany, 1997:33.
60. Schetter C, Heilbronn R. A recombinant herpesvirus expressing AAV Rep and Cap for efficient production of AAV vectors. VIIth International Parvovirus Workshop, Heidelberg, Germany, 1997, 3.2.
61. Grimm D, Rittner K, Kleinschmidt JA. Helpervirus-free packaging of adeno-associated virus derived vectors. VIIth International Parvovirus Workshop, Heidelberg, Germany, 1997:3.3.
62. Zhou SZ, Ladner M, Escobedo JA, Dwarki V. Recombinant adeno-associated virus preparation without the use of adenovirus: A novel triple transfection protocol. VIIth International Parvovirus Workshop, Heidelberg, Germany, 1997, 30.
63. Ferrari FK, Xiao X, McCarty D, Samulski RJ. New developments in the generation of Ad-free, high-titer rAAV gene therapy vectors. Nature Med 1997; 3:1295-1297.
64. Burstein H, Rogers LC. Stable split packaging cell lines for rAAV vectors based on Cre-LoxP system. VIIth International Parvovirus Workshop, Heidelberg, Germany, 1997:3.4.
65. Li J, Samulski RJ, and Xiao X. Role for highly regulated rep gene expression in adeno-associated virus vector production. J Virol 1997; 71(7):5236-5243.
66. Flottte TR, Barraza-Oritz X, Solow R et al. An improved system for packaging recombinant adeno-associated virus vectors capable of in vivo transduction. Gene Therapy 1995; 2:29-37.
67. Pereira DJ, McCarty DM, Muzyczka N. The adeno-associated virus (AAV) Rep protein acts as both a repressor and an activator to regulate AAV transcription during a productive infection. J Virol 1997; 71(2):1079-1088.
68. Pereira DJ, Muzyczka N. The adeno-associatedvirus type 2 p40 promoter requires a proximal Sp1 interaction and a p19 CArG-like element to facilitate Rep transactivation. J Virol 1997; 71(6):4300-4309.
69. Kube, DM, Ponnazhagan S, Srivastava A. Encapsidation of adeno-associated virus type 2 Rep proteins in wild-type and recombinant progeny virions: Rep-mediated growth inhibition of primary human cells. J Virol 1997; 71(10):7361-7371.
70. Kaplitt, MG., Leone P, Samulski RJ et al. Long-term gene expression and phenotypic correction using adeno-associated virus vectors in the mammalian brain. Nature Genetics 1994; 8:148-153.
71. Koeberl DD, Alexander IE, Halbert CL et al. Persistent expression of human clotting factor IX from mouse liver after intravenous injection of adeno-associated virus vectors. Proc Natl Acad Sci USA 1997; 94 (4):1426-1431.
72. Ponnazhagan S, Mukherjee P, Yoder MC et al. Adeno-associated virus2-mediated gene transfer in vivo: Organ-tropism and expression of transduced sequences in mice. Gene 1997; 190:203-210.
73. Rosenfeld MR, Bergman I, Schramm L et al. Adeno-associated viral vector gene transfer into leptomeningeal xenografts. J Neurooncol 1997; 34(2):139-144.
74. Yu M, Leavitt MC, Maruyama M et al. Intracellular immunization of human fetal cord blood stem/progenitor cells with a ribozyme against human immunodeficiency virus type 1. Proc Natl Acad Sci USA 1995; 92:699-703.
75. Hirt, B. Selective extraction of polyoma DNA from infected mouse cell cultures. J Mol Biol 1967; 26:365-369.

Section III
Ribozyme Targets for Gene Therapy

CHAPTER 9

Applications of Anti-Oncogene Ribozymes for the Treatment of Bladder Cancer

Akira Irie and Eric J. Small

Overview of Bladder Cancer

Bladder cancer is the fifth most common malignancy in the United States. Approximately 54,500 patients will be diagnosed in 1997, with nearly 12,000 deaths attributed to this disease.[1] Despite improved diagnostic and therapeutic modalities, the incidence of bladder cancer is increasing, and the overall mortality from bladder cancer has not decreased dramatically over the last decade. In the US, more than 90% of bladder cancers are transitional cell carcinoma; squamous carcinoma and adenocarcinoma constitute the remainder.[2] Bladder tumors are graded based on the degree of the anaplasia of the tumor cells. A correlation exists between tumor grade and tumor stage, i.e., well-differentiated tumors are more likely to be superficial, and poorly differentiated tumors are more likely to be muscle-invasive.

Bladder cancers can be characterized into two groups with considerably different natural histories, i.e., superficial tumors confined to the mucosa and muscle-invasive tumors, which penetrate the muscularis mucosa. Approximately 70% of bladder cancers are superficial tumors at the time of clinical presentation.[3] Superficial bladder cancers are primarily treated by transurethral resection (TUR). Despite complete resection of visible tumors, about 60% of patients will develop a recurrence within 5 years. Intravesical instillation of chemotherapeutic agents such as doxorubicin, thiotepa, and mitomycin or immunological agents such as bacillus Calmette-Guerin (BCG) has been shown to reduce the likelihood of recurrence or progression after TUR. One third of patients will have a tumor recurrence in spite of intravesical therapy. Progression of the disease, i.e., development of a more advanced stage, will be recognized in 10% of patients and is of more concern in carcinoma in situ (CIS), particularly if it is high grade or extensive and multifocal. Intravesical therapy is not without complications such as pyrexia, hematuria, cystitis, and irritative voiding symptoms. Severe adverse events are very uncommon but include BCG sepsis and massive hemorrhage.

Bladder cancer invades through the lamina propria into the submucosa, muscle layer, and perivesical fat. Also, it spreads hematogenously and via lymphatics to regional lymph nodes and distant metastatic sites. Clinical stage and depth of invasion correlate well with the risk of subsequent relapse even if local therapy has been undertaken. Regional lymph nodes, liver, lung, and bone are the most common sites of metastases. Approximately 30% of bladder cancer patients are characterized by muscle invasion and/or node positive disease

---

Ribozymes in the Gene Therapy of Cancer, edited by Kevin J. Scanlon and Mohammed Kashani-Sabet.
©1998 R.G. Landes Company.

at initial diagnosis. Radical cystectomy is generally recommended for treatment of muscle invasive non-metastatic bladder cancer, with or without adjuvant therapies.[4] Bladder preserving therapy with chemoradiotherapy may be appropriate in selected patients.[5] Recurrence after cystectomy is attributed to the presence of micrometastatic disease. Only a small percentage (20% or less) of patients with metastatic disease can obtain long term disease free survival with systemic chemotherapy.

Novel approaches are needed for the treatment of bladder cancer, both for recurrent superficial tumors and for muscle-invasive and metastatic disease. A biologically based approach designed to reverse the invasive and/or metastatic phenotype is attractive in this regard. Recently, molecular-based strategies have been investigated extensively for treatment of bladder cancer, including anti-oncogene agents such as antisense oligonucleotides and ribozymes, and restoration of tumor suppressor gene function.[6-12]

Molecular Genetics of Bladder Cancer

Many genetic alterations have been identified in bladder cancers. As in other malignancies, the pathogenesis of bladder cancer appears to involve a multi-step process of carcinogenesis and disease progression.[13-15] These genetic alterations include activation of oncogenes, inappropriate expression of growth factors and their receptors, and loss or inactivation of tumor suppressor genes. The role of these alterations with respect to tumorigenicity and their relation to clinical features have also been investigated. The *ras* family has been extensively investigated in bladder cancers. The *ras* family consists of H-*ras*, K-*ras*, and N-*ras*, and are important components of the signal transduction pathway.[16] Mutated *ras* oncogenes activate downstream proteins such as Raf, MAP kinase and MEK, resulting in uncontrolled phosphorylation of transcription factors that regulate gene expression. Once a Ras protein is activated, it loses its ability to return to its inactive form, and continues to stimulate cell proliferation. Recent studies have demonstrated that the activation of the Ras stimulates the expression of the transcription factor c-Fos. The expression of c-Fos is thought to be one of the downstream effects of Ras-regulated signal transduction.[17] Increased c-Fos expression is crucial for cell transformation, and activation of tumor growth. The H-*ras* oncogene has also been reported to stimulate tumor angiogenesis by activation of vascular endothelial growth factor (VEGF) and inactivation of angiogenesis inhibitors.[18,19] Neovascularization permits rapid expansion of tumor growth and may increase its metastatic ability.

The *erbB-2* gene is part of the epidermal growth factor receptor family and possesses tyrosine kinase activity. Overexpression of *erbB-2* has been observed in 20-40% bladder cancers, and the activation of *erbB-2* has been correlated with the stage and grade of the tumor.[20] Three oncogenes, *int-2*, *hst1* and *bcl-1* are located on the long arm of chromosome 11, a portion of which appears to be amplified in various epithelial tumors including bladder cancer.[21] *int-2* and *hst1* genes are members of the fibroblast growth factor family, and *bcl-1* is involved in the apoptotic pathway. These genes are thought to be related to bladder cancer tumorigenesis. Bcl-2 is known to be an inhibitor of apoptosis. Overexpression of Bcl-2 has been identified in approximately 30% of bladder tumors.[22,23] The relationship between expression of Bcl-2 and tumor grade or between Bcl-2 expression and patient survival is controversial. Epidermal growth factor (EGF) is a cellular mitogen which is excreted into the urine at high levels, and initiates the events of cell replication through the EGF-receptor (EGFR). Amplification or overexpression of EGFR is frequently present in bladder cancer, and has been shown to correlate with the stage of the tumor.[24]

Several tumor suppressor genes such as *p53*, the retinoblastoma (*Rb*) gene, *p16/CDKN2* and *DCC*, are thought to be related to tumorigenesis and/or progression of bladder cancers. Altered expression of *p53* has been described in up to 50% of bladder cancers.[14] Inactivation of *p53* can occur by point mutation at many sites, and these mutations are accompanied by the loss of the wild type allele of *p53*. Some *p53* mutations have a transdominant effect, even in the presence of wild type *p53*.[25] Also, some *p53* mutations are thought to have transforming ability and to act as oncogenes.[26] Mutations of the *p53* gene and nuclear accumulation of p53 protein are associated with grade and stage of bladder cancers. The detection of nuclear mutant p53 is associated with a higher risk of recurrence after radical cystectomy, and with lower overall survival.[27] *p53* mutations are presumed to play an important role in the multistep progression of bladder cancer. Rb is a nuclear phosphoprotein which negatively downregulates transcription. Mutation of *Rb* has been observed in 30-40% of invasive bladder cancers. Patients with absent or heterogeneous expression of Rb have a decreased survival compared to that of patients with positive Rb expression.[28,29] Furthermore, it has been shown that the introduction of *Rb* into *Rb*-negative cell lines decreases tumorigenicity and tumor growth in vitro and in vivo.[11,12] The *p16/CDKN2* gene is located at 9p21, and the deletion of 9p21 has been reported in up to 50% of bladder cancers. CDKN2 is an inhibitor of the cyclin/CDK complexes needed for Rb phosphorylation, and the loss of CDKN2 results in inactivation of Rb. p16/CDKN2 has been thought to be involved in the pathogenesis of bladder cancer.[30]

H-*ras* Oncogene in Bladder Cancer

The H-*ras* oncogene was initially discovered as the transforming gene of the T24 human bladder carcinoma cell line.[31,32] Subsequent studies have confirmed that the H-*ras* oncogene is activated by a point mutation resulting in the substitution of the encoding amino acid.[33-35] Codons 12, 13 and 61 of the H-*ras* gene are thought to be "hot spots" for point mutations.[36-38] Extensive studies have reported the prevalence and potential role of activated H-*ras* genes in bladder cancer. Overall, the frequency of H-*ras* mutations has been reported to range from 3 to 76% in primary bladder tumors, with no consensus to its relationship to tumor grade and stage.[39-48] These discordant results may reflect studies with small sample sizes, varying assay sensitivities and methodology. One of the technical problems associated with studies analyzing archived samples is the isolation of pure tumor cells and the potential for contamination with normal tissue. In addition, the potential coexistence of both wild type and mutated cells in a single tumor may further affect the reported incidence of H-*ras* mutations.

Recent reports which have studied the incidence of H-*ras* mutations in bladder cancer by molecular-based analyses are summarized in Table 9.1. A 45% incidence of a point mutation in codon 12 of H-*ras* (GGC to GTC) has been reported, using polymerase chain reaction (PCR)-based analysis.[40] Specifically, there were no H-*ras* mutants in grade I tumors, with a sharp increase to 44% in grade II, and 65% in grade III tumors. These results suggest a reasonably high frequency of H-*ras* mutations in bladder cancer when molecular based analyses are utilized, as well as a possible association of these mutations with increasing aggressiveness. A second study has also demonstrated the high incidence (67%) of mutations at H-*ras* codon 12 by PCR after the digestion with the restriction enzyme specific to the wild type codon 12.[41] In this study, mutations of H-*ras* were also detectable in 48% of urine samples. Furthermore, Fitzgerald et al[42] have shown that 44% (44/100) of urine samples demonstrate mutations in exon I of the H-*ras* gene by single-strand conformation polymorphism (SSCP) and sequencing. However, not all studies have shown such a high prevalence of H-*ras* mutations in bladder cancer patients. In one study, 9 of 152 samples evaluated by SSCP and digested restriction fragment length polymorphism (RFLP) were found to have a point mutation, none of which was a GGC to GTC mutation.[43] No correlation was found between tumor grade or stage and the presence of H-*ras* mutations in this study. By contrast, using SSCP and RFLP, Levesque et al[44] have demonstrated that 30% of specimens

Table 9.1. Incidence of H-ras mutation in bladder cancer

Methods of Detection	Number of Cases Examined	Number of Cases with Mutation (%)	GGC to GTC Mutation at Codon 12	Refs.
PCR-based Hybridization	67	30 (45)	30/30	40
RFLP	21	14 (67)	14/14	41
RFLP	21*	12 (48)	12/12	41
RFLP+SSCP	152	9 (6)	0/9	43
RFLP+SSCP	111	33 (30)	26/33	44
PCR+Sequencing	50	9 (18)	8/9	45
PCR	97	46 (47)	46/46	46
SSCP+Sequencing	100*	44 (44)	ND	42
SSCP+Sequencing	39	1 (3)	0/1	47
RFLP-PCR	50	6 (12)	0/6	48

PCR: polymerase chain reaction
RFLP: restriction fragment length polymorphism
SSCP: single-strand conformation polymorphism
* : urine samples
ND: not defined

harbored H-*ras* point mutations, with 26 out of 30 cases having a GGC to GTC mutation. Another study demonstrated a GGC to GTC mutation at codon 12 in 8 out of 9 mutations by a PCR-based assay.[45] In another study, 46 out of 97 (47%) specimens had mutations at H-*ras* codon 12, as detected by a hemi-nested, non-isotopic, allele-specific PCR.[46] The simultaneous presence of wild type and mutated H-*ras* codon 12 was seen in 44 cases out of 46 cases (96%) in this study. Two recent reports have demonstrated a 3% and 12% mutation incidence of H-*ras* codon 12 respectively, and none of these were a GGT to GTC mutation.[47,48]

The exact incidence of H-*ras* gene mutations in bladder cancer remains controversial, but the oncogenic role of mutated H-*ras* has been demonstrated. Increased tumorigenic and metastatic properties of NIH/3T3 murine fibroblast cells and the RT4 non-invasive bladder cancer cells have been demonstrated upon transfection of the activated H-*ras* gene into these cells.[49,50] The mutated H-*ras* oncogene has also been shown to have the ability to activate other tumor growth regulation factors such as c-Fos, VEGF, and EGFR.[51]

Anti-Oncogene Ribozymes Against Bladder Cancer

Cancers develop from a multi-step process, and several genes have already been identified in this process. The reversion of the malignant phenotype by elimination of a single activated oncogene or by restoration of a single tumor suppressor gene has been demonstrated.[6-12] Any disease in which a specific gene or protein appears to be important in its pathogenesis can be targeted with ribozymes. In cancer, oncogenes are obvious potential targets for ribozyme strategies. The mutated H-*ras* oncogene might be an appropriate target for ribozyme-mediated gene therapy, because the ribozyme might have a specific cleavage ability, leaving the normal proto-oncogene unaffected.[52] A hammerhead ribozyme targeted to the mutated H-*ras* oncogene has been designed, and has been studied in the bladder cancer cell line EJ, which contains a GTC mutation at codon 12 (Fig. 9.1). Initial attempts to examine the cellular effects of an anti-H-*ras* ribozyme have relied on stable transfection of eukaryotic plasmids encoding the ribozyme in EJ cells.[8] In one study, the anti-H-*ras* ribozyme was cloned into the mammalian expression vector pHβ Apr-1-neo, under the expression of a β-actin promoter. Following transfection of the vector into EJ cells, anti-H-*ras* ribozyme expression resulted in the decrease of H-*ras* mRNA and p21 protein levels. Moreover, clones with higher ribozyme expression exhibited greater reduction of H-*ras* mRNA and p21 protein. This reduction of H-*ras* gene expression led to altered morphology, cell growth inhibition, and decreased DNA synthesis in vitro. In vivo studies with these clones have demonstrated suppressed tumorigenicity, decreased invasive properties, and improved survival of nude mice. This anti-tumor efficacy was not seen in control EJ cells transfected with the empty plasmid which did not express the ribozyme. The anti-tumor properties of this anti-H-*ras* ribozyme have also been studied in NIH3T3 murine fibroblast cells transfected with a mutated H-*ras* gene.[53] When the anti-H-*ras* ribozyme vector was introduced in parent NIH3T3 cells and in the activated H-*ras* transformed NIH3T3 cells, cell growth was inhibited only in the mutated H-*ras* transfected NIH3T3 cells and not in the parent NIH3T3 cells. These findings demonstrated the ability of a ribozyme to discriminate between a normal and a mutated H-*ras* transcript, resulting in no deleterious effect on the normal H-*ras* proto-oncogene. The anti-tumor activity of a mutant ribozyme which does not possess cleavage ability was also examined. The results demonstrated the superior anti-tumor efficacy of the active anti-H-*ras* ribozyme compared to the inactive mutant ribozyme.[9] These studies have established the anti-H-*ras* ribozyme as a viable strategy for inhibiting the malignant phenotype of bladder cancer cells.

Although the potential utility of an anti-H-*ras* ribozyme has been demonstrated in cell-based assays, efficient delivery systems will be required for future clinical trials. Recently, a recombinant adenovirus encoding the anti-H-*ras* ribozyme was constructed and tested in EJ cells.[54,55] An anti-H-*ras* ribozyme sequence was cloned into an E1 deleted adenovirus type 5. The resultant replication-deficient recombinant adenovirus expressing the anti-H-*ras* ribozyme was infected into EJ cells. Downregulation of H-*ras* gene expression was demonstrated by Northern blot analysis in EJ cells infected by this recombinant adenovirus compared to the control adenoviral vectors lacking expression of the ribozyme. Further, treatment with the anti-H-*ras* ribozyme-expressing adenovirus resulted in growth inhibition and reduced viability of EJ cells, while these anti-tumor effects were not observed in the cells infected with control adenoviruses. This decreased tumorigenicity has also been demonstrated in mice by subcutaneous injection of EJ cells infected by adenoviruses expressing an anti-H*ras* ribozyme. In another study, tumor growth inhibition was demonstrated in athymic mice after intralesional injection of adenovirus expressing an anti-H-*ras* ribozyme.[55]

Because of its ability to activate cell proliferation and tumor growth, the c-*fos* oncogene is thought to be a suitable target for the treatment of cancers. Also, the expression of c-*fos* is thought to be partially regulated by Ras related signal transduction. The tumor inhibition efficacy of an anti-c-*fos* ribozyme has been investigated in the EJ cell line.[56] The anti-c-*fos* ribozyme was cloned into the plasmid pMAMneo, which contains a dexamethasone-inducible mouse mammary tumor virus promoter and Rous sarcoma virus-long terminal repeat. EJ cells were transfected with this anti-c-*fos* ribozyme-expressing plasmid, and the resultant transformants were tested with or without dexamethasone. Increased expression of an anti-*fos* ribozyme in transfected cells was seen by the addition of dexamethasone. Downregulation of c-*fos* RNA expression was seen in the ribozyme-expressing transfectants, along with changes of cell morphology. The parent EJ cells exhibit a spindled shape and spread rapidly, whereas cells with anti-c-*fos* ribozyme expression were rounded in shape and tended to grow in patches. Also, the downregulation of c-*fos* expression decreased DNA synthesis and inhibited cell growth. These results demonstrate the potential utility of anti-oncogene ribozymes as therapeutics against bladder cancer.

Fig. 9.1. Hammerhead ribozyme targeted to mutated H-*ras* oncogene. The H-*ras* gene is frequently activated by a point mutation at codon 12, which converts a GGC sequence encoding glycine to a GUC sequence encoding valine. The hammerhead ribozyme has been designed to cleave the 3' end of the mutated codon 12.

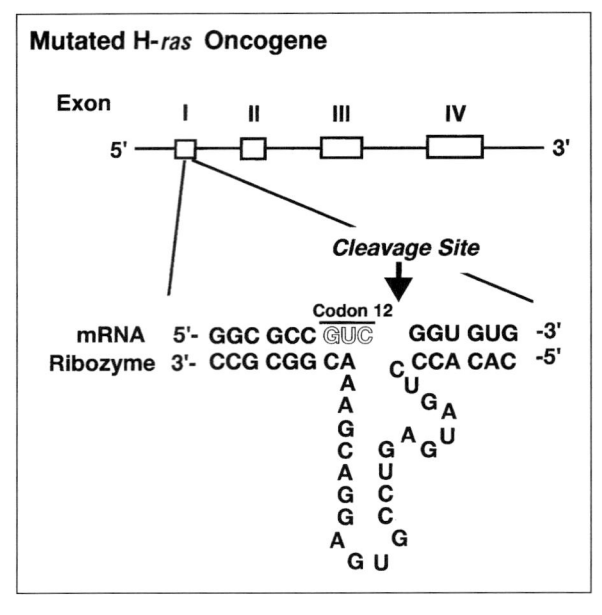

Delivery of Ribozymes to Bladder Tumors

Efficient ribozyme delivery to a tissue target remains one of the key obstacles to the development of ribozyme-based therapeutics. Adenoviral vectors are currently being used in several clinical trials and hold promise as an efficient delivery system for gene therapy.[57] Adenoviruses have advantages as a delivery system for urothelial cancer, because of their tropism for the lower genitourinary epithelium, and are said to infect epithelial cells with high frequency.[58] Successful adenoviral-mediated gene transfer to the bladder epithelium has been demonstrated.[59-61] Human adenovirus type 5 is one of the most well characterized and utilized for production of a replication-defective adenovirus. The viral genome can be divided into 4 noncontiguous early regions (E1-E4) and the continuous late regions (L1-L5).[62] Deletion of an early region causes a defect in viral DNA replication, and allows for the accommodation of a DNA insert.[63] Wild type adenovirus type 5 can accommodate 2 kb of insert DNA, and deletion of the E1 region increases the potential insert size an additional 3 kb. Therefore, approximately 5 kb of DNA can be inserted following the deletion of the E1 region.

The efficacy of gene transfer into bladder epithelium and bladder cancer cells has been studied with the adenoviral vector expressing a marker gene in vitro and in vivo. In one study, the adenoviral vector expressing the *Escherichia coli* β-galactosidase gene was inoculated into the rat bladder.[59] The expression of the marker gene was seen in excised bladder wall specimens both by histological staining and PCR based analysis of DNA and RNA. The maximal expression of the marker gene was detected at 24 hours after the adenoviral inoculation, with progressive decline thereafter. In another study, the transfection efficacy of adenovirus into bladder cancer cells was tested in vitro using adenovirus expressing the firefly luciferase marker gene.[60] The adenovirus was simply added to the cultured cells and incubated for 2 hours. The expression of the marker gene was seen in all 3 transitional carcinoma cell lines tested (HT1197, HT1376, and T24), and persisted for 7 days. Other investigators utilized orthotopic and peritoneal murine bladder tumors which were treated with intravesical or intraperitoneal inoculation of the adenovirus expressing β-galactosidase, respectively.[61] Gene transduction into bladder mucosa and tumors was confirmed by histology and PCR. Taken together, these results indicate that gene transfer into the bladder epithelium or bladder tumor can be achieved by topical administration of an adenoviral vector, and increase the potential utility of a replication-defective adenovirus as a delivery system of ribozymes against bladder cancer.

Conclusions

Novel therapies are clearly required both for muscle-invasive and metastatic bladder tumors, as well as for recurrent superficial tumors. A molecular-based approach may be an ideal strategy to reverse the malignant phenotype. Tumor specific oncogenes are suitable targets for ribozyme strategy. To date, efficient tumor inhibition by anti-oncogene ribozymes targeting H-*ras* and c-*fos* has been demonstrated in vitro and in vivo in bladder cancer models. However, any gene related to the oncogenesis of bladder cancer, including other oncogenes, growth factors, their receptors, and mutated tumor suppressor genes might also be suitable targets for a ribozyme-based therapeutic strategy. The delivery of ribozymes into bladder cancer cells remains a critical issue for future clinical applications. Because of their anatomy and pathophysiology, bladder tumors are well suited for delivery of genes by either intravesical instillation or intralesional injection at high concentrations. However, the development of an effective delivery system will be required to develop anti-bladder cancer therapeutics based on ribozymes.

References

1. Parker SL, Tong T, Bolden S et al. Cancer Statistics, 1997. CA Cancer J Clin 1997; 47:5-27.
2. Lamm DL, Torti FM. Bladder cancer, 1996. CA Cancer J Clin 1996; 46:93-112.
3. Raghavan D, Shipley WU, Garnick MB et al. Biology and management of bladder cancer. New Engl J Med 1990; 322:1129-1138.
4. Holmang S, Hedelin H, Anderstrom C et al. Long-term followup of all patients with muscle invasive (stages T2, T3 and T4) bladder carcinoma in a geographical region. J Urol 1997; 158:389-392.
5. Kaufman DS, Shipley WU, Griffin PP et al. Selective bladder preservation by combination treatment of invasive bladder cancer. N Engl J Med 1993; 329:1377-1382.
6. Schwab G, Chavany C, Duroux I et al. Antisense oligonucleotides adsorbed to polyalkylcyanoacrylate nanoparticles specifically inhibit mutated Ha-*ras* mediated cell proliferation and tumorigenicity in nude mice. Proc Natl Acad Sci USA 1994; 91:10460-10464.
7. Gray GD, Hernandez OM, Hebel D et al. Antisense DNA inhibition of tumor growth induced by c-Ha-*ras* oncogene in nude mice. Cancer Res 1993; 53:577-580.
8. Kashani-Sabet M, Funato T, Tone T et al. Reversal of the malignant phenotype by an anti-*ras* ribozyme. Antisense Res Develop 1992; 2:3-15.
9. Tone T, Kashani-Sabet M, Funato T et al. Suppression of EJ cells tumorigenicity. in vivo 1993; 7:471-476.
10. Werthman PE, Drazan KE, Rosenthal JT et al. Adenoviral-p53 gene transfer to orthotopic and peritoneal murine bladder cancer. J Urol 1996; 155:753-756.
11. Goodrich DW, Chen Y, Scully P et al. Expression of the retinoblastoma gene product in bladder carcinoma cells associates with a low frequency of tumor formation. Cancer Res 1992; 52:1968-1973.
12. Takahashi R, Hashimoto T, Xu HJ et al. The retinoblastoma gene functions as a growth and tumor suppressor in human bladder carcinoma cells. Proc Natl Acad Sci USA 1991; 88:5257-5261.
13. Strohmeyer TG, Slamon DJ. Proto-oncogenes and tumor suppressor genes in human urological malignancies. J Urol 1994; 151:1479-1497.
14. Reznikoff CA, Belair CD, Yeager TR et al. A molecular genetic model of human bladder cancer pathogenesis. Semi Oncol 1996; 23:571-584.

15. Sandberg AA, Berger CS. Review of chromosome study in urological tumors. II. Cytogenetics and molecular genetics of bladder cancer. J Urol 1994; 151:545-560.
16. Egan SE, Weinberg RA. The pathway to signal achievement. Nature 1993; 365:781-783.
17. Ledwith BJ, Manam S, Kraynak AR et al. Antisense-fos RNA causes partial reversion of the transformed phenotypes induced by the c-Ha-*ras* oncogene. Mol Cell Biol 1990; 10:1545-1555.
18. Rak J, Mitsuhasi Y, Bayko L et al. Mutant *ras* oncogenes upregulate VEGF/VPF expression: Implication for induction and inhibition of tumor angiogenesis. Cancer Res 1995; 55:4575-4580.
19. Arbiser JL, Moses MA, Fernandez CA et al. Oncogenic H-*ras* stimulates tumor angiogenesis by two distinct pathways. Proc Natl Acad Sci USA 1997; 94:861-866.
20. Moriyama M, Akiyama T, Yamamoto T et al. Expression of c-erbB-2 gene product in urinary bladder cancer. J Urol 1991; 145:423-427
21. Proctor AJ, Coombs LM, Cairns JP et al. Amplification at chromosome 11q13 in transitional cell tumours of the bladder. Oncogene 1991; 6:789-795.
22. Glick SH, Howell LP, Devere White RW. Relationship of p53 and bcl-2 to prognosis in muscle-invasive transitional cell carcinoma of the bladder. J Urol 1996; 155:1754-1757.
23. King J, Matteson J, Jacobs SC et al. Incidence of apoptosis, cell proliferation and bcl-2 expression in transitional cell carcinoma of the bladder: Association with tumor progression. J Urol 1996; 155:316-320.
24. Neal DE, Sharples L, Smith K et al. The epidermal growth factor receptor and the prognosis of bladder cancer. Cancer 1990; 65:1619-1625.
25. Harvey M, Vogel H, Morris D et al. A mutant p53 transgene accelerates tumor development in heterozygous but not nullizygous p53-deficient mice. Nat Genet 1995; 9:305-311.
26. Dittmer D, Pati S, Zambetti G et al. Gain of function mutations in p53. Nat Genet 1993; 4:42-46.
27. Esrig D, Elmajian D, Groshen S et al. Accumulation of nuclear p53 and tumor progression in bladder cancer. New Engl J Med 1994; 331:1259-1264.
28. Cordon-Cardo C, Wartinger D, Petrylak D et al. Altered expression of the retinoblastoma gene product: Prognostic indicator in bladder cancer. J Natl Cancer Inst 1992; 84:1251-1256.
29. Logothetis CJ, Xu HJ, Ro JY et al. Altered expression of retinoblastoma protein and known prognostic variables in locally advanced bladder cancer. J Natl Cancer Inst 1992; 84:1256-1261.
30. Wu Q, Possati L, Montesi M et al. Growth arrest and suppression of tumorigenicity of bladder-carcinoma cell lines induced by the p16/CDKN2 (p16INK4A, MTS1) gene and other loci on chromosome 9. Int J Cancer 1996; 65:840-846.
31. Goldfarb M, Shimizu K, Perucho M et al. Isolation and preliminary characterization of a transforming gene from T24 bladder carcinoma cells. Nature 1982; 296:404-409.
32. Shih C, Weinberg RA. Isolation and transforming sequence from a human bladder carcinoma cell line. Cell 1982; 29:161-169.
33. Tabin CJ, Bradley SM, Bargmann CI et al. Mechanism of activation of a human oncogene. Nature 1982; 300:143-149.
34. Reddy EP, Reynolds RK, Santos E et al. A point mutation is responsible for the acquisition of transforming properties by the T24 human bladder carcinoma oncogene. Nature 1982; 300:149-152.
35. Taparowsky E, Suard Y, Fasano O et al. Activation of the T24 bladder carcinoma transforming gene is linked to a single amino acid change. Nature 1982; 300:762-765.
36. Fujita J, Srivastava SK, Kraus MH et al. Frequency of molecular alterations affecting *ras* proto-oncogenes in human urinary tract tumors. Proc Natl Acad Sci USA 1985; 82: 3879-3853.
37. Fujita J, Yoshida O, Yuasa Y et al. Ha-*ras* oncogenes are activated by somatic alteration in human urinary tract tumors. Nature 1984; 309: 464-466
38. Visvanathan KU, Pocock RD, Summerhayes IC. Preferential and novel activation of H-*ras* in human bladder carcinomas. Oncol Res 1988; 53: 133-139.

39. Burchill SA, Lunec J, Mellon K et al. Analysis of Ha-*ras* mutations in primary human bladder tumors. Br J Cancer 1991; 63 (supp):162
40. Czerniak B, Cohen GL, Etkind P et al. Concurrent mutation of coding and regulatory sequences of the Ha-*ras* gene in urinary bladder carcinomas. Hum Pathol 1992; 23:1199-1204.
41. Haliassos A, Liloglou T, Likourinas M et al. H-*ras* oncogene mutations in the urine of patients with bladder tumors: Description of a non-invasive method for the detection of neoplasia. Int J Oncol 1992; 1:731-734.
42. Fitzgerald JM, Ramchurren N, Rieger K et al. Identification of H-*ras* mutations in urine sediments complements cytology in the detection of bladder tumors. J Natl Cancer Inst 1995; 87:129-133.
43. Knowles MA, Williamson M. Mutation of H-*ras* is infrequent in bladder cancer: Confirmation by single-strand conformation polymorphism analysis, designed restriction fragment length polymorphisms, and direct sequencing. Cancer Res 1993; 53: 133-139.
44. Levesque P, Ramchurren N, Saini K et al. Sequencing of human bladder tumors and urine sediments for the presence of H-*ras* mutations. Int J Cancer 1993; 55: 785-790.
45. Burchill SA, Neal DE, Lunec J. Frequency of H-*ras* mutations in human bladder cancer detected by direct sequencing. Br J Urol 1994; 73:516-521.
46. Ooi A, Herz F, Ii S et al. Ha-*ras* codon 12 mutation in papillary tumors of the urinary bladder. A retrospective study. Int J Oncol 1994; 4:85-90.
47. Uchida T, Wada C, Ishida H et al. Infrequent involvement of mutations on neurofibromatosis type 1, H-*ras*, K-*ras* and N-*ras* in urothelial tumors. Urol Int 1995; 55: 63-67.
48. Saito S, Hata M, Fukuyama R et al. Screening of H-*ras* gene point mutations in 50 cases of bladder carcinoma. Int J Urol 1997; 4:178-185.
49. Greig RG, Koestler TP, Trainer DL et al. Tumorigenic and metastatic properties of "normal" and *ras*-transfected NIH/3T3 cells. Proc Natl Acad Sci USA 1985; 82:3698-3701.
50. Theodorescu D, Cornil I, Fernandez BJ et al. Overexpression of normal and mutated forms of HRAS induces orthotopic bladder invasion in a human transitional cell carcinoma. Proc Natl Acad Sci USA 1990; 87:9047-9051.
51. Theodorescu D, Cornil I, Sheehan C et al. Ha-*ras* induction of the invasive phenotype results in up-regulation of epidermal growth factor receptors and altered responsiveness to epidermal growth factor in human papillary transitional cell carcinoma cells. Cancer Res 1991; 51:4486-4491.
52. Koizumi M, Hayase Y, Iwai S et al. Design of RNA enzymes distinguishing a single base mutation in RNA. Nucleic Acids Res 1989; 17:7059-7071.
53. Funato T, Shitara T, Tone T et al. Suppression of H-*ras*-mediated transformation in NIH 3T3 cells by a *ras* ribozyme. Biochem Pharmacol 1994; 48:1471-1475.
54. Feng M, Carbrera G, Deshane J et al. Neoplastic reversion accomplished by high efficiency adenoviral-mediated delivery of anti-*ras* ribozyme. Cancer Res 1995; 55:2024-2028.
55. Irie A, Scanlon KJ. Gene therapy for experimental carcinomas using antioncogene ribozymes. Cancer Invest 1997; 15 suppl 1:79-80.
56. Shitara T, Scanlon KJ. Suppression of the human carcinoma phenotype by an antioncogene ribozyme. In: Robbins PD, ed. Gene therapy protocols. New Jersey: Humana press, 1997:391-401.
57. Weitzman MD, Wilson JM, Eck SL. Adenovirus vectors in cancer gene therapy. In: Sobol RE, Scanlon KJ (eds) The internet book of gene therapy. Stamford: Appleton & Lange, 1995:17-25.
58. Mufson MA, Belshe RB. A review of adenoviruses in the etiology of acute hemorrhagic cystitis. J Urol 1976; 115:191-194.
59. Morris BD, Drazan KE, Csete ME et al. Adenoviral-mediated gene transfer to bladder in vivo. J Urol 1994; 153: 506-509.
60. Bass C, Cabrera G, Elgavish A et al. Recombinant adenoviral-mediated gene transfer to genitourinary epithelium in vitro and in vivo. Cancer Gene Ther 1995; 2: 97-104.
61. Werthman PE, Drazan KE, Rosenthal JT et al. Adenoviral-p53 gene transfer to orthotopic and peritoneal murine bladder cancer. J Urol 1996; 155: 753-756.

62. Berkner KL. Development of adenovirus vectors for the expression of heterologous genes. Biotech 1988; 6:616-629.
63. Bett AD, Prevec L, Graham FL. Packaging capacity of human adenovirus type 5 vectors. J Virol 1993; 67:5911-5921.

CHAPTER 10

Gene Therapy of Breast Cancer

T. Suzuki and B. Anderegg

Introduction

Breast cancer is the most common cancer among women in the United States and the western world. It is estimated to be responsible for 15–20% of all female cancer related deaths in 1997.[1] Although the mortality rate from breast cancer has been declining since 1989, about a third of all new cancer cases diagnosed in women are localized to the breast.[2] Whereas node-negative patients with tumors 1.0 to 2.0 cm in diameter have a good prognosis with an average five-year disease-free survival of 85%, this rate decreases dramatically to approximately 45% in patients with four or more positive nodes.[3]

Among oncogenes and tumor-suppressor genes, c-erbB2 is an important prognostic factor in breast cancer.[4] In addition, it is probably linked to neoplastic transformation itself and/or to its promotion.[5] Therefore, it is a potential target gene for gene therapy of breast cancer. In this chapter, the application of ribozymes in the field of breast cancer gene therapy is discussed based on results regarding the anti-c-erbB-2 ribozyme. Recently, it has been shown that the growth of breast cancer cells can be efficiently inhibited by anti-c-erbB-2 hammerhead ribozymes.[6-8]

Anti-c-*erb*B-2 Ribozyme Strategy

Anti-Oncogene Ribozymes

The utility of catalytic RNAs (hammerhead ribozymes, hairpin ribozymes, etc.) to attenuate mRNA expression has been well documented in a variety of tumors and its application to cancer gene therapy has been demonstrated.[9,10] Ribozymes have the ability to cleave RNA species in trans and prevent them from subsequent translation. It has been demonstrated that anti-oncogene ribozymes of the hammerhead type are effective in reversing the malignant phenotype of cancer cells in EJ human bladder cancer cells,[11-13] FEM human malignant melanoma cells,[14-16] Capan-1 human pancreatic cancer cells,[17] and NIH3T3 mouse fibroblast cells transformed by mutated H-*ras*.[18,19]

A critical step in designing any ribozyme is the selection of a suitable target gene. EJ and FEM cells have a H-*ras* gene mutated at codon 12 which has been implicated in their malignant phenotype. An anti-H-*ras* ribozyme targeting this mutation was introduced into EJ cells, FEM cells, and NIH3T3 cells transformed by mutated H-*ras*. The ribozyme was shown to cleave only the mutated H-*ras* mRNA containing the GUC mutation at codon 12 without affecting the normal counterpart containing GGC at this site. The ribozyme was shown to downregulate H-*ras* expression and reverse the malignant phenotype of the EJ and FEM cells.

Ribozymes in the Gene Therapy of Cancer, edited by Kevin J. Scanlon and Mohammed Kashani-Sabet.
©1998 R.G. Landes Company.

Mutated K-*ras* is another good target gene for ribozyme cleavage. An anti-K-*ras* ribozyme designed against the K-*ras* mutation found in Capan-1 cells (GUU at codon 12) has already been shown to downregulate K-*ras* expression and reverse the malignant phenotype effectively.[17]

The c-erbB-2 Gene

The c-*erb*B-2 proto-oncogene (also called *HER-2/neu*) encodes a 185 kDa tyrosine kinase type transmembrane receptor homologous with the epidermal growth factor receptor (EGFR).[20,21] EGFR is known to transform mouse NIH3T3 cells only in the presence of ligand and receptor[22] while the c-*erb*B-2 protein is constitutively phosphorylated and demonstrates tyrosine kinase activity without the presence of ligand when overexpressed in NIH3T3 cells.[14] Thus, c-*erb*B-2 overexpressing NIH3T3 cells can be transformed in a ligand-independent manner.[23-25] A growth stimulatory role for c-*erb*B-2 in human breast and ovarian cancer has been postulated through its amplification and overexpression.[5] c-*erb*B-2 overexpression occurs in approximately 30% of all tumors examined.[26,27] High levels of c-*erb*B-2 expression and poor clinical outcome seem to be correlated, especially in patients with positive axillary lymph nodes.[28-30] c-*erb*B-2 also has been implicated in the metastatic phenotype.[31]

Since the c-*erb*B-2 protein is not expressed in most normal human tissues,[32,33] downregulating c-*erb*B-2 expression at the level of DNA, mRNA, or protein may be a realistic strategy for cancer gene therapy (Table 10.1). Downregulation at the DNA level has been performed using triplex forming oligonucleotides against c-*erb*B-2 genomic DNA.[34,35] Inhibition at the protein level has been achieved by monoclonal antibodies[36-39] and intracellular expression of single chain antibodies.[40-43] In fact, a monoclonal antibody targeting c-*erb*B-2 protein has been tested in clinical trials of breast cancer.[44] Antisense oligonucleotides targeting c-*erb*B-2 mRNA have been utilized to downregulate the c-*erb*B-2 mRNA level.[45-47] Finally, suppression of gene expression at the mRNA level can be further optimized by utilizing an anti-c-*erb*B-2 ribozyme.

Designing anti-c-erbB-2 Ribozymes

Since specific c-*erb*B-2 mutations have not been found in breast cancer,[48] an anti-c-*erb*B-2 ribozyme was designed to cleave normal c-*erb*B-2 mRNA. Two different anti-c-*erb*B-2 hammerhead ribozymes targeting the GUC sequences at codon 663/664,[8] and at the translation initiation site at codon 71/72,[7] respectively, were designed. In vitro studies revealed the anti-oncogenic potential of these ribozymes in ovarian[8] and breast cancer cells[7,8] overexpressing the c-*erb*B-2 gene. The ribozyme targeting codon 71/72 was even capable of downregulating the growth of breast cancer MCF-7 cells which show low c-*erb*B-2 protein levels.[7]

Anti-c-*erb*B-2 Ribozyme Expression

Plasmid-Mediated Anti-c-erbB-2 Ribozyme Expression In Vitro

The effect of plasmid-mediated anti-c-*erb*B-2 ribozyme expression was evaluated by using stable transformants expressing the anti-c-*erb*B-2 ribozyme. The anti-c-*erb*B-2 ribozyme was cloned into the pHβ APr-1-neo expression plasmid and transfected into BT-474 or MCF-7 breast carcinoma cells by electroporation.[7] The doubling time of the ribozyme expressing cells was significantly longer than that of controls.[6,7] Anti-c-*erb-B*-2 ribozyme expression reversed the phenotype of transformed cells when the ribozyme was expressed in stable transformants, probably by blocking aberrant growth signals from the receptor to the nucleus. The in vitro expression of a significant amount of anti-c-*erb*B-2 ribozyme driven

Table 10.1. Mechanisms of inhibition of c-erbB-2 expression

Method of Inhibition	References	Comments
monoclonal antibodies	36-39	effective in breast cancer cells overexpressing c-erbB-2; successful immunological stimulation in vitro
single chain antibodies	40-43	selective growth inhibition in ovarian and breast cancer cells overexpressing c-erbB-2; intracellular expression of the antibody
triplex formation	34, 35	effective and specific transcriptional inhibition in vitro; polypurine:polypyrimidine target sequence or linker molecule required
antisense strategies	45-47	successful growth inhibition of ovarian and breast cancer cells overexpressing c-erbB-2 in vitro; inhibition of serum induced cell spreading
ribozyme strategies	6-8	successful growth inhibition of ovarian and breast cancer cells independent of the c-erbB-2 expression level; adenoviral delivery and expression demonstrated in vitro, in vivo

by the β-actin promoter and downregulation of the steady state c-erbB-2 mRNA level were clearly correlated.[6]

Adenovirus-Mediated Anti-c-erbB-2 Ribozyme Expression In Vitro

In order to achieve more efficient gene delivery and expression, a replication deficient recombinant adenovirus was prepared encoding the anti-c-erbB-2 ribozyme driven by the CMV promoter (rAdEB2Rz[7]). The growth of MCF-7 and BT-474 cells was efficiently inhibited by transduction with 500 plaque forming units (PFU)/cell of rAdEB2Rz.[7] The control vector rAdCMVLacZ expressing the LacZ gene instead of the ribozyme did not suppress tumor growth in vitro, although the transduction efficiency was virtually 100% as analyzed by X-gal staining.[7]

The specificity of the growth inhibitory effect produced by the ribozyme on breast cancer cells was confirmed by transducing several types of recombinant control adenoviruses into BT-474 cells. Only the recombinant adenovirus expressing an anti-c-erbB-2 antisense oligonucleotide inhibited breast cancer cell growth, although the effect was not as strong as that of rAdEB2Rz.[7] Northern blot analysis revealed that the anti-c-erbB-2 ribozyme in fact cleaved c-erbB-2 mRNA and, thus, downregulated c-erbB-2 expression.[7]

In a recent study, Czubayko et al also used a recombinant adenoviral vector to drive expression of a hammerhead ribozyme targeting c-erbB-2 at codon 1991.[8] In vitro studies suggested ribozyme expression peaked three days after adenoviral infection and was undetectable by day 10. Moreover, a dose dependent increase in ribozyme expression was noted in vitro with increasing viral titer. Recombinant adenoviral infection of SK-OV-3 ovarian cancer cells at a dose of 100 MOI resulted in downregulation of c-erbB-2 mRNA by 75%.

Decreased c-*erb*B-2 protein levels were demonstrated using fluorescence activated cell sorter analysis in MDA-MB-361 breast cancer cells. However, no effects of ribozyme expression on in vitro cell growth of these tumor cell lines were reported.

Adenovirus-Mediated Anti-c-erbB-2 Ribozyme Expression In Vivo

The effects of rAdEB2Rz treatment were examined by subcutaneous inoculation of BT-474 cells into the flanks of nude mice and subsequent administration of 10 MOI of rAdEB2Rz or the control vector rAdCMVLacZ into the tumor nodules. The tumorigenicity was significantly reduced by rAdEB2Rz treatment in comparison with rAdCMVLacZ application.[7]

Repeated administration of 10 MOI of rAdEB2Rz inhibited the growth of BT-474 nodules to 20% of the size of control PBS-treated tumors.[7] Treatment of the nodules with a recombinant adenovirus encoding an anti-c-*erb*B-2 antisense oligonucleotide also inhibited tumor growth, but the effect was weaker than that achieved by rAdEB2Rz. Other adenoviral control vectors did not show any significant growth inhibitory effect. rAdEB2Rz injection also inhibited the tumor growth of MCF-7 cells effectively and specifically and appeared to be superior to the antisense-expressing construct, whereas none of the control vectors showed any significant effect. The results indicate that the c-*erb*B-2 protein may be a critical factor for growth of breast cancer cells in general.

Mechanisms of Ribozyme Action

The mechanisms underlying the inhibition of tumor cell growth by ribozyme-mediated cleavage of c-*erb*B-2 mRNA remain unknown. Pathological analysis of the adenovirus-treated tumors showed that there was neither obvious induction of differentiation nor inflammatory cell infiltration.[7] Reduction of c-*erb*B-2 expression by a ribozyme may lead to a shift to alternative signal transduction pathways which slow down cell growth or induce apoptosis, as reported for single chain antibody-treated cells.[43] However, complete responses were not obtained even by the administration of the rather high viral dose of 500 MOI of rAdEB2Rz.[7] This is probably partially due to the presence of other members of the type I growth factor receptor family, such as EGFR/c-*erb*B-1,[49] c-*erb*B-3,[50] or c-*erb*B-4,[51] which may complement the role of c-*erb*B-2 in cell growth signaling.[52] Alternatively, the half life of c-*erb*B-2 mRNA may be too long to achieve complete suppression of gene expression in the model system reported here.

Future Prospects

Although treatment with rAdEB2Rz alone may not be strong enough to eradicate breast cancer cells completely, it can be expected to enhance the antitumor efficacy of conventional therapeutic modalities. It is especially intriguing to investigate the combination of anti-c-*erb*B-2 treatment and cytostatic drugs such as tamoxifen or cis-diamminedichloroplatinum (cisplatin): c-*erb*B-2 overexpression is known to be associated with tamoxifen resistance,[53,54] but a monoclonal antibody raised against c-*erb*B-2 protein was reported to enhance cisplatin cytotoxicity in nude mice.[55] Similarly, downregulation of c-*erb*B-2 by rAdEB2Rz may enhance the cytotoxicity of tamoxifen and, possibly, cisplatin also.

As an alternative to the addition of ribozyme therapy to conventional hormonal and/or chemotherapies, combination gene therapy should be considered. The contribution of tumor suppressor genes such as *BRCA1*,[56] *BRCA2*,[57] and *p53*[58] to the pathogenesis of breast cancer has been postulated. Coexpression of these tumor suppressor genes and anti-c-*erb*B-2 ribozyme may lead to further reduction or even complete eradication of breast cancer cells in vivo. Moreover, the inhibition of c-*erb*B-2 may be coupled with cell cycle interruption, whether through the expression of genes such as p21waf^1 or inhibition of the cyclins D1 and E.[59-62]

Conclusions

Expression of a hammerhead ribozyme targeting c-*erb*B-2 can suppress human breast cancer cell growth effectively both in vitro and in vivo. c-*erb*B-2 expression seems to be critical for breast cancer growth, especially since inhibition of cell growth can be achieved irrespective of the basal level of c-*erb*B-2 expression by the tumor cells. In this respect the ribozyme approach might be superior to the antisense, triplex, or antibody-based assays; it remains to be shown that the latter are also sufficient for targeting cells not overexpressing c-*erb*B-2. The reported results suggest ribozyme-mediated downregulation of c-*erb*B-2 as a reasonable strategy for gene therapy of breast cancer.

Acknowledgments

T. Suzuki is supported by the grant from Uehara Memorial Foundation for Research of Life Science, Japan.

References

1. Parker SL, Tong T, Bolden S, Wingo PA. Cancer Statistics, 1997. CA Cancer J Clin 1997; 47:5-27.
2. Ries LAG, Kosary CL, Hankey BF et al. SEER Cancer Statistics Review, 1973-1993: Tables and Graphs (NIH Pub. 96-2789). Bethesda, Md. National Cancer Institute, 1995.
3. Donegan WL. Tumor-related prognostic factors for breast cancer. CA Cancer J Clin 1997; 47:28-51.
4. Marks JR, Humphrey PA, Wu K et al. Overexpression of p53 and HER-2/neu proteins as prognostic markers in early stage breast cancer. Ann Surg 1994; 219:332-341.
5. Gusterson BA. Identification and interpretation of epidermal growth factor and c-*erb*B-2 overexpression. Eur J Cancer 1992; 28:263-267.
6. Suzuki T, Tsai J, Curcio LD et al. Anti-c-*erb*B-2 ribozyme for breast cancer. In: Scanlon KJ, ed. Therapeutic Application of Ribozymes. Totowa: Humana Press, 1998: (in press).
7. Suzuki T, Ohkawa T, Anderegg B et al. A recombinant adenovirus encoding a ribozyme targeting c-*erb*B-2 inhibits tumorigenicity and growth of human breast cancer cells in vivo. 1997; (submitted).
8. Czubayko F, Downing SG, Hsieh SS et al. Adenovirus-mediated transduction of ribozymes abrogates HER-2/neu and pleiotrophin expression and inhibits tumor cell proliferation. Gene Ther 1997; 4:943-949.
9. Scanlon KJ, Ohta Y, Ishida H et al. Oligonucleotide-mediated modulation of mammalian gene expression. FASEB J 1995; 9:1288-1296.
10. Irie A, Kijima H, Ohkawa T et al. Anti-oncogene ribozymes for cancer gene therapy. In: Gene Therapy. August JT, ed. San Diego: Academic Press, 1997:207-257.
11. Kashani-Sabet M, Funato T, Tone T et al. Reversal of the malignant phenotype by an anti-*ras* ribozyme. Antisense Res Dev 1992; 2:3-15.
12. Feng M, Cabrera G, Deshane J et al. Neoplastic reversion accomplished by high efficiency adenoviral-mediated delivery of an anti-*ras* ribozyme. Cancer Res 1995; 55:2024-2028.
13. Tone T, Kashani-Sabet M, Funato T et al. Suppression of EJ cells tumorigenicity. IN VIVO 1993; 7:471-476.
14. Ohta Y, Tone T, Shitara T et al. H-*ras* ribozyme-mediated alteration of the human melanoma phenotype. Ann NY Acad Sci USA 1994; 716:242-253.
15. Ohta Y, Kijima H, Kashani-Sabet M et al. Suppression of the malignant phenotype of melanoma cells by anti-oncogene ribozymes. J Invest Dermatol 1996; 106:275-280.
16. Ohta Y, Kijima H, Ohkawa T et al. Tissue-specific expression of an anti-*ras* ribozyme inhibits proliferation of human malignant melanoma cells. Nucleic Acids Res 1996; 24:938-942.

17. Kijima H, Bouffard DY, Scanlon KJ. Ribozyme-mediated reversal of human pancreatic carcinoma phenotype. In: Ikehara S, Takaku F, Good RA, eds. Proceedings of International Symposium on Bone Marrow Transplantation. Berlin: Springer, 1996:153-164.
18. Kashani-Sabet M, Funato T, Florenes VA et al. Suppression of the neoplastic phenotype in vivo by an anti-*ras* ribozyme. Cancer Res 1994; 54:900-902.
19. Funato T, Shitara T, Tone T et al. Suppression of H-*ras*-mediated transformation in NIH3T3 cells by a *ras* ribozyme. Biochem Pharmacol 1994; 48:1471-1475.
20. Bargmann CI, Hung M-C, Weinberg RA. The *neu* oncogene encodes an epidermal growth factor receptor-related protein. Nature (Lond.) 1986; 319:226-230.
21. Yamamoto T, Ikawa S, Akiyama T et al. Similarity of protein encoded by the human c-*erb*B-2 gene to epidermal growth factor receptor. Nature (Lond.) 1986; 319:230-234.
22. Di Fiore PP, Pierce JH, Fleming TB et al. Overexpression of the human EGF receptor confers an EGF-dependent transformed phenotype to NIH 3T3 cells. Cell 1987; 51:1063-1070.
23. Lonardo F, Di Marco E, King CR et al. The normal *erb*B-2 product is an atypical receptor-like tyrosine kinase with constitutive activity in the absence of ligand. New Biol 1990; 2:992-1003.
24. Hudziak RM, Schlessinger J, Ullrich A. Increased expression of the putative growth factor receptor p185HER^2 causes transformation and tumorigenesis of NIH3T3 cells. Proc Natl Acad Sci USA 1987; 84:7159-7163.
25. Di Fiore PP, Pierce JH, Kraus MH et al. *erb*B-2 is a potent oncogene when overexpressed in NIH/3T3 cells. Science (Washington, DC) 1987; 237:178-182.
26. Slamon DJ, Godolphin W, Jones LA et al. Studies of the *HER-2/neu* proto-oncogene in human breast and ovarian cancer. Science (Washington, DC) 1989; 244:707-712.
27. Slamon, DJ, Clark GM, Wong SG et al. Human breast cancer: Correlation of relapse and survival with amplification of the *HER-2/neu* oncogene. Science (Washington, DC) 1987; 235:177-182.
28. Perren TJ. c-*erb*B-2 oncogene as a prognostic marker in breast cancer (Editorial). Br J Cancer 1991; 63:328-332.
29. Gullick WJ, Love SB, Wright C et al. c-*erb*B-2 protein overexpression in breast cancer is a risk factor in patients with involved and uninvolved lymph nodes. Br J Cancer 1991; 63:434-438.
30. Muss HB, Thor AD, Berry DA et al. C-*erb*B-2 expression and response to adjuvant therapy in women with node-positive early breast cancer. N Eng J Med 1994; 330:1260-1266.
31. Tan M, Yu D. Overexpression of the c-*erb*B-2 gene enhanced intrinsic metastasis potential in human breast cancer cells without increasing their transformation abilities. Cancer Res 1997; 57:1199-1205.
32. Pier GN, Nicortra MR, Bigotti A et al. Expression of the p185 encoded by *HER2* oncogene in normal and transformed human tissues. Int J Cancer 1990; 45:457-461.
33. Press MF, Cordon-Cardo C, Slamon D. Expression of the *HER-2/neu* proto-oncogene in normal human adult and fetal tissues. Oncogen 1990; 5:953-962.
34. Ebbinghaus SW, Gee JE, Roudu B et al. Triplex formation inhibits *HER-2/neu* transcription in vitro. J Clin Invest 1993; 92:2433-2439.
35. Noonberb SB, Scott GK, Hunt CA et al. Inhibition of transcription factor binding to the *HER2* promoter by triplex-forming oligodeoxyribonucleotides. Gene 1994; 149:123-126.
36. Hudziak RM, Lewis GD, Winget M et al. p185HER^{-2} monoclonal antibody has antiproliferative effects in vitro and sensitized human breast cancer cells to tumor necrosis factor. Mol Cell Biol 1989; 9:1165-1172.
37. Fendly BM, Winget M, Hudziak RM et al. The extracellular domain of *HER2/neu* is a potential immunogen for active specific immunotherapy of breast cancer. Cancer Res 1990; 50:1550-1558.
38. Shepard HM, Lewis GD, Sarup JC et al. Monoclonal antibody therapy of human cancer: Taking the *HER2* proto-oncogene to the clinic. J Clin Immunol 1991; 11:117-127.
39. Lewis GD, Figari I, Fendly B et al. Differential responses of human tumor cell lines to anti-p185HER^2 monoclonal antibodies. Cancer Immunol Immunother 1993; 37:255-263.

40. Beerli RR, Wels W, Hynes NE. Intracellular expression of single chain antibodies reverts *erb*B2 transformation. J Biol Chem 1994; 269:23931-23936.
41. Deshane J, Loechel F, Conry RM et al. Intracellular single-chain antibody directed against *erb*B2 down-regulated cell surface *erb*B2 and exhibits a selective anti-proliferative effect in *erb*B2 overexpressing cancer cell lines. Gene Therapy 1994; 1:332-337.
42. Deshane J, Grim J, Loechel L et al. Intracellular antibody against *erb*B-2 mediates targeted tumor cell eradication by apoptosis. Cancer Gene Ther 1996; 3:89-98.
43. Deshane J, Siegel GP, Alvarez RD et al. Targeted tumor killing via an intracellular antibody against *erb*B-2. J Clin Invest 1995; 96:2980-2989.
44. Baselga J, Tripathy D, Mendelsohn J et al. Phase II study of weekly intravenous recombinant humanized anti-p185 HER2 monoclonal antibody in patients with HER2/neu-overexpressiong metastatic breast cancer. J Clin Oncol 14:737-744.
45. Vaughn JP, Igelehart JD, Demirdji S et al. Antisense DNA downregulation of the *ERBB*2 oncogene measured by a flow cytometric assay. Proc Natl Acad Sci USA 1995; 92:8338-8342.
46. Wiechen K, Dietel M. c-*erb*B-2 anti-sense phosphorothioate oligodeoxynucleotides inhibit growth and serum-induced cell spreading of p185$^{c-erbB-2}$ overexpressing ovarian carcinoma cells. Int J Cancer 1995; 63:604-608.
47. Liu X and Pogo B. Inhibition of *erb*B-2-positive breast cancer cell growth by *erb*B-2 antisense oligonucleotides. Antisense Res Dev 1996; 6:9-16.
48. Pier GN, Nicortra MR, Bigotti A et al. Expression of the p185 encoded by *HER*2 oncogene in normal and transformed human tissues. Int J Cancer 1990; 45:457-461.
49. Ullrich A, Coussens L, Hayflick JS et al. Human epidermal growth factor receptor cDNA sequence and aberrant expression of the amplified gene in A431 epidermoid carcinoma cells. Nature (Lond.) 1984; 309:418-425.
50. Kraus MH., Issing W, Miki T et al. Isolation and characterization of *ERB*-B-3, a third member of the *ERB*B/epidermal growth factor receptor family: evidence for overexpression in a subset of human mammary tumors. Proc Natl Acad Sci USA 1989; 86:9193-9197.
51. Plowman GD, Culouscou JM, Whitney GS et al. Ligand-specific activation of *HER*4/p180 (*erb*B4), a 4th member of the epidermal growth factor receptor family. Proc Natl Acad Sci USA 1993; 90:1746-1750.
52. Kokai Y, Myers JN, Wada T et al. Synergistic interaction of p185c-neu and the EGF receptor leads to transformation of rodent fibroblast. Cell 1989; 58:287-292.
53. Borg A, Baldetorp B, Ferno M et al. *Erb*B2 amplification is associated with tamoxifen resistance in steroid-receptor positive breast cancer. Cancer Lett 1994; 81:137-144.
54. Pietras RJ, Arboleda J, Reese DM. *HER*-2 tyrosine kinase pathway targets estrogen receptor and promotes hormone-independent growth in human breast cancer cells. Oncogene 1995; 10:2435-2446.
55. Hancock MC, Langton BC, Chan T et al. A monoclonal antibody against the c-*erb*B-2 protein enhances the cytotoxity of cis-diamminedichloroplatinum against human breast and ovarian tumor cells. Cancer Res 1991; 51:4575-4580.
56. Miki Y, Swensen J, Shattuck-Eidens D et al. A strong candidate for the breast and ovarian cancer susceptibility gene *BRCA*1. Science (Washington, DC) 1994; 266:66-71.
57. Wooster R, Bignell G, Lancaster J et al. Identification of the breast cancer susceptibility gene *BRCA*2. Nature (Lond.) 1995; 378:789-792.
58. Malkin D, Li FP, Strong LC et al. Germ line p53 mutations in a familial syndrome of breast cancer, sarcomas, and other neoplasms. Science (Wash. DC) 1990; 250:1233-1238.
59. Katayose D, Wersto R, Cowan KH et al. Effects of a recombinant adenovirus expressing WAF/Cip1 on cell growth, cell cycle, and apoptosis. Cell Growth Differ 1995; 6:1207-1212.
60. Buckley MF, Sweeney KJE, Hamilton JA et al. Expression and amplification of cyclin genes in human breast cancer. Oncogene 1993; 8:2127-2133.
61. Lammie GA, Fantl V, Smith R et al. *D11S287*, a putative oncogene on chromosome 11q13, is amplified and expressed in squamous cell and mammary carcinomas and linked to BCL-1. Oncogene 1991; 6:439-444.
62. Keyomarsi K, O'Leary N, Molnar G et al. Cyclin E, a potential prognostic marker for breast cancer. Cancer Res 1994; 54:380-385.

CHAPTER 11

Therapeutic Application of an Anti-ras Ribozyme in Human Pancreatic Cancer

Hiroshi Kijima and Kevin J. Scanlon

Abstract

Pancreatic cancer is one of the most lethal human cancers, and development of new therapeutic strategies is urgently required. Point mutation in the K-*ras* gene is observed at a high incidence in human pancreatic carcinomas. These alterations can be used as potential targets for specific ribozyme-mediated reversal of the malignant phenotype. We have demonstrated previously the efficacy of a hammerhead ribozyme directed against codon 12 of the activated K-*ras* gene in a Capan-1 human pancreatic carcinoma cell line. To develop this strategy into a therapeutic application, we designed a recombinant adenovirus encoding a gene cassette for the anti-K-*ras* ribozyme. By using this recombinant adenovirus in a murine model system, it was possible to accomplish efficient reversion of the malignant phenotype in human pancreatic tumors with K-*ras* gene mutations. The high efficiency adenoviral-mediated delivery of anti-oncogene ribozyme could emerge as a significant gene therapy strategy against human malignancies.

Introduction

Pancreatic cancer is a lethal human malignancy with a less than 10% 3-year survival.[1,2] The factors which account for this poor prognosis include:
1. difficulty of early diagnosis due to anatomical location and lack of early symptoms;
2. limitation of conventional cancer therapy, including surgery, chemotherapy, radiation therapy or immune therapy;
3. rapid tumor spread to the surrounding organs, causing obstructive jaundice; and
4. frequent incidence of metastasis from even a small primary tumor less than 2 cm in diameter.[3-5]

Pancreatic cancer ranks fifth as a cause of cancer-related mortality in the United States, as well as Japan. Development of a new therapeutic strategy such as gene therapy for pancreatic cancer represents one of the most pressing issues in medicine today.[6,7]

Cancer cells have been shown to have alterations of oncogene expression such as point mutation, amplification or overexpression.[8,9] A point mutation of the *ras* oncogene family activates the p21 gene products affecting cancer cell growth and the malignant phenotype.[10] Characteristically, K-*ras* gene mutations have been found in approximately 90% of human

---

Ribozymes in the Gene Therapy of Cancer, edited by Kevin J. Scanlon and Mohammed Kashani-Sabet. ©1998 R.G. Landes Company.

pancreatic adenocarcinomas.[11-17] Most of the tumors examined harbored activated K-*ras* genes with mutations at codon 12. The K-*ras* mutation could occur in the early phase of pancreatic ductal carcinogenesis because this mutation has also been found in some pancreatic precancerous lesions, such as mucous cell hyperplasia.[18-20] However, the activated *ras* oncogene products are thought to alter the cellular signal transduction pathways and to affect neoplastic growth of the pancreatic cells.

Recent advances in the understanding of the genetic mechanisms of carcinogenesis and the manipulation of gene expression have introduced new therapeutics for cancer including gene therapy. Specific gene modulation using oligonucleotides have been developed and defined as a plausible strategy for suppressing activated oncogenes.[21-24] Oligonucleotides modulating target gene expression include triplex DNA, antisense DNA/RNA and ribozymes (catalytic RNA).[21] Antisense oligonucleotides are capable of altering the intermediary metabolism of mRNA and inhibiting the transfer of information from gene to protein. Antisense-mediated gene modulation has been shown to be effective for gene therapy.[25-27] In contrast, ribozymes have been characterized as RNA molecules having site-specific catalytic activity.[28,29] Trans-acting ribozyme molecules, such as "hammerhead" and "hairpin" ribozymes, include catalytic core and flanking sequences which bind the target RNA. Ribozymes are modified antisense molecules with site-specific cleavage activity and catalytic potential.[22,30-34] In recent years, researchers have demonstrated the efficacy of ribozymes against various oncogenes (e.g., *ras*, *c-fos*, *BCR-ABL*),[35] the drug resistance genes (e.g., *mdr*1)[36,37] and the human immunodeficiency virus type 1.[31,38,39] We have previously demonstrated that anti-oncogene ribozymes effectively suppress the expression of targeted genes and result in reversal of the malignant phenotype in human cancer cells.[40-47] Because of their in vitro efficacy, the anti-oncogene ribozymes have been proposed to have future clinical utilities as anticancer agents.

In a recent study, we investigated the in vivo efficacy of a hammerhead ribozyme against activated K-*ras* gene transcripts in human pancreatic carcinoma cells. For future clinical trials of cancer gene therapy using ribozymes, we have evaluated an efficient adenoviral-mediated delivery system of the anti-K-*ras* ribozyme as a therapeutic agent against human pancreatic carcinoma.

Results

Double-stranded DNA cycle sequencing of genomic DNA isolated from Capan-1 human pancreatic cancer cells exhibited a GTT homozygous mutation of the K-*ras* oncogene at codon 12 which encodes a valine (data not shown). This sequence is recognized by the anti-K-*ras* hammerhead ribozyme which we have designed for this study (Fig. 11.1). For expressing the anti-K-*ras* ribozyme, oligonucleotides KrasRz-1 and -2 were synthesized and cloned into an adenoviral shuttle vector, the pACCMVpLpA plasmid. The methodology for recombinant adenovirus construction is based on in vivo homologous recombination between the adenoviral shuttle vector pACCMVpLpA and the adenoviral packaging plasmid pJM17. The adenoviral vector Ad-K*ras* Rz contains the anti-K-*ras* ribozyme expression cassette inserted in place of the deleted adenoviral E1 region. The PCR assay of viral DNA demonstrated the presence of the anti-K-*ras* ribozyme in the recombinant adenovirus (data not shown).

In a tissue culture study, the Capan-1 cells infected with Ad-K*ras* Rz exhibited expression of the anti-K-*ras* ribozyme and decreased K-*ras* gene expression (data not shown). In the Capan-1 cells infected with Ad-K*ras* Rz, the generation time was significantly longer by 4.3 times compared to the parental cells (Table 11.1). Also, the Capan-1 cells infected with Ad-K*ras* Rz showed 47% and 83% decrease in [^{3}H] thymidine incorporation and soft agar colony formation, respectively.

Anit-K-ras ribozyme against mutant K-ras (codon 12)

```
                    cleavage site
          codon        |
           12          ↓
      5'- A GCU GUU GGC GUA -3'
      3'- U CGA C A    CCG CAU -5'
                 A   C
                 A    U
                 A     G
                 G      A
                 C  G A  U
                 A    G G
                 A  U
                 G  C
                 G  C         K-ras codon 12
                 A    G       (GUU), oncogene (valine)
                   G U        (GGU), proto oncogene (glycine)
```

Insert anti-K-ras ribozyme sequences

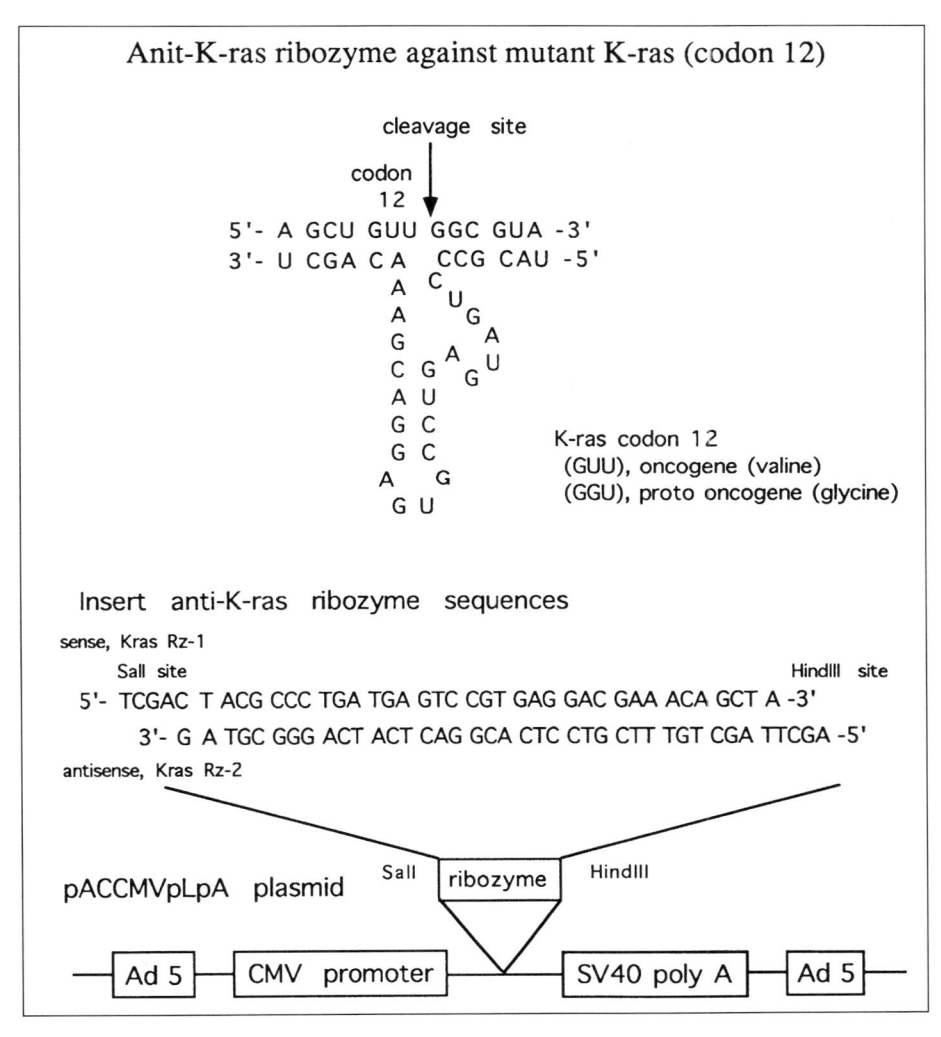

sense, Kras Rz-1
  Sall site   HindIII site
5'- TCGAC T ACG CCC TGA TGA GTC CGT GAG GAC GAA ACA GCT A -3'
    3'- G A TGC GGG ACT ACT CAG GCA CTC CTG CTT TGT CGA TTCGA -5'
antisense, Kras Rz-2

pACCMVpLpA plasmid — Sall [ribozyme] HindIII

— Ad 5 — CMV promoter — SV40 poly A — Ad 5 —

Fig. 11.1. Design of the recombinant adenovirus encoding the anti-K-*ras* ribozyme. The hammerhead ribozyme against K-*ras* targets the GUU mutant mRNA sequence of K-*ras* codon 12, which encodes valine (top of the figure). The GGU wild type sequence encoding glycine is not cleaved by the ribozyme. The pACCMVpLpA shuttle vector of the recombinant adenovirus is driven by the cytomegalovirus (CMV) promoter (bottom of the figure). The insert containing the anti-K-*ras* ribozyme sequence is cloned between the promoter and SV40 poly A.

In an in vivo system, inoculation of 1×10^6 Capan-1 cells subcutaneously into the flanks of athymic mice resulted in the rapid development of progressively enlarging tumors (Fig. 11.2). The efficacy of Ad-K*ras*Rz was investigated using a single intralesional injection of the ribozyme-encoding adenovirus at a viral dose of 1×10^8 PFU when the tumor volume reached 100 mm³. Overall, treatment with Ad-K*ras*Rz resulted in profound suppression of Capan-1 cell growth in vivo (Fig. 11.2), with the average tumor volume on day 40 approximately one-third that of control tumors. Significantly, of the 20 mouse tumors treated with

Table 11.1. Growth characteristics of the Capan-1 pancreatic carcinoma cells

Cell Line	GT[1]	[³H]Thd[2]	SAC[3]
Capan-1 (parent)	100% (59 hrs)	100%	100% (121)
Capan-1 / Ad dl312 (E1-)	102	99	92
Capan-1 / Ad anti-K-ras Rz	432	53	17

[1] GT, generation time (hours);
[2] [³H]Thd, the rate of [³H]-labeled thymidine incorporation compared to parental cells
[3] SAC, the rate of soft agar colony formation assay with 20% fetal bovine serum compared to parental cells (colony number provided in parentheses).
[1-3] Experiments were performed at least twice in duplicate. Standard deviation was less than 10%.

Fig. 11.2. Effect of adenovirus-mediated anti-K-*ras* ribozyme (Ad-K*ras* Rz) treatment on growth inhibition of Capan-1 tumors in athymic nude mice. Injection of the Ad-K*ras* Rz suppressed tumor growth of the Capan-1 cells, compared to the untreated control cells or the Capan-1 cells injected with the irrelevant adenovirus (Ad dl312; Ad-vector only). The graph shows data regarding thirteen Capan-1 tumors injected with Ad-K*ras* Rz; the other seven Capan-1 tumors completely regressed after Ad-K*ras* Rz treatment.

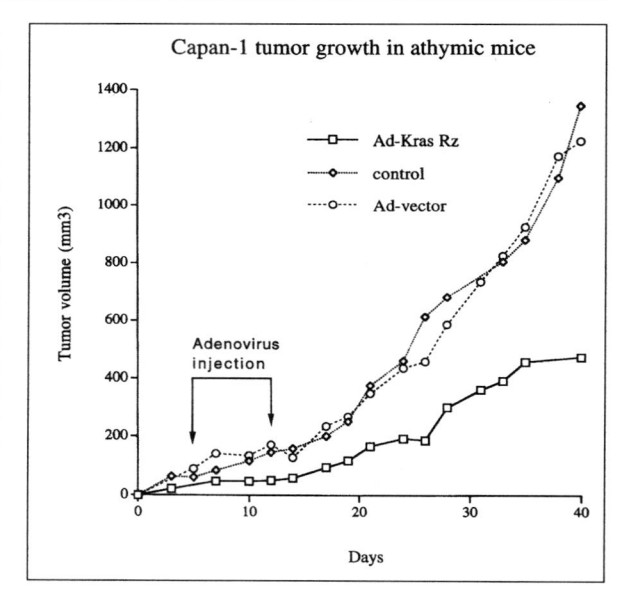

Ad-K*ras*Rz, seven regressed completely. Finally, the effects of vector-mediated cytotoxicity were investigated using an irrelevant adenovirus (Ad dl312). Treatment of Capan-1 tumors in vivo with Ad dl312 using an identical schedule to that of Ad-K*ras*Rz had little effect on the rate of tumor growth (Fig. 11.2).

Discussion

In the present study, we have demonstrated the efficacy of a hammerhead ribozyme against the mutant K-*ras* gene in the Capan-1 human pancreatic carcinoma cell line. Recently, other groups have reported the efficacy of antisense molecules against the K-*ras* gene to suppress human pancreatic tumor growth in vitro and in vivo in mouse models.[48,49] Potential advantages of ribozyme-mediated gene modulation include its catalytic activity, site-specific cleavage and ability to discriminate a single base mutation.[21,22,50] For examination of ribozyme-mediated strategies, investigators should take into account determinants of an effective ribozyme, such as the target gene, cleavage site, flanking sequences, ribozyme stability and delivery systems.[22,31,36,51]

Point mutations of the K-*ras* gene at codon 12 are found in approximately 90% of human pancreatic carcinomas, and activate its oncogene product.[10-17] This mutant mRNA can be a candidate for ribozyme-mediated gene modulation. The hammerhead ribozyme targeting the mutant K-*ras* gene we have designed could cleave mutant but not wild type mRNA.[51] The ultimate goal of this study is therapeutic application of the anti-K-*ras* ribozyme in human pancreatic cancer.[6,30,52-55] Therefore, to express the anti-K-*ras* ribozyme in Capan-1 tumors in a mouse model, we have cloned it into the adenoviral vector and generated Ad-K*ras* Rz. The adenoviral vector is driven by a cytomegalovirus early promoter/enhancer and polyadenylation signals from SV40. This system has been shown to express high amounts of the inserted transgene in human cells.[46,56]

In a tissue culture study, we demonstrated the efficacy of Ad-K*ras* Rz in inhibiting human pancreatic cancer cell proliferation.[6] The Capan-1 pancreatic carcinoma cells were effectively infected with Ad-K*ras* Rz, and their generation time was ≤.3 times longer than control cells. The anti-K-*ras* ribozyme affected not only the generation time, but also other growth characteristics, such as thymidine incorporation into DNA and soft agar colony formation. Thus the sequence-specific modulation of mutant K-*ras* mRNA by the hammerhead ribozyme was capable of reversing the malignant phenotype of human pancreatic carcinoma cells.

In our in vivo system, xenograft implantation of the Capan-1 cells in athymic mice resulted in the rapid development of subcutaneous tumors. The Capan-1 tumor nodules injected with the irrelevant adenovirus (Ad dl312) result in a similar pattern of rapid tumor progression, suggesting lack of vector-associated toxicity. Injection of the Ad-K*ras* Rz suppressed the rapid tumor growth effectively. These results indicated that adenovirus-mediated anti-K-*ras* ribozyme targeted mutant K-*ras* mRNA transcripts and was capable of inhibiting neoplastic progression of pancreatic cancer in vivo.

In this study using a recombinant adenoviral vector, we demonstrated high-efficiency in vivo delivery of the anti-K-*ras* ribozyme to human pancreatic carcinoma cells. However, the adenovirus we used was driven by the cytomegalovirus early promoter/enhancer, and not by a tissue-specific promoter.[22,57,58] For future clinical application of ribozyme-mediated gene modulation, tissue-specific promoters will be investigated. One potential promoter is the carcinoembryonic antigen (CEA) promoter, because pancreatic carcinomas frequently produce high amounts of CEA.[59,60] When targeting a tumor-selective gene expressed in a tissue-specific manner, ribozymes may offer minimal toxicity for the application of cancer gene therapy.

Conclusion

The anti-K-*ras* ribozyme is an effective modulator of mutant K-*ras* gene expression because of its site-specific cleavage activity. Adenovirus-mediated ribozyme expression suppressed tumor growth of the target pancreatic carcinoma in the in vivo system. Further studies of an optimal vector with a tissue-specific promoter are required to advance the anti-K-*ras* ribozyme toward clinical application of pancreatic cancer gene therapy.

Acknowledgments

This work was supported in part by Grants-in-Aid for Scientific Research from the Ministry of Education, Science and Culture of Japan (H.K.) and Tokai University School of Medicine Research Aid (H.K.).

References

1. Warshaw AL, Fernandez-del Castillo C. Pancreatic carcinoma. N Engl J Med 1992; 326:455-456.
2. Yamaguchi K, Enjoji E. Carcinoma of the pancreas: A clinicopathologic study of 96 cases with immunohistochemical observations. Jpn J Clin Oncol 1989; 19:14-22.
3. Ozaki H. Improvement of pancreatic cancer treatment from the Japanese experience in the 1980's. Int J Pancreatol 1992; 12:5-9.
4. Arbuck SG. Overview of chemotherapy for pancreatic cancer. Int J Pancreatol 1990; 7:209-222.
5. Cohn I Jr. Overview of pancreatic cancer, 1989. Int J Pancreatol 1990; 7:1-11.
6. Kijima H, Bouffard DY, Scanlon KJ. Ribozyme-mediated reversal of human pancreatic carcinoma phenotype. In: Ikehara S, Takaku F, Good RA, eds. Bone Marrow Transplantation—Basic and Clinical Studies. Tokyo: Springer, 1996:153-163.
7. Kijima H, Bouffard DY, Scanlon KJ. Ribozymes as a novel approach for the treatment of human pancreatic carcinoma. Methods Mol Med 1998; 11:193-208.
8. Egan SE, Weinberg RA. The pathway to signal achievement. Nature 1993; 365:781-783.
9. Slamon DJ, deKernion JB, Verma IM, Cline MJ. Expression of cellular oncogenes in human malignancies. Science 1984; 224:256-262.
10. Barbacid M. *ras* genes. Annu Rev Biochem 1987; 56:779-827.
11. Bos JL. *ras* oncogenes in human cancer: A review. Cancer Res 1989; 49:4682-4689.
12. Almoguera C, Shibata D, Forrester K, Martin J, Arnheim N, Perucho M. Most human carcinomas of the exocrine pancreas contain mutant c-K-*ras* genes. Cell 1988; 53:549-554.
13. Smit VTHBM, Boot AJM, Smit AMM, Fleuren GJ, Cornelisse CJ, Bos JL. Kras codon 12 mutations occur very frequently in pancreatic adenocarcinomas. Nucleic Acids Res 1988; 16:7773-7782.
14. Grunewald K, Lyons J, Frohlich A, Feichtinger H, Weger RA, Schwab G, Janssen JWG, Bartram CR. High frequency of Ki-*ras* codon 12 mutations in pancreatic adenocarcinomas. Int J Cancer 1989; 43:1037-1041.
15. Mariyama M, Kishi K, Nakamura, K, Obata H, Nishimura S. Frequency and types of point mutation at the 12th codon of the c-Ki-*ras* gene found in pancreatic cancers from Japanese patients. Jpn J Cancer Res 1989; 80:622-626.
16. Tada M, Yokosuka O, Omata M, Ohto M, Isono K. Analysis of *ras* gene mutations in biliary and pancreatic tumors by polymerase chain reaction and direct sequencing. Cancer 1990; 66:930-935.
17. Nagata Y, Abe M, Motoshima K, Nakayama E, Shiku H. Frequent glycine-to-aspartic acid mutations at codon 12 of c-Ki-*ras* gene in human pancreatic cancer in Japanese. Jpn J Cancer Res 1990; 81:135-140.
18. Yanagisawa A, Ohtake K, Ohashi K, Hori M, Kitagawa T, Sugano H, Kato Y. Frequent c-K-*ras* oncogene activation in mucous cell hyperplasia of pancreas suffering from chronic inflammation. Cancer Res 1993; 53:953-956.
19. DiGiuseppe JA, Hruban RH, Offerhaus GJ, Clement MJ, van den Berg FM, Cameron JL, van Mansfeld ADM. Detection of K-*ras* mutations in mucinous pancreatic duct hyperplasia from a patient with a family history of pancreatic carcinoma. Am J Pathol 1994; 144:889-895.
20. Tada M, Ohashi M, Shiratori Y, Okudaira T, Komatsu Y, Kawabe T, Yoshida H, Machinami R, Kishi K, Omata M. Analysis of K-*ras* gene mutation in hyperplastic duct cells of the pancreas without pancreatic disease. Gastroenterol 1997; 110:227-231.
21. Scanlon KJ, Ohta Y, Ishida H, Kijima H, Ohkawa T, Kaminski A, Tsai J, Horng G, Kashani-Sabet M. Oligonucleotide-meiated modulation of mammalian gene expression. FASEB J 1995; 6:1288-1296.
22. Kashani-Sabet M, Scanlon KJ. Application of ribozymes to cancer gene therapy. Cancer Gene Ther 1995; 2:213-221.
23. Christoffersen RE, Marr JJ. Ribozymes as human therapeutic agents. J Med Chem 1995; 38:2023-2037.

24. Helene C. Control of oncogene expression by antisense nucleic acids. Eur J Cancer 1994; 30A:1721-1726.
25. Georges RN, Mukhopadhyay T, Zhang Y, Yen N, Roth JA. Prevention of orthotopic human lung cancer growth by intratracheal instillation of a retroviral antisense K-*ras* construct. Cancer Res 1993; 53:1743-1746.
26. Zhang Y, Mukhopadhyay T, Donehower LA, Georges RN, Roth JA. Retroviral vector-mediated transduction of K-*ras* antisense RNA into human lung cancer inhibits expression of the malignant phenotype. Human Gene Ther 1993; 4:451-460.
27. Mercola D, Cohen JS. Antisense approach to cancer gene therapy. Cancer Gene Ther 1995; 2:47-59.
28. Castanotto D, Rossi JJ, Sarver N. Antisense catalytic RNAs as therapeutic agents. Adv Pharmacol 1994; 25:289-317.
29. Symons RH. Ribozymes. Curr Opin Structural Biol 1994; 4:322-330.
30. Kijima H, Ishida H, Ohkawa T, Kashani-Sabet M, Scanlon KJ. Therapeutic applications of ribozymes. Pharmacol Ther 1995; 68:247-267.
31. Irie A, Kijima H, Ohkawa T, Bouffard DY, Suzuki T, Curcio LD, Holm PS, Sassani A, Scanlon KJ. Anti-oncogene ribozymes for cancer gene therapy. Adv Pharmacol 1997; 40:207-257.
32. Pley HW, Flaherty KM, McKay DB. Three-dimensional structure of a hammerhead ribozyme. Nature 1994; 372:68-74.
33. Uhlenbeck OC. A small catalytic oligonucleotide. Nature 1987; 328:596-600.
34. Fujita S, Koguma T, Ohkawa J, Mori K, Kohda T, Kise H, Nishikawa S, Iwakuma M, Taira K. Discrimination of a single base change in a ribozyme using the gene for dihydrofolate reductase as a selective marker in Escherichia coli. Proc Natl Acad Sci USA 1997; 94:391-396.
35. Bouffard DY, Ohkawa T, Kijima H, Irie A, Suzuki T, Curcio LD, Holm PS, Sassani A, Scanlon KJ. Oligonucleotide modulation of multidrug resistance. Eur J Cancer 1996; 32A:1010-1018.
36. Ohkawa T, Kijima H, Irie A, Horng, G, Kaminski A, Tsai J, Kashfian BI, Scanlon KJ. Oligonucleotide modulation of multidrug resistance gene expression. In: Gupta S, Tsuruo T, eds. Multidrug Resistance in Cancer Cells. England: Wiley & Sons, 1996:413-433.
37. Sarver N, Cantin EM, Chang PS, Zaia JA, Ladne PA, Stephens DA, Rossi JJ. Ribozymes as potential anti-HIV-1 therapeutic agents. Science 1990; 247:1222-1225.
38. Yu M, Ojwang J, Yamada O, Hample A, Rapapport J, Looney D, Wong-Staal F. A hairpin ribozyme inhibits expression of diverse strains of human immunodeficiency virus type-1. Proc Natl Acad Sci USA 1993; 87:6340-6344.
39. Scanlon KJ, Jiao L, Funato T, Wang W, Tone T, Rossi JJ, Kashani-Sabet M. Ribozyme-mediated cleavage of c-fos mRNA reduces gene expression of DNA synthesis enzymes and metallothionein. Proc Natl Acad Sci USA 1991; 88:10591-10595.
40. Kashani-Sabet M, Funato T, Tone T, Jiao L, Wang W, Yoshida E, Kashfian BI, Shitara T, Wu AM, Moreno JG, Traweek ST, Ahlering TE, Scanlon KJ. Reversal of the malignant phenotype by an anti-*ras* ribozyme. Antisense Res Dev 1992; 2:3-15.
41. Tone T, Kashani-Sabet M, Funato T, Shitara T, Yoshida E, Kashfian BI, Horng M, Fodstad O, Scanlon KJ. Suppression of EJ cells tumorigenicity. In Vivo 1993; 7:471-476.
42. Funato T, Shitara T, Tone T, Jiao L, Kashani-Sabet M, Scanlon KJ. Suppression of H-*ras*-mediated transformation in NIH3T3 cells by a *ras* ribozyme. Biochem Pharmacol 1994; 48:1471-1475.
43. Ohta Y, Tone T, Shitara T, Funato T, Jiao L, Kashfian BI, Yoshida E, Horng M, Tsai P, Lauterbach K, Kashani-Sabet M, Florenes VA, Fodstad O, Scanlon KJ. H-*ras* ribozyme-mediated alteration of the human melanoma phenotype. Ann NY Acad Sci 1994; 716:242-253.
44. Kashani-Sabet M, Funato T, Florenes VA, Fodstad O, Scanlon KJ. Suppression of the neoplastic phenotype in vivo by an anti-*ras* ribozyme. Cancer Res 1994; 54:900-902.
45. Scanlon KJ, Ishida H, Kashani-Sabet M. Ribozyme-mediated reversal of the multidrug-resistant phenotype. Proc Natl Acad Sci USA 1994; 91:11123-11127.

46. Feng M, Cabrera G, Deshane J, Scanlon KJ, Curiel DT. Neoplastic reversion accomplished by high efficiency adenoviral-mediated delivery of an anti-*ras* ribozyme. Cancer Res 1995; 55:2024-2028.
47. Ohta Y, Kijima H, Kashani-Sabet M, Scanlon KJ. Suppression of the malignant phenotype of melanoma cells by anti-oncogene ribozymes. J Invest Dermatol 1996; 106:275-280.
48. Carter G, Gilbert C, Lemoine NR. Effects of antisense oligonucleotides targeting K-*ras* expression in pancreatic cancer cell lines. Int J Oncol 1995; 6:1105-1112.
49. Aoki K, Yoshida T, Sugimura T, Terada M. Liposome-mediated in vivo gene transfer of antisense K-*ras* construct inhibits pancreatic tumor dissemination in the murine peritoneal cavity. Cancer Res 1995; 55:3810-3816.
50. Koizumi M, Hayase Y, Iwai S, Kamiya H, Inoue H, Ohtsuka E. Design of RNA enzymes distinguishing a single base mutation in RNA. Nucleic Acids Res 1989; 17:7059-7071.
51. Cech TR, Uhlenbeck OC. Hammerhead nailed down. Nature 1994; 372:39-40.
52. Jolly D. Viral vector systems for gene therapy. Cancer Gene Ther 1994; 1:51-64.
53. Hodgson CP. The vector void in gene therapy. Biotechnology 1995; 13:222-225.
54. Anderson WF. Human gene therapy. Science 1992; 256:808-813.
55. Thompson JD, Macejak D, Couture L, Stinchcomb DT. Ribozymes in gene therapy. Nature Med 1995; 1:277-278.
56. Lieber A, Kay MA. Adenovirus-mediated expression of ribozymes in mice. J Virol 1996; 70:3153-3158.
57. Ohta Y, Kijima H, Kashani-Sabet M, Scanlon KJ. Tissue-specific expression of an anti-*ras* ribozyme inhibits proliferation of human malignant melanoma cells. Nucleic Acids Res 1996; 24:938-942.
58. Lan K-H, Kanai F, Shiratori Y, Ohashi M, Tanaka T, Okudaira T, Yoshida Y, Hamada H, Omata M. In vivo selective gene expression and therapy mediated by adenoviral vectors for human carcinoembryonic antigen-producing gastric carcinoma. Cancer Res 1997; 57:4279-4284.
59. Schrewe H, Thompson J, Bona M, Hefta LA, Maruya A, Hassauer, M, Shively JH, von Kleist S, Zimmermann W. Cloning of the complete gene for carcinoembryonic antigen: Analysis of its promoter indicates a region conveying cell type-specific expression. Mol Cell Biol 1990; 10:2738-2748.
60. Hauck W, Stanners CP. Transcriptional regulation of the carcinoembryonic antigen gene. J Biol Chem 1995; 270:3602-3610.

CHAPTER 12

The Use of Ribozymes for Gene Therapy of Lung Cancer

Alex W. Tong, Yu-An Zhang, David Y. Bouffard, John Nemunaitis

Summary

The adverse prognosis of patients having common oncogene mutations (*ras*, *p53*, c-*erbB-2*) suggests that these genetic lesions contribute to tumor pathogenesis. Currently, the majority of lung cancer gene therapy makes use of antisense oligonucleotides (AS-ODN) or expression vectors (such as a viral vector construct) that deliver the antisense sequence to inactivate the mutant oncogene. The specific targeting of *ras*, c-*myc*, L-*myc*, *bcl-2*, c-*kit*, and mutant *p53* by AS-ODNs collaterally suppressed lung cancer cell growth in vitro by 40-90%. Ribozymes present a viable alternative in antisense therapy by virtue of their renewable catalytic capability for site-specific RNA cleavage. We recently examined the growth-modulating effect of a hammerhead ribozyme that is specific for the K-*ras* codon 12 mutant sequence GUU, given the findings that:

1. in the United States, approximately 30% of human non-small cell lung cancers (NSCLC) express K-*ras* oncogene mutations, nearly all of which reside in codon 12;
2. anti-K-*ras*, anti-H- as well as anti-N-*ras* hammerhead ribozymes are potent growth inhibitors in various human cancers tested; and
3. in vitro and animal model studies suggest that ribozymes directed at oncoproteins (K- and H-Ras, c-Fos, BCR-ABL) or human immunodeficiency viral proteins are more effective than their antisense counterpart.

We examined the growth inhibitory effect of a K-*ras* ribozyme, using the human lung adenocarcinoma cell line H1725 with a heterozygous GGT→GTT mutation at K-*ras* codon 12. H1725 cell growth was reduced by 81% following treatment with a pHb Apr-1-neo plasmid construct with the relevant ribozyme (KRbz) sequence against GTT, whereas the growth rate of mock-transfected cultures was reduced by less than 15%. By contrast, KRbz did not significantly affect the growth of the NSCLC cell line H460, which lacks the relevant K-*ras* mutation. Further studies with a KRbz-adenoviral (ADV) vector construct (pACCMVpLpA) inhibited H1725 cell growth by >90%, based on enumeration of viable cell numbers and [^{3}H]-thymidine uptake. KRbz-ADV-treated cells had a correspondingly lower K-*ras* expression. These findings indicate that KRbz-ADV is potentially useful for controlling the growth of lung tumor cells having the relevant K-*ras* mutation. Additional measures that could further improve ribozyme efficacy are discussed, including biochemical modifications of the ribozyme backbone, and the simultaneous targeting of multiple oncogene/tumor suppressor genes.

Ribozymes in the Gene Therapy of Cancer, edited by Kevin J. Scanlon and Mohammed Kashani-Sabet. ©1998 R.G. Landes Company.

Introduction

The increasing incidence of lung cancer is estimated to reach 2,000,000 cases worldwide by the year 2000. Lung cancer is currently the leading cause of cancer death for men and women in the United States,[1] with a 5 year survival rate of <15% for newly diagnosed cases. With the improved understanding in lung cancer molecular pathogenesis, numerous studies have explored the applicability of reversing oncogenetic mutation-related defects as a means of controlling lung tumor cell growth.

Perhaps as many as 10-20 genetic mutations have occurred by the time lung cancer becomes clinically evident. Controlled normal cell growth and differentiation depend on the balanced functions of two groups of cellular genes, collectively known as proto-oncogenes and tumor suppressor genes (reviewed in refs. 2-5). Tumorigenesis may involve the activation of dominant oncogenes (such as *ras*, *c-erbB-2*, *myc*, *raf*, *jun*, *myb*, *fms*, *fur*), recessive mutations that lead to loss of tumor suppresser/negative regulator function (such as *p53* or retinoblastoma [*rb*]), or both.[2-4] Most genetic lesions associated with lung cancer occur across small cell (SCLC) and non-small cell (NSCLC, including large cell, adenocarcinoma, and squamous cell) histologic types. Exceptions are mutations in the *ras* gene family, which occur in 30% of adenocarcinomas but are not present in SCLCs, and *rb* gene mutations that are found in >95% of SCLC but in only 20-30% of NSCLC cancers (Table 12.1). The contribution of each genetic lesion in lung cancer growth alteration is undefined, although clinical data suggest that *ras*, *p53* and *c-erbB-2* mutations are associated with adverse survival and are likely to play a role in tumor pathogenesis.[5-8]

Growth Inhibition by Antisense Oligonucleotides (AS-ODN)

The current armamentarium for modulating gene expression includes triplex DNA, antisense RNA/DNA and ribozymes (catalytic RNA).[9] A majority of lung cancer gene therapy studies make use of antisense oligonucleotides (AS-ODN) or expression vectors (such as a viral vector construct) for delivering the antisense sequence to inactivate mutant oncogenes. AS-ODNs are short, gene-specific nucleic acid sequences, typically 15-25 bases in length. They bind to mRNA, or single/double stranded DNA via base pairing to form double-stranded mRNA:DNA, mRNA:RNA or triple-stranded DNA, thereby stopping the translation or transcription of targeted genes via degradation by specific RNase.

In vitro studies show that AS-ODNs are effective for inhibiting human lung tumor cell growth (Table 12.2). AS-ODNs specific for the translation initiation codon of *c-myc* mRNA reduced NSCLC cell line growth by 32-72%, and inhibited cell adhesion and *c-myc* expression.[10] *c-myc*, *bcl-2*, and mutant *p53* specific AS-ODNs were equally effective in lowering the corresponding oncoprotein expression, and reduced the growth of NSCLC cell lines by up to 40%.[11] Other effective targets for AS-ODN inhibition of NSCLC growth include growth factor receptors (IGF-IR and IL-8 R1)[12,13] and the cell cycle protein cyclin D1 that regulates phosphorylation of the Rb gene product.[14] Similarly, L-Myc and c-Kit oncoprotein expression in SCLC cell lines were downregulated by the relevant AS-ODNs, which also decreased cell growth by 58% and 40%, respectively.[15,16]

AS-ODN viral vector constructs similarly inhibit lung tumor cell growth in vitro, and provide a highly effective means for the delivery of AS-ODN in vivo.[17-19] Retroviral (LNSX)[17] or adenoviral[20] constructs with a 2 kb K-*ras* gene antisense DNA insert specifically inhibited expression of the codon 61-mutated K-Ras p21 protein in NSCLC H460a cells, and reduced in vitro growth by up to 90%. Intratracheal instillation of this construct similarly inhibited the growth of the cell line xenograft in 87% of inoculated animals (Table 12.2).[18]

These observations indicate that specific targeting of oncogenetic defects can collaterally suppress lung cancer cell growth. The introduction of phosphorothioate linkage improves the stability of AS-ODNs.[10,16,21] Nevertheless, their capacity to inhibit lung tumor

Table 12.1. Clinically relevant oncogenetic alterations in lung cancer

Aberrations	NSCLC	SCLC
Proto-oncogene/ oncogene	K-*ras* (activating point mutation) c-*erbB-2* (altered transcription)	c-*myc* (gene amplification)
Tumor Suppressor gene	*p53* (point mutation+deletion) *rb* (point mutation+deletion) 3p deletion	*rb* 3p deletion *p53*
Growth Factor/receptors	Insulin-like growth factor I (IGF-I) Transforming growth factor-α (TGFα) c-*jun*, c-*fos* IGF-I receptor c-*erbB-1* receptor (EGFR)	Bombesin/gastric-releasing peptide-neuroendocrine peptides Transferrin

[a]NSCLC: non-small cell lung cancer; SCLC: small cell lung cancer; *rb*: retinoblastoma

cell growth ranges from 40-90%. Contributing factors may include tumor heterogeneity with respect to the oncogene defect; incomplete penetration by the vector delivery system; a limited role of the targeted oncoprotein in cancer pathophysiology; stoichiometric limitations on the reversible interactions between the antisense reagent and the targeted genetic message; or dependence on endogenous RNase H, which may be required to release the bound antisense molecule while destroying the target mRNA.[22]

Growth Inhibition by Ribozyme

Ribozymes (catalytic RNAs, RNA enzymes) are RNAs with intrinsic site-specific RNA cleavage or ligation activities (reviewed in refs. 23, 24). Originally discovered in the pre-rRNA of *Tetrahymena thermophilia*,[25] seven types of naturally occurring RNA catalytic motifs have now been identified, and trans-cleaving variants based on these motifs have been constructed.[26] Trans-cleaving ribozymes are appealing agents for gene therapy, in view of their ability to irreversibly inactivate their targets and their regenerative catalytic activity. By cloning specific antisense sequences into a basic ribozyme motif, it is feasible to design ribozymes that discriminate substrate RNAs with a single base mutation [27] as well as closely-related RNAs.[28]

The hammerhead ribozyme motif is widely utilized in gene therapy ribozyme design.[23] Hammerhead ribozymes were originally identified in the plus (+) strand of satellite RNA of tobacco ringspot virus (sTobRV). They represent the smallest ribozyme motif (30 nucleotides) and are best characterized with respect to target sequence, requirement for the catalytic core, and kinetics. As described in detail in other chapters of this monograph, the secondary structure of the ribozyme-substrate complex consists of three helical stems emanating from the catalytic core.[9] The RNA substrate binds to the hammerhead ribozyme through two helices/stems (helix I and III). The catalytic core is comprised of an unpaired connector loop and helix II, which is made up of 8 internally complementary nucleotides. Based on early mutational analysis, interaction between the hammerhead ribozyme and its substrate requires an "NUH" triplet sequence 3' of the cleavage site, with N being any nucleotide and H being A,C, or U. The GUC triplet is frequently chosen as a cleavage substrate because of its wide occurrence in natural ribozyme motifs.[29] Substrates containing GUA, GUU, UUC or CUC triplets are also efficiently cleaved, whereas GAC, GUG, AUC, CGC,

Table 12.2. Targets of gene therapy in human lung cancer

Cell Type	Target[a]	Agent (Reference)	Efficacy In Vitro	Efficacy In Vivo
NSCLC[a]				
H460a line	K-ras codon 61 mutant	AS-ADV (18,20)	47-90% ↓ growth	NT
H460 line	K-ras codon 61	AS-RTV (17)	up to 90% ↓ growth	87% of treated (vs. 10% untreated) mice are tumor-free
H596 line	mutant p53	AS-ODN (59)	potentiates apoptosis	NT
A549 line	c-myc	4G-AS-ODN (10)	62-72% ↓ growth	NT
A427, SKMES-1, A549	c-myc bcl-2 mutant p53	AS-ODN (11)	40% ↓ growth	NT
H460, SCC5	IGF-IR IL-8 Receptor B	AS-ADV (12) AS-ODN (13)	84% ↓ clonogenicity Reversible growth inhibition	Prolonged survival NT
SCLC				
SBC-1 line	c-kit proto-oncogene	AS-ADV (15)	40% ↓ growth	NT
H209, H510, H82	L-myc	AS-ODN (16)	70% ↓ growth	NT
Drug-resistant SCLC lines	MRP[a]	AS-ODN (21)	>90% ↓ expression	NT

[a]NSCLC: non-small cell lung cancer; SCLC: small cell lung cancer; IGF-IR: insulin growth factor-I receptor; MRP: multidrug resistant protein; AS: antisense; RTV: retroviral vector; ODN: oligodeoxynucleotides; ADV: adenoviral vector; NT: not tested.

GGC, AGC or UGC triplet sequences are poorly cleaved. Sense-anti-sense complementation by flanking sequences (helix I or helix III of the ribozyme but probably not both)[30] ensures sequence specificity of the cleavage reaction and juxtaposes the conserved 13 nucleotide-catalytic core across from the cleavage site. Hammerhead ribozymes are recognized as metalloenzymes, since divalent cations (Mg^{2+}) are captured by the catalytic domain and play an integral role in the multiple turnover site-specific trans-cleavage process by non-hydrolytic transesterification.[31] Efficacy of cleavage is dependent on the length of the complementary flanking sequence (optimal length, 12-13 nt), and composition and accessibility of the cleavage site.[32,33] Based on the current understanding of the ribozyme cleavage reaction, the criteria for efficient functioning of ribozyme within a cell are:

1. the target RNA sequence must be accessible for ribozyme hybridization;
2. the ribozyme and target RNAs must be present in the same subcellular compartment;
3. the ribozyme must be stable in order to attain a high ribozyme RNA:target RNA ratio; and
4. the ribozyme should be able to access all the target cells within a particular tissue,[30,34] except in circumstances where downregulation of the target RNA has a "bystander" effect on neighboring cells.

Ribozymes that target the expression products of mutant or amplified genes have been used to modulate growth and/or drug-resistance activities of human cancer cells.[24] The *ras*-encoded p21*ras* protein is a guanine nucleotide binding GTPase.[35,36] Activating *ras* mutations, invariably found in the GTP binding regions of p21*ras*, produce a constitutively activated GTP-locked p21*ras* which is believed to contribute to uncontrolled malignant growth. The mutant *ras* oncogene is an attractive target for ribozyme-mediated gene modulation, in view of its high mutation incidence, the restricted localization in the *ras* gene, and the crucial role of *ras* in signal transduction during neoplastic growth. Treatment with a hammerhead ribozyme against the H-*ras* codon 12 mutation (GGC→GUC) inhibited H-*ras* mutant tumor cell growth and partially reverted the malignant phenotype in human bladder carcinoma, human melanoma, and murine NIH3T3 models, while normal H-*ras* proto-oncogene function was unaffected.[37] In vivo treatment similarly reduced tumorigenicity of the H-*ras* mutant bladder carcinoma xenograft with no identifiable toxicity.[38] By comparison, mutant ribozymes that lack cleavage activity did not exert a tumor-suppressive effect, despite having the appropriate complementary antisense sequence.[37] Thus cleavage function appears integral to the ribozyme's ability to alter H-*ras* gene expression and cell growth.

Approximately 30% of NSCLCs carry a *ras* mutation, which occur primarily in lung adenocarcinomas and small numbers of large cell undifferentiated and squamous cell lung carcinomas. NSCLC patients with *ras* mutation and/or p21*ras* overexpression have a significantly poorer prognosis (reviewed in refs. 5, 8). In US and European studies, nearly all mutations occur in the K-*ras* gene, although N-*ras* and H-*ras* mutations have been detected occasionally.[8] K-*ras* mutations occur predominantly in codon 12 with a G→T transversion (Table 12.3). Roth and coworkers have demonstrated that K-*ras* AS-viral constructs are effective for inhibiting human NSCLC cell growth in vitro and in vivo.[17,20] However, these studies are based on the H460a cell line model, which has a homozygous K-*ras* codon 61 mutation.

We recently examined the growth-modulating effect of a hammerhead ribozyme that is specific for the K-*ras* codon 12 mutant sequence GUU, given the findings that

1. nearly all NSCLC *ras* mutations occur in K-*ras* codon 12 in the United States (Table 12.3; also ref. 8);
2. anti-K-*ras*, anti-H- as well as anti-N-*ras* hammerhead ribozymes are potent growth inhibitors in various human cancers tested;[24,39-42] and

Table 12.3. K-ras mutations and potential ribozyme substrate sites in non-small cell lung cancers

Mutation* Codon	Sequence	Corresponding Ribozyme Substrate Sequence	% of Total Mutations
12	TGT	UGU	55
12	GAT	GAU	18
12	GTT	GUU	12
12	GCT	GCU	3
12	AGT	AGU	3
12	TTT	UUU	3
13	TGC	UGC	6

*wild type sequence is GGT for codon 12, GGC for codon 13. Mutation was determined by PCR/gene sequencing with 10³ paraffin-embedded, formalin-fixed archived specimens of histologically proven lung cancer.[6]
Reprinted with permission from Tong AW et al. In: Scanlon K, ed. Therapeutic Applications of Ribozymes. Methods in Molecular Medicine, 1997.

3. comparative studies show that ribozymes directed at oncogenes (K- and H-*ras*, c-*fos*, *BCR-ABL*) or viral proteins are more effective than their antisense counterpart;[43]

Double-stranded DNA dideoxy end-label sequencing of the human lung adenocarcinoma cell line H1725 genome DNA demonstrated a heterozygous GGT/GTT mutation at codon 12 of the K-*ras* gene.[44] This cell line is relevant in the study of mutant *ras* gene modulation, since the point mutation resulting in a heterozygous single base pair mismatch is expected to be more prevalent than homozygous *ras* mutations.

Earlier transfection studies were performed using this ribozyme construct (KRbz) cloned into the pHβ Apr-1-neo plasmid and transfected into H1725 cells by electroporation.[44,45] Expression of the transgene was demonstrated in isolated G418-resistant clones by RT-PCR. The growth rate of KRbz-transfected H1725 cells was reduced by 81% as compared with less than 15% decrease in growth rate for mock-transfected cultures, based on cell number determinations at day 8 (Fig. 12.1, Table 12.4). Parent monolayer culture cells were of irregular morphology with long, spindly processes that rapidly spread and overlap one another. By contrast, KRbz-transfected cells were round, had fewer spindly processes and tended to grow in patches, suggesting a reversion of the malignant phenotype. Culture doubling time was substantially longer for KRbz-treated H1725 cells (>45 hours) as compared with untreated H1725 cells (28 hours; Table 12.4). By contrast, KRbz did not significantly affect the growth of the NSCLC cell line H460 (Table 12.4), which lacks the relevant K-*ras* mutation.[44] These observations suggest that KRbz treatment is effective in inhibiting the growth of lung adenocarcinoma cells carrying the relevant heterozygous K-*ras* codon 12 mutation.

For potential in vivo applications, it is necessary that the ribozyme be delivered effectively to the desired tissue in a non-toxic manner. Recent studies have utilized plasmids, retroviruses, adenoviruses, adeno-associated viruses (AAV), and cationic lipids for ribozyme delivery. A problem of lipofection (cationic liposome) is its high toxicity in currently available formulations.[46] Among the various viral vectors, the adenovirus is preferred because of its high efficacy of gene transfer in many types of human cancers and its ability to infect both dividing and non-dividing cells. Adenoviruses are stable and can be obtained, in many systems, in higher titer than retrovirus (10^{10} vs. 10^8 PFU/ml, respectively), which is advantageous in clinical situations that require large quantities of viral particles. Adenoviral vector

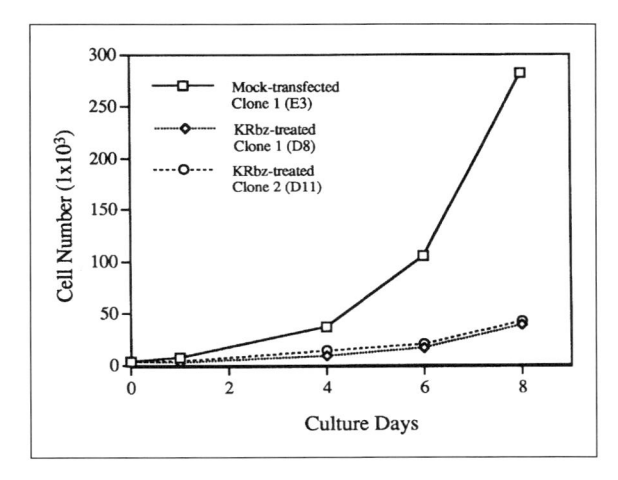

Fig. 12.1. Growth inhibition of NSCLC H1725 Cells by the KRbz-Plasmid vector. H1725 cells were transfected with KRbz-pHβ Apr-1 or pHβ Apr-1 empty cassette by electroporation (200 V, 960 µFd). Transfected cells were selected and cloned in presence of G418. Growth rate of KRbz-treated and mock-transfected cultures was compared by the number of viable cells determined at a given day. Duplicate variations are <20%.

Table 12.4. Cell culture doubling time following transfection with pHβ vector or pHβ KRbz[a]

Cell Line	Treatment	Clones	Avg. Doubling Time (hours)[b]	% Change[c]
H1725	Untreated		28.0	
	pHβ	E3	32.4	15.7
	pHβ Rbz	D8	45.9	63.9
	pHβ Rbz	D11	50.9	81.8
H460	Untreated		20.3	
	pHβ	D4	24.3	19.7
	pHβ Rbz	B7	20.6	1.2
	pHβ Rbz	D5	20.6	1.2

[a]Cells were transfected with pHβ K-*ras* or pHβ mock vector, cloned, and selected by G418 for 2 months before evaluation.
[b]Cell generation number (N) is calculated by the formula: $N = 3.32 \times (\log_{10} Cy - \log_{10} Cx)$ where Cy is cell number on day 8 and Cx is the cell number on day 1. Doubling time = $1/N \times 24$ hours;
[c]($N_{treated\ culture} - N_{untreated\ culture} / N_{untreated\ culture}$) × 100.

constructs are expected to have a transient (episomal) mode of expression. Nevertheless, the recombinant adenoviral:ribozyme construct (pACCMVpLpA/KRbz) was more effective in suppressing K-*ras* gene expression in pancreatic cancer cells as compared with its retroviral (pLNCX) or plasmid (pHβ) counterpart.[39] In light of its natural tropism for respiratory tissues, the adenovirus vector is particularly appropriate for delivery to lung cancers. Within each vector construct, an optimal promoter/enhancer system is crucial for stable and efficient expression of the ribozyme. Certain ribozymes could be designed with an inducible and/or tissue-specific enhancer/promoter for exclusive expression in diseased tissue.[40] Such a sequence is currently not available for lung cancer applications.

Based on these considerations, we have constructed a replication-deficient adenoviral vector encoding the anti-K-*ras* ribozyme(KRbz-ADV) under a cytomegalovirus promoter/enhancer element and an SV40 polyadenylation signal. Oligonucleotides encoding the sequence of the ribozyme were cloned into the polylinker of the shuttle pACCMVpLpA.[45] pACCMVpLpA contains a constitutive CMV promoter insert for high levels of ribozyme RNA production.[38,39] The resultant plasmid and the pJM17 packaging plasmid were cotransfected into the E1 transcomplementing cell line HEK293 using a cationic liposome (DOTAP), where the anti-K-*ras* ribozyme was generated via homologous recombination between pACCMVpLpA-KRbz and pJM17 (Fig. 12.2).[38] The purified adenoviral vector preparation is predicted to contain the anti-K-*ras* ribozyme expression cassette inserted in place of the deleted adenoviral E1 sequence. The presence of contaminating replication-competent (wild type) adenoviruses was ruled out by PCR analysis, using specific primers to the E1A region (Fig. 12.3).

The adenoviral-mediated suppression of H1725 cell growth was evaluated in absence of any selection pressure, following infection with pretitered concentrations of KRbz-ADV. KRbz-ADV infected H1725 cells expressed the KRbz and had an approximately 25% decrease in p21*ras* expression, based on semi-quantitative immunohistochemical analysis (Table 12.5). The decreased Ras expression parallels a dose-dependent growth inhibition that ranged from 54% (50 PFU/cell) to 92% (500 PFU/cell) in KRbz-ADV-treated H1725 cells at day 11 post-infection. [^{3}H]-thymidine uptake assays showed that KRbz-ADV (250 PFU/cell) significantly inhibited DNA synthesis of H1725 cells (Table 12.6). Significantly prolonged generation time was observed following KRbz-ADV. The growth inhibitory effect of KRbz-ADV increased with time.[45] These findings suggest that the KRbz-ADV vector can effectively inhibit H1725 lung cancer cell growth, despite the transient expression characteristics of ADV vectors. Tumor cell growth appears to be more dependent on oncogenic Ras protein function as compared with that of normal p21*ras*.[47] This may explain our observation that moderate decreases in overall p21*ras* expression (but preferential depletion of oncogenic *ras* by KRbz) can lead to >90% growth inhibition in the K-*ras* codon 12 heterozygous mutant H1725 cells.

Future Considerations

Our observations confirm that the mutant *ras* gene could serve as a specific target for cancer gene modulation.[9,24,38] Ribozymes directed at N-, H- and K-*ras* has been shown to selectively discriminate mutated oncogenes from proto-oncogenes and reversed the transformed phenotype of human melanoma, pancreatic and bladder carcinomas.[37,38,40,48] The moderate suppression of p21*ras* expression in KRbz-treated cultures may be explained by the heterozygous genotype of H1725 cells, where normal p21*ras* may continue to be expressed and unaffected by KRbz treatment. Nevertheless, modulation of K-*ras* codon 12 mutant gene expression by plasmid or ADV was effective in suppressing >90% of lung cancer cell growth. Thus the same treatment may be potentially applicable for the treatment of lung cancers having the same single base pair substitution in K-*ras* codon 12. We plan further studies to verify the enhanced growth-inhibitory efficacy of this KRbz-Adv vector in comparison with K-*ras* AS-ODNs of the same specificity.

Based on kinetic studies, we have optimized the anti-K-*ras* ribozyme with a 12 base optimal length flanking sequence to maximize the turnover rate of the ribozyme and to enhance its efficacy. Recent studies suggest that modifications of the hammerhead ribozyme basic structure may further enhance its efficacy. 2'-fluoro-2'-deoxyuridine/cytidine-substituted N-*ras* ribozymes have prolonged stability in vitro and comparable catalytic activity as their unmodified counterpart.[41] The introduction of terminal phosphorothioate groups may further improve stability without loss of efficacy.[41] Alternatively, oligonucleotide facili-

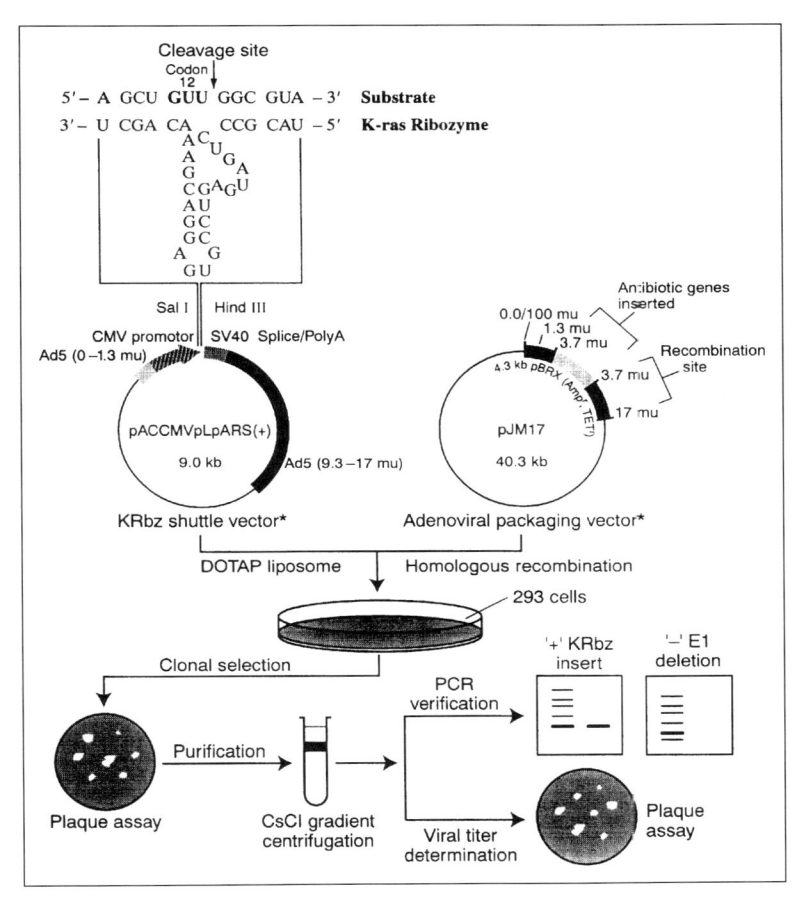

Fig. 12.2. Generation of KRbz-ADV. The K-*ras* ribozyme hammerhead sequence targets the GUU mutant mRNA sequence of K-*ras* codon 12. The ribozyme sequence was subcloned into the *Hind*III and *Sal*I site of pACCMVpLpARS (+) to form the shuttle plasmid KRbz-pACCMVpLpA. This ribozyme expression shuttle vector and the adenoviral packaging plasmid pJM17 were cotransfected into HEK293 cells to generate the KRbz-ADV by homologous recombination. Standard protocols were used for purification of viral vectors from transfected cultures, verification of KRbz insert in viral DNA and determination of viral stock titer.[60]

tators that are inserted at 3' and 5' ends of the flanking sequence can potentially pre-form the substrate for ribozyme attack,[49] thereby promoting ribozyme-substrate association as well as the cleavage rate. These facilitators produce the most pronounced improvements for long substrates (>900 bp) cleavage, although short substrate (<40 bp) cleavage was also improved by 4-fold.[50] Minizymes, hammerhead ribozymes with short oligonucleotide linkers instead of stem-loop II, have been produced with high specific activity. Minizymes form dimeric structures with a common stem II which endow homodimers with a biphasic cleavage activity, and allow heterodimers to simultaneously cleave a substrate at two different sites.[51,52] These mechanisms account for the higher catalytic activity of minizymes as

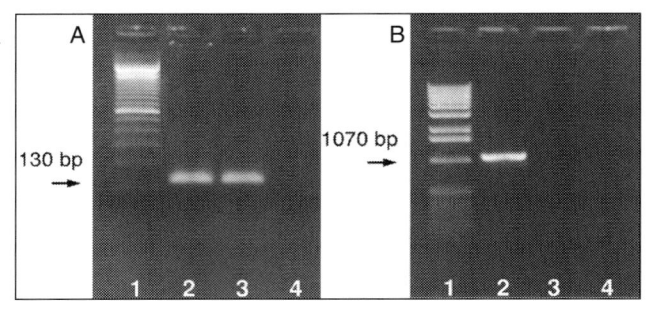

Fig. 12.3. PCR analysis of the KRbz-ADV vector. Purity of KRbz-ADV preparations was determined by PCR, using KRbz sequence-specific primers (A) and primers for detecting the presence of wt adenoviral DNA (E1 region) sequence (B).

(A): Lane 1, DNA Marker; Lane 2, pACCMVpLpA KRbz plasmid (positive control); Lane 3, KRbz-ADV vector; Lane 4, water control. Primers used are: 5'-primer: 5'-GCGTGTACGGTGGGAGGTCT-3' (CMV promoter); 3'-primer: 5'-GTTTCGTCC-TCACGGACTCAT-3' (KRbz insert); for 32 cycles of amplification. (B): Lane 1, DNA Marker; Lane 2, wt adenovirus type 2 DNA (positive control); Lane 3, KRbz-ADV vector; Lane 4, water control. 5'-primer: 5'-ATTACCGAAGAA-ATGGCCGC (1.64 mu); 3'-primer: 5'-CCCATTTAACACGCCATGCA (4.60 mu); for 29 cycles of amplification. Sensitivity of wt adenoviral DNA (E1A) detection is ≥ 1 pg.

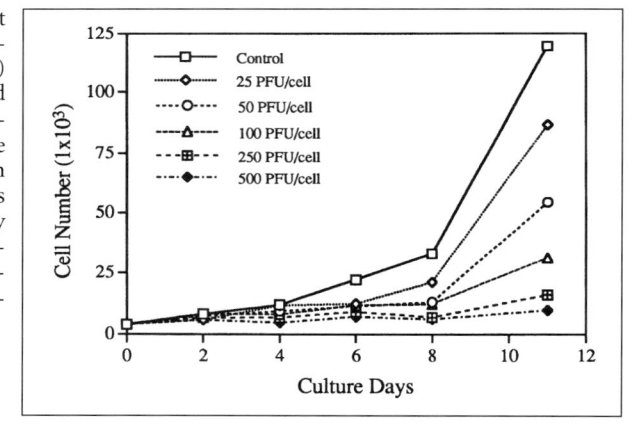

Fig. 12.4. Dose-dependent growth inhibition by KRbz-ADV. H1725 cells (4 x 10³/well) were infected with graded doses of KRbz-ADV (25-500 PFU/cell; 90 min). The average (n = 2) cell numbers in treated and control cultures were determined through day 11 post-infection. Control cultures were treated with medium alone. Duplicate variations are <20%.

compared with the parent hammerhead ribozyme. Such structural modifications presumably may be combined with approaches that upregulate the activity of ribozyme-activating proteins in vivo.[53,54]

Finally, KRbz growth inhibition may be enhanced by concomitant targeting of other oncogene/tumor suppressor gene candidates. Subsequent to establishing the patient's tumor oncogenetic phenotype (Table 12.1), administration of multiple relevant ribozyme/minizyme agents of proven efficacy could conceivably produce an additive/synergistic growth inhibitory effect. The reconstitution of wild type (wt) *p53* function induced either growth suppression or apoptosis in *p53*-mutant NSCLC cells.[55] This *p53*-targeted gene modulation approach appears more effective than ribozymes directed at endogenous mutant *p53* pre-messenger RNAs.[56] Serial direct injection of a wt *p53*-retroviral similarly produced tumor regression in previously chemorefractory NSCLC patients.[57,58] Thus the suppression of mutant K-*ras* expression by the K-*ras* ribozyme, together with wt *p53* gene replacement, represents a promising combination gene therapy approach for NSCLC.

Table 12.6. Decreased [³H]-Thymidine uptake in KRbz-ADV-treated H1725 cell cultures[a]

Experiment no.	% Inhibition ± SD[b]
1	60 ± 12
2	78 ± 12
3	56 ± 4
Mean	65 ± 9

[a]H1725 cells (1 x 10⁴/well) were infected by KRbz-ADV (25C PFU/cell) and cultured for 48 hours. [³H]-thymidine (0.15 µCi/well) was added for additional 16 hours. Value represents mean of 3 to 6 replicas.
[b]compared with culture with medium only; SD: standard deviation.

Table 12.5. Decrease in p21^{ras} expression in KRbz-ADV-treated cultures[a]

	% Total (Mean ± SD)[b]		
	Strongly Reactive	**Moderate/ Weakly Reactive**	**Non-Reactive**
Untreated	74.2 ± 5.0	20.2 ± 4.8	5.6 ± 2.0
KRbz-treated	44.4 ± 9.2 **	31.2 ± 5.9 *	24.6 ± 7.5 **

[a]determined with cytospin preparations at 48 hours after transfection, using the pan-Ras monoclonal antibody Ab-3 (Oncogene Science) and the immunoperoxidase technique (Ventana Automated Systems).[6]
[b]differs statistically from untreated sample (student's t test; * $p < 0.05$, ** $p < 0.001$).

Acknowledgments

This work was supported in part by the Robert Schanbaum Memorial Fund, the Edward and Ruth Wilkof Foundation and the Tri Delta Cancer Research Fund.

References

1. Ginsberg R, Vokes E, Raben A. Non-small cell lung cancer. In: DeVita VJ, Hellman S, Rosenberg S, eds. Cancer: Principles and Practice of Oncology. 5th ed. Philadelphia: Lippincott-Raven, 1997:858-911.
2. Bishop J. Molecular themes in oncogenes. Cell 1991; 64:235-248.
3. Hunter T. Cooperation between oncogenes. Cell 1991; 64:249-270.
4. Levin W, Press M, Gaynor R et al. Expression patterns of immediate early transcription factors in human non-small cell lung cancer. Oncogene 1995; 11(7):1261-1269.
5. Strauss GM, Kwiatkowski DJ, Harpole DH, Lynch TJ, Skarin AT, Sugarbaker DJ. Molecular and pathologic markers in stage I non-small-cell carcinoma of the lung. J Clin Oncol 1995; 13:1265-1279.
6. Nemunaitis J, Klemow S, Tong A et al. Prognostic value of K-*ras* mutations, *ras* oncoprotein and c-erb B-2 oncoprotein expression in adenocarcinoma of the lung. Am J Clin Oncol 1997; 21:155-160.
7. Minna J. The molecular biology of lung cancer pathogenesis. Chest 1993; 103:445S-456S.

8. Rodenhuis S. Ras oncogenes and human lung cancer. In: Pass H, Mitchell J, Johnson D, Turrisi A, eds. Lung Cancer: Principles and Practice. Philadelphia: Lippincott-Raven, 1996:73-82.
9. Scanlon K, Ohta Y, Ishida H et al. Oligoncleotide-mediated modulation of mammalian gene expression. FASEB J 1995; 9(13):1288-1296.
10. Saijo Y, Uchiyama B, Abe T, Satoh K, Nukiwa T. Contiguous four-guanosine sequence in c-myc antisense phosphorothioate olognucleotides inhibits cell growth on human lung cancer cells: possible involvement of cell adhesion inhibition. Jpn J Cancer Res 1997; 88(1):26-33.
11. Robinson L, Smith L, Fontaine M, Kay H, Mountjoy C, Pirrucello S. c-myc antisense oligodeoxyribonucleotides inhibit proliferation of non-small cell lung cancer. Ann Thorac Surg 1995; 60(6):1583-1591.
12. Lee C, Wu S, Gabrilovich D et al. Antitumor effects of an adenovirus expressing antisense insulin-like growth factor I receptor on human lung cancer cell lines. Cancer Res 1996; 56(13):3038-3041.
13. Olbina G, Cieslak D, Ruzdijic S et al. Reversible inhibition of IL-8 receptor B mRNA expression and proliferation in non-small cell lung cancer by antisense oligonucleotides. Anti-Cancer Res 1996; 16(6B):3525-3530.
14. Schrump D, Chen A, Consoli U. Inhibition of lung cancer proliferation by antisense cyclin D. Cancer Gene Ther 1996; 3(2):131-135.
15. Yamanishi Y, Maeda H, Hiyama K, Ishioka S, Yamakido M. Specific growth inhibition of small cell lung cancer cells by adenovirus vector expressing antisense c-kit transcripts. Jpn J Cancer Res 1996; 87(5):534-542.
16. Dosaka-Akita H, Akie K, Hiroumi H, Kinoshita I, Kawakami Y, Murakami A. Inhibition of proliferation by L-myc antisense DNA for the translational initiation site in human small cell lung cancer. Cancer Res 1995; 55(7):1559-1564.
17. Zhang W, Roth J. Anti-oncogene and tumor suppressor gene therapy-examples from a lung cancer animal model. In Vivo 1994; 8(5):755-769.
18. Georges R, Mukhopadhyay T, Zhang Y, Yen N, Roth J. Prevention of orthotopic human lung cancer growth by intratracheal instillation of a retroviral antisense K-*ras* construct. Cancer Res 1993; 53(8):1743-1746.
19. Mukhopadhyay T, Roth J. A codon 248 p53 mutation retains tumor suppressor function as shown by enhancement of tumor growth by antisense p53. Cancer Res 1993; 53(18):4362-4366.
20. Alemany R, Ruan S, Kataoka M et al. Growth inhibitory effect of anti-K-*ras* adenovirus on lung cancer cells. Cancer Gene Ther 1996; 3(5):296-301.
21. Stewart A, Canitrot Y, Baracchini E, Dean N, Deeley R, Cole S. Reduction of expression of the multidrug resistance protein (MRP) in human tumor cells by antisense phosphorothioate oligonucleotides. Biochem Pharmacol 1996; 51(4):461-469.
22. Agrawal S, Jiang Z, Zhao Q et al. Mixed-backbone oligonucleotides as second generation antisense oligonucleotidess: in vitro and in vivo studies. Proc Natl Acad Sci USA 1997; 94(6):2620-2625.
23. Cech TR, Uhlenbeck OC. Hammerhead nailed down. Nature 1994; 372:39-40.
24. Kijima H, Ishida H, Ohkawa T, Kashani-Sabet M, KJ S. Theraputic applications of ribozymes. Pharmacol Therap 1995; 68:247-267.
25. Cech T. Self-splicing of group I introns. Ann Rev Biochem 1990; 59:543-568.
26. Uhlenbeck O. A small catalytic oligonribonucleotide. Nature 1987; 328:596-600.
27. Koizumi M, Kamiya H, Ohtsuka E. Ribozyme designed to inhibit transformation of NIH3T3 cells by the activated c-Ha-*ras* gene. Gene 1992; 117:179-184.
28. Bennett M, Cullimore J. Selective cleavage of closely related mRNAs by synthetic ribozymes. Nuc Acids Res 1992; 20:831-837.
29. Haseloff J, Gerlach WL. Simple RNA enzymes with new and highly specific endoribonuclease activities. Nature 1988; 334:585-591.
30. Kronenwett R, Haas R, Sczakiel G. Kinetic selectivity of complementary nucleic acids: bcr-abl-directed antisense RNA and ribozymes. J Mol Biol 1996; 259(4):632-644.

31. Ohkawa J, Koguma T, Kohda T, Taira K. Ribozymes: From mechanistic studies to applications in vivo. J Biochem 1995; 118:251-258.
32. Ruffner DE, Stormo GD, Uhlenbeck OC. Sequence requirements of the hammerhead RNA self-cleavage reaction. Biochemistry 1990; 29:10695-10702.
33. Bertrand E, Castanotto D, Zhou C et al. The expression cassette determines the functional activity of ribozymes in mammalian cells by controlling their intracellular localization. RNA 1997; 3(1):75-88.
34. Lieber A, Kay M. Adenovirus-mediated expression of ribozymes in mice. J Virol 1996; 70(5):3153-3158.
35. McCormick F. Signal transduction: How receptors turn ras on. Nature 1993; 363:15-16.
36. Sun J, Qian Y, Hamilton A, Sebti S. Ras CAAX peptidomimetic FTI276 selectively blocks tumor growth in nude mice of a human lung carcinoma with K-ras mutation and p53 deletion. Cancer Res 1995; 55:4243-4247.
37. Funato T, Shitara T, Tone T, Jiao L, Kashani-Sabet M, Scanlon KJ. Suppression of H-ras-mediated transformation in NIH3T3 cells by a ras ribozyme. Biochem Pharmacol 1994; 48:1471-1475.
38. Feng M, Cabrera G, Desane J, Scanlon KJ, Curiel DT. Neoplastic reversion accomplished by high efficiency adenoviral-mediated delivery of an anti-ras ribozyme. Cancer Res 1995; 55: 2024-2028.
39. Kijima H, Bouffard D, Scanlon K. Ribozyme-mediated reversal of human pancreatic carcinoma phenotype. In: Ikehara S, Takaku F, Good R, eds. Proceedings of International Symposium on Bone Marrow Transplantation. Tokyo: Springer-Verlag, 1996:153-163.
40. Ohta Y, Kijima H, Kashani-Sabet M, Scanlon K. Suppression of the malignant phenotype of melanoma cells by anti-oncogene ribozymes. J Invest Dermatol 1996; 106(2):275-280.
41. Scherr M, Grez M, Ganser A, Engels J. Specific hammerhead ribozyme-mediated cleavage of mutant N-ras mRNA in vitro and ex vivo. Oligoribonucleotides as therapeutic agents. J Biol Chem 1997; 272(22):14304-14313.
42. Eastham J, Ahlering T. Use of an anti-ras ribozyme to alter the malignant phenotype of a human bladder cancer cell line. J Urol 1996; 156(3):1186-1188.
43. Kashani-Sabet, M., Scanlon KJ. Application of ribozymes to cancer gene therapy. Cancer Gene Therapy 1995; 2:213-223.
44. Zhang Y, Nemunaitis J, Mues G, Scanlon K, Tong A. In vitro suppression of human non-small cell lung cancer (NSCLC) cell growth by an anti-K-ras ribozyme. FASEB J 1996; 10(6):A1409.
45. Zhang Y, Mues G, Nemunaitis J, Scanlon K, Tong A. Inhibition of human non-small cell lung cancer growth in vitro by a recombinant anti-K-ras adenoviral vector. AACR Proceedings 1997; 38:6.
46. Snyder DS, Wu Y, Wang JL et al. Ribozyme-mediated inhibition of bcr-abl gene expression in a Philadelphia chromosome-positive cell line. Blood 1993; 82:600-605.
47. James G, Goldstein J, Brown M et al. Benzodizepine petidomimetics: Potent inhibitors of ras farnesylation in animal cells. Science 1993; 260:1937-1942.
48. Kashani-Sabet M, Funato T, Tone T et al. Reversal of the malignant phenotype by anti-ras ribozyme. Antisense Res & Develop 1992; 2:3-15.
49. Dedman R. Facilitator oligonucleotides increase ribozyme RNA binding to full-length RNA substrates in vitro. FEBS Letters 1996; 382:116-120.
50. Jankowsky E, Schwenzer B. Efficient improvement of hammerhead ribozyme mediated cleavage of long substrates by oligonucleotide facilitators. Biochemistry 1996; 35(48):15313-15321.
51. Amontov S, Nishikawa S, Taira K. Dependence on Mg++ ions of the activities of dimeric hammerhead minizymes. FEBS Lett 1996; 386(2-3):99-102.
52. Kuwabara T, Amontov S, Warashina M, Ohkawa J, Taira K. Characterization of several kines of dimer minizyme: Simultaneous cleavage at two sites in HIV-1 tat mRNA by dimer minizymes. Nucleic Acids Res 1996; 24(12):2302-2310.
53. Kiehntofp M, Esquivel E, Brach M, Herrman F. Ribozymes: Biology, biochemistry, and implications for clinical medicine. J Mol Med 1995; 73:65-71.

54. Herschlag D, Khosla M, Tsuchihashi Z, Karpel R. An RNA chaperone activity of non-specific RNA binding proteins in hammerhead ribozyme catalysis. EMBO J 1994; 13:2913-2924.
55. Fujiwara T, Kagawa S, Ogawa N et al. Recombinant virus-mediated transfer of the wild-type p53 gene is a potent therapeutic strategy for human cancer. Hum Cell 1996; 9(1):25-30.
56. Cai D, Mukhopadhyay T, Roth J. Suppression of lung cancer cell growth by ribozyme-mediated modification of p53 pre-mRNA. Cancer Gene Ther 1995; 2(3):199-205.
57. Roth J, Nguyen D, Lawrence D et al. Retrovirus-mediated wild-type p53 gene transfer to tumors of patients with lung cancer. Nature Med 1996; 2(9):985-991.
58. Swisher S, Roth J, Lawrence D et al. Persistent transgene expression following repeated injections of a recombinant adenovirus containing the p53 wildtype gene in patients with non-small cell lung cancer. AACR Proceedings 1997; 38:342.
59. Murayama Y, Horiuchi S. Antisense oligonucleotides to p53 tumor suppressor suppress the induction of apoptosis by epidermal growth factor in NCI-H596 human lung cancer cells. Antisense Nucleic Acid Drug Dev 1997; 7(2):109-114.
60. Tong A, Zhang Y, Nemunaitis J, Mues G. K-*ras* ribozyme for lung cancer. In: Scanlon K, ed. Theraputic Application of Ribozymes. Methods in Molecular Medicine. vol. II; Totowa (NJ): Humana 1998:209-222.

CHAPTER 13

Ribozymes in Gene Therapy of Prostate Cancer

Dale J. Voeks, Gary A. Clawson, and James S. Norris

Introduction

Since the discovery of naturally occurring catalytic RNA,[1,2] research in ribozyme design and its implementation in therapy has expanded exponentially. Ribozyme-mediated inhibition of gene expression at the message level allows the mRNA of nearly any gene to be targeted for destruction. Possible applications are limited only by knowledge of the disease. The greatest part of ribozyme utility in therapy thus far has centered on HIV and cancer. Use in HIV protocols has been widespread due to the wealth of targets offered by a well-characterized retroviral genome. In cancer, oncogenes are often overexpressed or mutated in the signal transduction pathway, leading to uncontrolled cell growth. Because the process works through an RNA intermediate, targets are readily available for ribozyme activity. The major focus of ribozymes in gene therapy of cancer has been on inhibition of specific oncogene expression in tumors having a relatively defined genetic basis. In these instances, ribozymes have demonstrated great therapeutic potential. Unfortunately, ribozyme protocols in prostate cancer have been restricted due to an uncertainty of targets.

Prostate Cancer Background

Prostate cancer is the most frequently diagnosed cancer in US males and the second leading cause of cancer death.[3] Although already a major health problem with predicted dramatic increases in incidence and mortality over the next 15 years, the molecular mechanisms behind the disease's initiation and progression remain largely a mystery. The overall value of screening and treatment also remains controversial. PSA is currently the most sensitive marker for screening and monitoring prostate cancer. However, questions of diagnostic accuracy hinder its predictive ability.[4] Therapeutic modalities are limited, mostly ineffective, and defined in large part by stage. Locally confined disease can be controlled with radical prostatectomy and radiation therapy. Treatment for disease with local advancement or distant metastasis includes watchful waiting, radiation therapy, hormonal therapy, and limited chemotherapy. Recurrence rates and mortality with non-localized disease are very high.[4] Further, approximately one-third of patients are in advanced stages of the disease at the time of diagnosis.[5] Additional therapeutic options are clearly necessary.

Gene Therapy in Prostate Cancer

Several prostate cancer gene therapy protocols have been approved for clinical trial. Immunotherapy trials involve either ex vivo gene delivery of interleukin-2 (IL-2) or

Ribozymes in the Gene Therapy of Cancer, edited by Kevin J. Scanlon and Mohammed Kashani-Sabet.
©1998 R.G. Landes Company.

granulocyte-macrophage stimulating factor (GM-CSF), or in vivo gene delivery of prostate-specific antigen (PSA).[6] GM-CSF and IL-2 cytokine-secreting tumor cells proved to have preclinical efficacy as therapeutic vaccines in the Dunning rat model of prostate cancer.[7,8] A tumor-specific host immune response can also be generated by in vivo transfer of the prostate tumor antigen gene.[9] In another clinical trial, transfer of herpes simplex virus thymidine kinase (HSV-tk) creates susceptibility to cytotoxic ganciclovir treatment.[10] The final approach targets c-*myc* by antisense technology for therapy of late stage androgen-resistant cancer.[11]

A large body of prostate cancer therapeutic research covering a wide range of strategies is currently in preclinical stages. Due to advances in vector biology, cytokine delivery in vivo has emerged as a viable alternative to ex vivo approaches.[7] In addition, a number of genes such as p53, Rb, E-cadherin and androgen receptor have been found mutated or with altered levels of expression in late stage prostate cancer.[12-15] Gene therapy strategies directed at these late stage changes have been developed. Delivery of cell adhesion molecules (CAMs) or an active form of the androgen receptor into advanced stage prostate cancer cells displaying decreased E-cadherin expression and androgen independence induced a strong antiproliferative response.[16,17] Introduction of the cell cycle and apoptosis regulatory genes p21 and p53 resulted in reduced tumorgenicity.[18,19] Similarly, transfection of Rb inhibited prostate tumor cell growth.[20] As the understanding of prostate cancer grows, so too will the number of potential gene therapy approaches.

Ribozymes in Prostate Cancer

With the explosion of ribozyme technology, their involvement in prostate cancer gene therapy remains conspicuously absent. A sequential series of activations and inactivations of oncogenes and tumor suppressor genes has not been elucidated in prostate cancer as they have, for example, in colon cancer.[21] Because specific genetic alterations are relatively unknown or represent only a limited number of the tumors, ribozyme strategies cannot rely solely on inhibition of oncogene expression. The target needs to be more universal, encompassing all prostate cancers rather than just a subset containing a specific oncogene or tumor suppressor gene dysfunction.

Ribozyme Target

RNA polymerase I (RNA pol I) is responsible for the transcription of ribosomal genes (rDNA). rDNA constitutes only 1% of the genome but accounts for 40% of total cellular transcription and 80% of the RNA content of the cell.[22] The ribosomal RNA (rRNA) is cleaved to mature rRNA, which interacts with ribosomal proteins to form the ribosome complex necessary for translation and protein synthesis. This immense undertaking is completely dependent on activated RNA pol I and its associated factors. A ribozyme targeted to this essential player in growth and viability would exert a profound impact on the cell. Indeed, Rb may repress cellular proliferation by disrupting RNA pol I-mediated transcription through interaction with its transcription factor UBF, which hinders formation of the initiation complex.[23,24]

A ribozyme was targeted to bind and cleave at a susceptible site in subunit AC40 of RNA pol I (Fig. 13.1). The AC40 subunit is highly conserved among distant eukaryotes, suggesting its importance as a core component of RNA pol I.[25] AC40 was also found to be a shared subunit with RNA polymerase III.[26] Therefore, a ribozyme targeted to this subunit may also interfere with tRNA production to further disrupt protein synthesis.

The RNA pol I targeted ribozyme was cloned between 5' and 3' autocatalytic ribozyme sequences to form a triple ribozyme (TR) (Fig. 13.2). The two cis-acting ribozymes undergo self-cleavage, releasing the internal RNA pol I targeted ribozyme as a short uniform

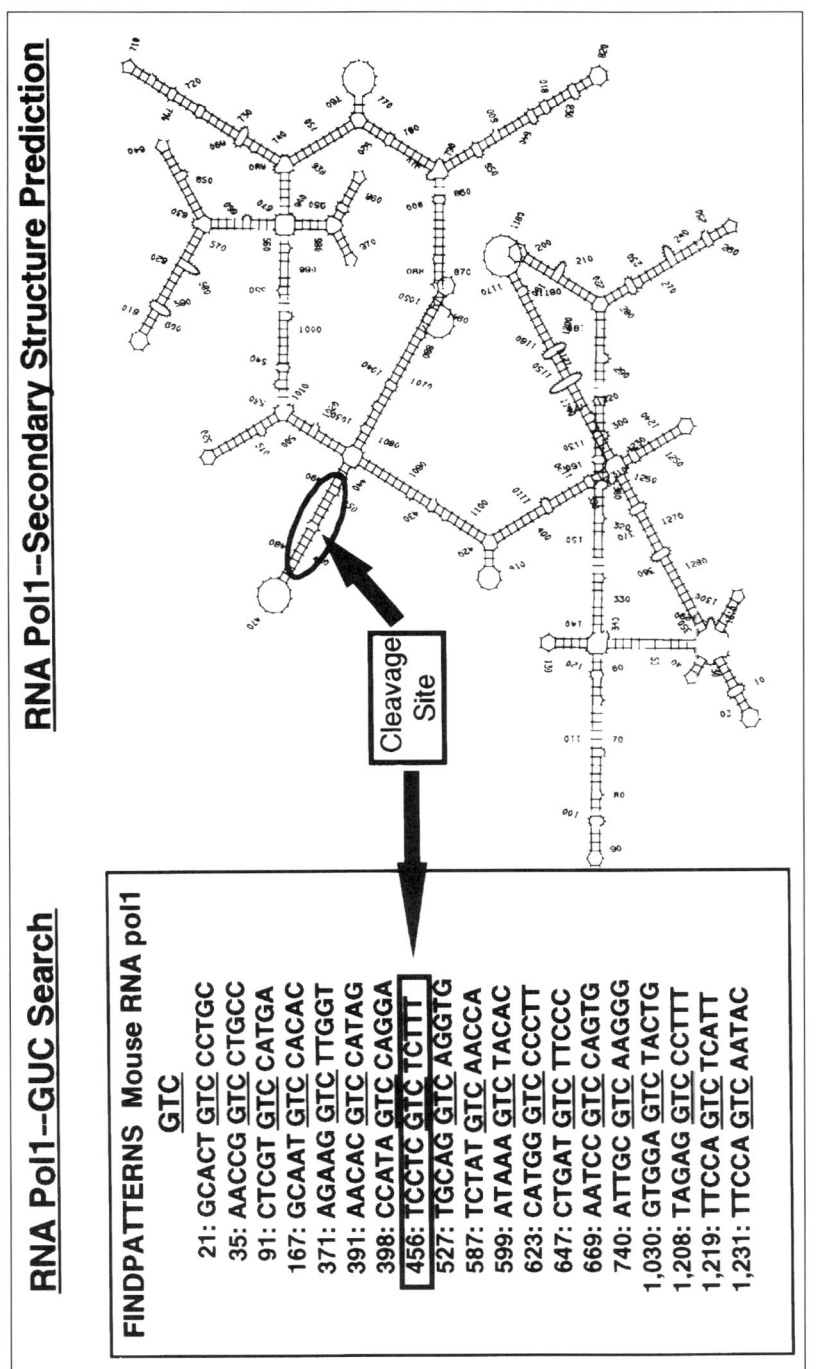

Fig. 13.1. Ribozyme target site (RNA polymerase I). To identify potential ribozyme cleavage sites, the sequence of mouse RNA pol I was searched for the presence of the nucleotide triplet GUC. Secondary RNA structure of the RNA pol I transcript was then predicted using the program MFOLD. Susceptible regions of the transcript sequence containing GUC were identified. The region at nucleotide 457–459 indicated by the arrow was chosen as the target cleavage site.

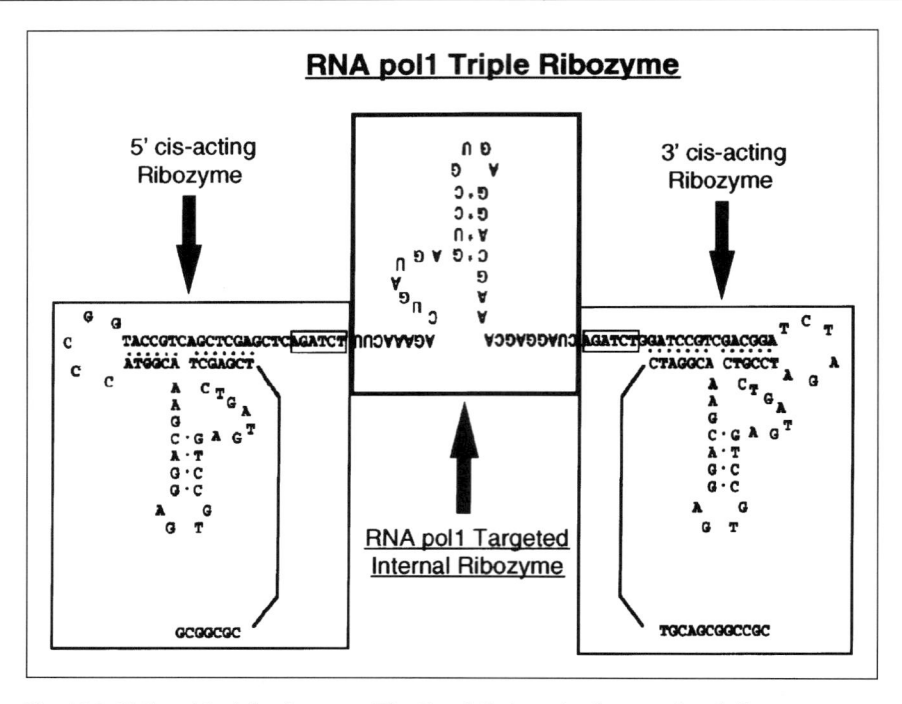

Fig. 13.2. RNA pol I triple ribozyme. The 5' and 3' cis-acting hammerhead ribozymes were designed to bind and undergo self-cleavage at GUC sequences by homology of 13 bases, thereby releasing the internal RNA pol I (subunit AC40) targeted ribozyme with defined 5' and 3' ends.

RNA to avoid compromised activity due to non-specific flanking sequences.[27] Transfection of TR into mouse fibroblast cells resulted in a 50% decrease in RNA pol I message levels (50% transfection efficiency).[27] The reduction of RNA pol I mRNA caused by the activity of the triple ribozyme was sufficient to markedly diminish cell population compared to a mutant non-catalytic version of the ribozyme acting in antisense fashion.[27] Hence, the ribozyme is able to decrease ribosomal gene transcription through knockout of the polymerase to a level significant enough to realize cell killing activity. However, application of the RNA pol I triple ribozyme to prostate cancer gene therapy requires highly restricted targeting of expression to the tissue of interest, to prevent collateral damage in other tissues.

Tissue Specificity

Tumors often sustain the ability to produce proteins specific for the tissue from which the neoplasm arose.[28] To exploit this transcriptional specificity, essential promoter regions can be defined and used to restrict expression of an exogenous gene of interest. Although transcriptional targeting is generally considered to be tissue-specific, a number of promoters can also be thought of as tumor-specific if the normal tissues are not essential for viability or accessible to the introduced DNA.[29] Prostate tissue can be technically considered nonessential, thereby defining prostate-specific promoters as both tissue-specific and tumor-specific.[29] The coupling of cytotoxic or apoptosis-inducing genes to prostate-specific promoters is a promising approach to prostate cancer gene therapy.

The expression of a number of proteins is strongly restricted to prostate tissue. PSA is the most notable example. PSA production is nearly exclusive to both normal and, in most cases, neoplastic luminal prostatic epithelial cells.[30] Its androgen regulated promoter region has been isolated and characterized.[31] A minimal PSA promoter segment was able to drive expression of a reporter gene in LNCaP cells (PSA-producing human prostate cancer cell line) without showing activity in lines of non-prostatic origin.[32] A larger 6 kb PSA promoter fragment containing an additional upstream enhancer region demonstrated prostate-specific expression of a reporter gene in transgenic mice mirroring the expression patterns seen in humans.[33] Research to further refine the promoter regulatory elements necessary for tissue specificity and maximum expression continues.[34,35] Nonetheless, the PSA promoter has already shown significant potential in prostate cancer gene therapy. The adenoviral gene E1A, DNA polymerase-α and topoisomerase IIα under transcriptional control of the PSA promoter displayed both specificity of expression and cytotoxicity in PSA-expressing cancer cells.[32,36]

Similarly, androgen regulated rat probasin production occurs predominantly in the dorsal and lateral regions of the prostate.[37] A minimal probasin promoter region driving expression of a reporter construct in transgenic mice displayed highly specific expression restricted to the lateral, dorsal and ventral lobes of the prostate, with very limited expression also observed in the anterior prostate and seminal vesicles but nowhere else in the body.[38] The highest level occurred in the mouse dorsolateral prostate, which correlates to the peripheral zone of the human prostate where the majority and most invasive forms of human cancer arise.[39] A larger promoter fragment containing both androgen and zinc regulatory regions was able to direct higher and more consistent levels of expression in subsequent research.[40] Expression patterns of the probasin promoter have yet to be determined in human tissue but, at minimum, the promoter sequence has utility in the transcriptional targeting of prostate cancer gene therapy constructs for evaluation of effect in animal model systems.

By coupling to the minimal probasin promoter, the cell killing effects of the RNA pol I targeted triple ribozyme can be highly restricted to prostatic epithelium and its neoplastic derivatives. The activity of the probasin-driven triple ribozyme (PBTR) construct was evaluated in a recently developed mouse prostate tumor cell line (TRAMP) (kindly provided by Norman M. Greenberg). Transient transfection of a probasin-driven Seap reporter construct showed that the probasin promoter was able to drive expression of a heterologous gene in this cell line. Initiation of maximal expression occurred between day one and two with slightly increasing intensity thereafter.[41] Transfection of PBTR into the prostate tumor cells reduced cellular proliferation beginning between day one and two as compared to control transfected cells (Fig. 13.3).[42] The span of decreased cell growth corresponded to a diminished level of RNA pol I (subunit AC40) as judged by Western blot analysis (unpublished). As these were transient transfections at low efficiency, a marked deviation in cell number occurred for several days only before returning to normalcy (presumably when the transduced cells were removed from the population following expression of the triple ribozyme).

For evaluation of therapeutic potential on tumor tissue in vivo (TRAMP xenografts), the PBTR construct was administered via intra-tumoral injection utilizing a cationic liposomal vehicle. Both single administration and repeated administration on three consecutive days demonstrated a consistent reduction in tumor growth between approximately day two and day six post-administration followed by a return to the normal tumor growth curve (Fig. 13.4)[42] compared to control injections (data not shown). Reporter construct delivery under the same conditions indicated extremely low liposomal gene transfer (unpublished). Still, the overall trend of reduced tumor burden displayed in a transient manner following

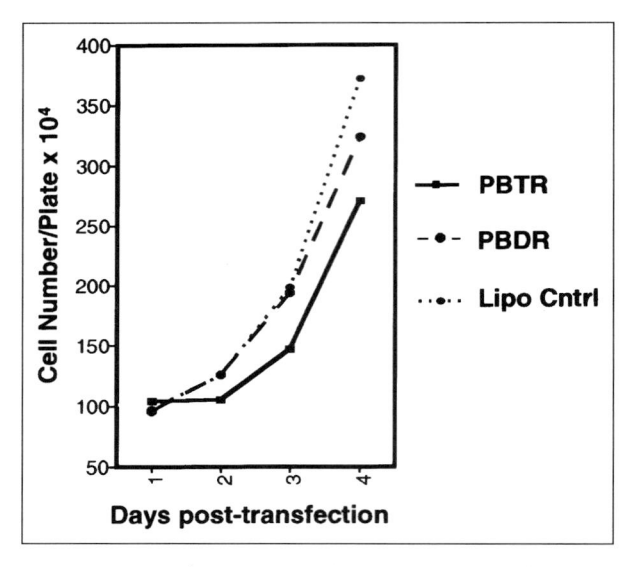

Fig. 13.3. Transfection assay (probasin-RNA pol I triple ribozyme). TRAMP cells were transfected with the probasin-driven RNA pol I targeted triple ribozyme (PBTR), the identical construct without the internal ribozyme (PBDR) or mock transfected with liposome only (Lipo Cntrl). Cell number was determined daily. Reprinted with permission, Cancer Gene Therapy. Savage LM, ed. Southborough, MA: International Business Communications, Inc. 1997.

injection of the probasin-driven triple ribozyme offers the promise of increased effectiveness through use of a more efficient delivery vehicle.

Conclusions

Ribozymes have displayed significant therapeutic potential in a number of malignancies. Due to the relatively poor understanding of the molecular events responsible for prostate cancer initiation and progression, target sites for ribozyme design are not overly clear. To overcome this and the variable genetics associated with each stage of prostate cancer, ribozymes can be designed to have universal cell killing effects if properly targeted to the tissue of interest. Prostate epithelial cell-specific knockout of a key gene in cellular growth and viability is capable of localized cell killing, with the potential for tracking metastasized tumor cells. The initial reduction in tumor burden caused by liposomal delivery of the probasin-driven RNA pol I triple ribozyme indicates the possible translation of a prostate-specific RNA pol I ribozyme therapy strategy to human cancer if increased levels of cell killing can be achieved with improved delivery. However, even with stronger research emphasis, delivery remains the major rate-limiting step in most gene therapy protocols. Besides improved efficiency, targeted delivery coupled with the expanding list of tissue-specific regulatory elements will allow both direct delivery to the tumor site and systemic delivery to treat metastatic sites. Also, increased molecular knowledge of malignancies will identify additional ribozyme targets. The potential of ribozymes in gene therapy, in general, and prostate cancer therapy, in particular, will eventually be realized if advances in ribozyme technology, delivery vectors, and the genetics of disease continue at the current rate.

Ribozymes in Gene Therapy of Prostate Cancer

Tumor Growth Curve

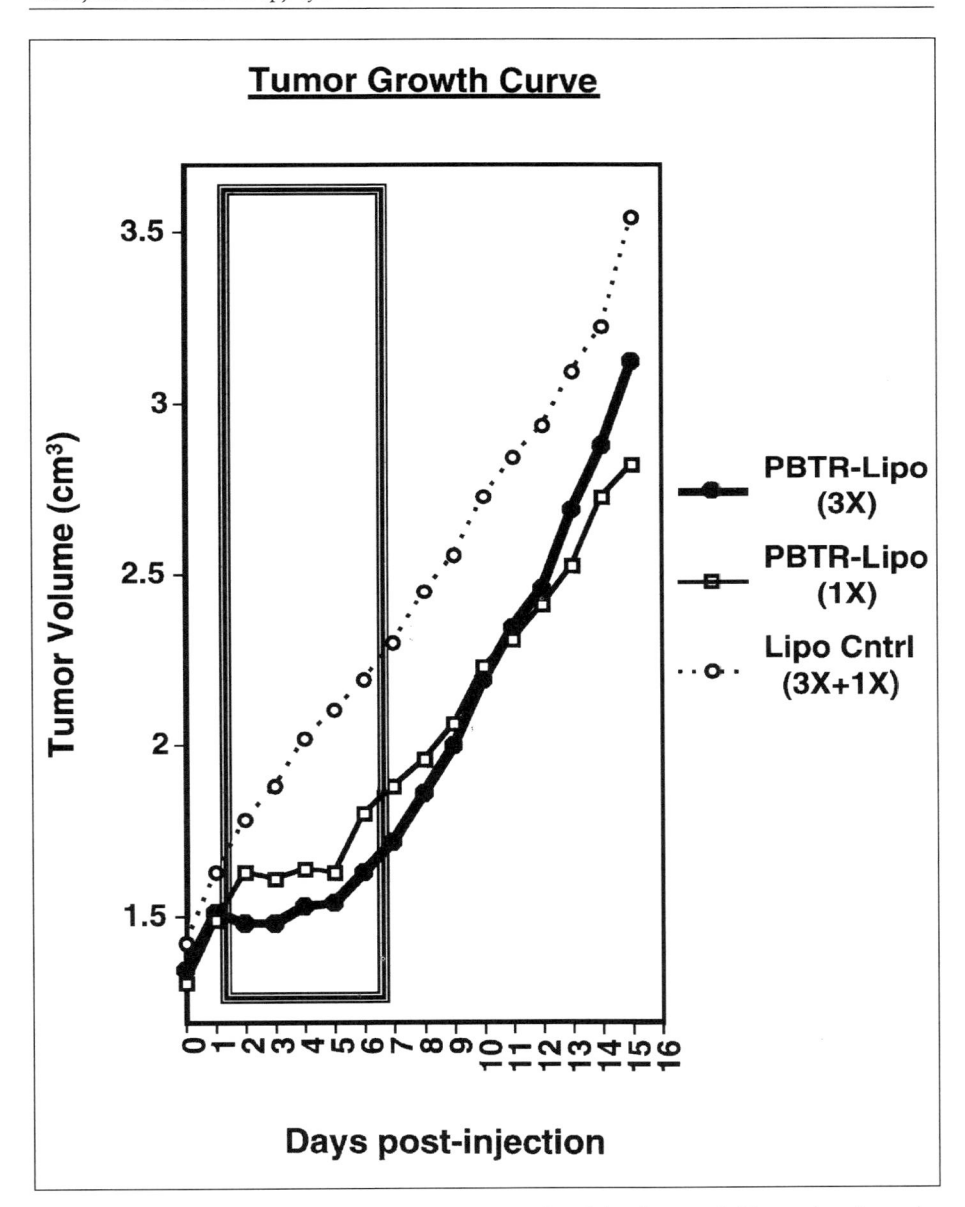

Fig. 13.4. Tumor grafting studies (probasin-RNA pol1 triple ribozyme). Tumor-bearing mice were generated by subcutaneous injection of TRAMP cells. Direct intra-tumoral injections of PBTR-liposome complexes (PBTR-Lipo) or liposome only (Lipo Cntrl) were performed as a single administration (1x) or a repeated administration on three consecutive days (3x). Tumor volume was calculated from standard caliper measurement. Lipo Cntrl showed no deviation from normal tumor growth curves. A consistent reduction in tumor growth was observed between ≈ day two and day six postadministration of PBTR.

References

1. Cech TR, Bass BL. Biological catalysis by RNA. Annu Rev Biochem 1986; 55:599-629.
2. Altman S. Ribonuclease P: an enzyme with a catalytic RNA subunit. Adv Enzymol Relat Areas Mol Biol 1989; 62:1-36.
3. Parker SL, Tong T, Bolden S et al. Cancer statistics. CA Cancer J Clin 1997; 47(1):5-27.
4. Cersosimo RJ, Carr D. Prostate cancer: Current and evolving strategies. Am J Health Syst Pharm 1996; 53(4):381-396.
5. Konety BR, Getzenberg RH. Novel therapies for advanced prostate cancer. Semin Urol Oncol 1997; 15(1):33-42.
6. Sanda MG. Biological principles and clinical development of prostate cancer gene therapy. Sem Urol Oncol 1997; 15(1):43-55.
7. Sanda MG, Ayyagari SR, Jaffee EM et al. Demonstration of a rational strategy for human prostate cancer gene therapy. J Urol 1994; 151(3):622-628.
8. Viewig J, Rosenthal FM, Bannerji R et al. Immunotherapy of prostate cancer in the Dunning rat model: Use of cytokine gene modified tumor vaccines. Cancer Res 1994; 54(7):1760-1765.
9. Xue BH, Zhang Y, Sosman JA et al. Induction of human cytotoxic T lymphocytes specific for prostate-specific antigen. Prostate 1997; 30(2):73-78.
10. Hall SJ, Mutchnik SE, Chen SH et al. Adenovirus-mediated herpes simplex virus thymidine kinase gene and ganciclovir therapy leads to systemic activity against spontaneous and induced metastasis in an orthotopic mouse model of prostate cancer. Int J Cancer 1997; 70(2):183-187.
11. Hrouda D, Dalgeish AG. Gene therapy for prostate cancer. Gene Ther 1996; 3(10):845-852.
12. Dahiya R, Deng G, Chen KM et al. p53 tumour-suppressor gene mutations are mainly localized on exon 7 in human primary and metastatic prostate cancer. Br J Cancer 1996; 74(2):264-268.
13. Kubota Y, Fujinami K, Uemura H et al. Retinoblastoma gene mutations in primary human prostate cancer. Prostate 1995; 27(6):314-320.
14. Umbas R, Schalken JA, Aalders TW et al. Expression of the cellular adhesion molecule E-cadherin is reduced or absent in high-grade prostate cancer. Cancer Res 1992; 52(18):5104-5109.
15. Tilley WD, Wilson CM, Morcelli M et al. Androgen receptor gene expression in human prostate carcinoma cell lines. Cancer Res 1990; 50(17):5382-5386.
16. Kleinerman DI, Zhang WW, Lin SH et al. Application of a tumor suppressor (C-CAM1)-expressing recombinant adenovirus in androgen-independent human prostate cancer therapy: a preclinical study. Cancer Res 1995; 55(13):2831-2836.
17. Yuan S, Trachtenberg J, Mills GB et al. Androgen-induced inhibition of cell proliferation in an androgen-insensitive prostate cancer cell line (PC-3) transfected with a human androgen receptor complementary DNA. Cancer Res 1993; 53(6):1304-1311.
18. Yang C, Cirielli C, Capogrossi MC et al. Adenovirus-mediated wild-type p53 expression induces apoptosis and suppresses tumorigenesis of prostatic tumor cells. Cancer Res 1995; 55(19):4210-4213.
19. Eastham JA, Hall SJ, Sehgal I et al. In vivo gene therapy with p53 or p21 adenovirus for prostate cancer. Cancer Res 1995; 55(22):5151-5155.
20. Bookstein R, Shew JY, Chen PH et al. Suppression of tumorigenicity of human prostate carcinoma cells by replacing a mutated RB gene. Science 1990; 247(4943):712-715.
21. Cho KR, Vogelstein B. Genetic alterations in the adenoma-carcinoma sequence. Cancer 1992; 70(6 suppl): 1727-1731.
22. Moss T, Stefanovsky VY. Promotion and regulation of ribosomal transcription in eukaryotes by RNA polymerase I. Prog Nucleic Acid Res Mol Biol 1995; 50:25-66.
23. Cavanaugh AH, Hempel WM, Taylor LJ et al. Activity of RNA polymerase I transcription factor UBF blocked by Rb gene product. Nature 1995; 374(6518):177-180.
24. Voit R, Schafer K, Grummit I. Mechanism of repression of RNA polymerase I transcription by retinoblastoma protein. Mol Cell Biol 1997; 17(8):4230-4237.

25. Song CZ, Hanada K, Yano K et al. High conservation of subunit compostion of RNA polymerase I(A) between yeast and mouse and the molecular cloning of mouse RNA polymerase I 40-kDa subunit RPA40. J Biol Chem 1994; 269(43):26976-26981.
26. Lanzendorfer M, Smid A, Klinger C et al. A shared subunit belongs to the eukaryotic core RNA polymerase. Gene Dev 1997; 11(8):1037-1047.
27. Clawson GA. (personal communciation).
28. Hart IR. Tissue specific promoters in targeting systemically delivered gene therapy. Semin Oncol 1996; 23(1):154-158.
29. Deonarain MP, Spooner RA, Epenetos AA. Genetic delivery of enzymes for cancer therapy. Gene Ther 1995; 2(4):235-244.
30. Peehl DM. Prostate specific antigen role and function. Cancer 1995; 75(7 suppl): 2021-2026.
31. Lundwall A. Characterization of the gene for prostate-specific antigen, a human glandular kallikrein. Biochem Biophys Res Commun 1989; 161(3):1151-1156.
32. Lee CH, Liu M, Sie KL et al. Prostate-specific antigen promoter driven gene therapy targeting DNA polymerase-α and topoisomerase IIα in prostate cancer. Anticancer Res 1996;16(4A):1805-1812.
33. Cleutjens KB, van der Korput HA, van Eekelen CC et al. A 6-kb promoter fragment mimics in transgenic mice the prostate-specific and androgen-regulated expression of the endogenous prostate-specific antigen gene in humans. Mol Endocrinol 1997; 11(9):1256-1264.
34. Zhang S, Murtha PE, Young CY. Defining a functional androgen responsive element in the 5' far upstream flanking region of the prostate-specific antigen gene. Biochem Biophys Res Commun 1997; 231(3):784-788.
35. Pang S, Dannull J, Kaboo R et al. Identification of a positive regulatory element responsible for tissue-specific expression of prostate-specific antigen. Cancer Res 1997; 57(3):495-499.
36. Rodriguez R, Schuur ER, Lim HY et al. Prostate attenuated replication competent adenovirus (ARCA) CN706: A selective cytotoxic for prostate-specific antigen-positive prostate cancer cells. Cancer Res 1997; 57(13):2559-2563.
37. Spence AM, Sheppard PC, Davie JR et al. Regulation of a bifunctional mRNA results in synthesis of secreted and nuclear probasin. Proc Natl Acad Sci USA 1989; 86(20):7843-7847.
38. Greenberg NM, DeMayo FJ, Sheppard PC et al. The rat probasin gene promoter directs hormonally and developmentally regulation of a heterologous gene specifically to the prostate in transgenic mice. Mol Endocrinol 1994; 8(2):230-239.
39. Price D. Comparative aspects of development and structure in the prostate. In: Vollmer EP, Kauffman G, eds. Biology of the Prostate and Related Tissues. Washington DC: US Government Printing Office, 1963:1-28.
40. Yan Y, Sheppard PC, Kasper S et al. A large fragment of the probasin promoter targets high levels of transgene expression to the prostate of transgenic mice. Prostate 1997; 32:129-139.
41. Voeks DJ, Clawson GA, Norris JS. Tissue-specific triple ribozyme vectors for prostate cancer gene therapy. Gene Ther Mol Biol 1998; 1:407-418.
42. Voeks DJ, Staley MC, Greenberg NM et al. Prostate cancer gene therapy using targeted expression of ribozymes against the AC40 subunit of RNA poll. In: Savage L, ed. Cancer Gene Therapy. IBC 1997:213-222.

CHAPTER 14

Ribozymes in Targeting Tumor Suppressor Genes

Tapas Mukhopadhyay and Jack A. Roth

A promising approach to gene therapy for cancer involves decreasing the level of abnormal proteins by specific interference with gene expression at the mRNA level. The expression of a specific mRNA can be suppressed using a number of antisense approaches, including ribozymes. Ribozymes are catalytic RNA molecules that can destroy the target RNA. Ribozymes have several advantages over other available antisense approaches. Ribozymes can inactivate the target RNA without relying on the host cell's machinery, and they can cleave more than one copy of the target RNA by dissociating from the cleavage products and binding to another target molecule. Furthermore, ribozymes are effective in modulating gene expression because of their simple structure, site-specific cleavage activity, and catalytic potential. The targets of ribozyme-mediated gene modulation range from cancer cells to foreign genes that cause infectious diseases, and additional target sites are being developed. The numerous genes against which ribozymes have been targeted include oncogenes (*ras*, *BCR-ABL*), telomeres, and drug-resistance genes (*mdr*1, *c-fos*). The demonstration that target RNA can be cleaved by cis ribozymes (catalytic RNAs, RNA enzymes) has potentially important therapeutic implications.

Introduction

Certain RNA molecules have enzymatic activity, as was first described for the autocatalytic removal of the intervening sequence from the large ribosomal RNA precursor of *Tetrahymena thermophila*. Catalytic RNAs have now been described in a number of systems ranging from bacteria to human. The ubiquity of catalytic RNA has prompted intense investigation into the understanding of its macromolecular function and potential application in the therapy of genetic diseases, including cancer.[1-3]

Tumor cells undergo profound genetic alterations before a malignant phenotype is established. Genetic changes such as mutation or overexpression can lead to oncogene activation, and these events are clearly important in the etiology of cancer. Structural and functional alterations in a number of vital genes have been associated with a high percentage of human cancers. Current experimental clinical approaches involve selectively killing cells with unique cancer-related phenotypes, such as cell surface antigens or growth factor receptors, or altering the host immune system to attack cancer cells. However, the key to specific cancer therapy is likely to be the identification and targeting of processes that are unique to the tumor. Cells expressing mutations in the oncoproteins that lead to the development of the cancer are therefore ideal targets for gene therapy.

Ribozymes in the Gene Therapy of Cancer, edited by Kevin J. Scanlon and Mohammed Kashani-Sabet.
©1998 R.G. Landes Company.

The inhibition of abnormally functioning oncogenes or tumor suppressor genes, and thus the alteration of the malignant phenotype of the cell,[4] is theoretically attractive, but such biological therapy is beset with major logistic difficulties. Mutations in the vital genes could lead to the production of faulty proteins with altered biological functions. During the multistep process of carcinogenesis, a number of such faulty gene products accumulate and provide a growth advantage to the cancer cells.

There are many ways to affect the activity of gene products: Ribozyme targeting of mRNA is one of them. Ribozymes are a group of catalytic RNA molecules that cleave targeted RNAs in a sequence-specific manner that is unique in their class. Ribozymes have the potential to cycle; that is, having cleaved one target RNA, they can move on to the next. For this reason, catalytic RNAs and their counterparts are being assessed as potential tools for future gene therapy.

General Considerations for Ribozyme Function

The demonstration that RNA can be cleaved by ribozymes (catalytic RNAs, RNA enzymes) may have important therapeutic implications. Ribozymes are suitable for the modulation of gene expression because of their simple structure, site-specific cleavage activity, and catalytic potential. Ribozymes, a class of antisense agents, are small catalytic RNAs that were initially discovered in a group-I self-splicing intron of the *Tetrahymena* pre-rRNA.[5] Examples of these types of catalytic RNAs have now been found in many plants and animals. Ribozymes are small oligo-ribonucleotides whose specific catalytic domain has endonuclease activity.[6-8] This activity can be directed against virtually any RNA target by the insertion of an antisense region into the ribozyme, but a GUC consensus sequence in the target RNA is required at the targeted cleavage site. A typically altered ribozyme, called a "hammerhead" ribozyme, is shown in Figure 14.1.

Despite so many promising attributes, ribozymes have their shortcomings. A major disadvantage is that, being an RNA, ribozymes are particularly sensitive to nuclease digestion. A number of modifications in ribozyme structure and function are currently under investigation.[9] One such strategy helps ribozymes achieve their delivery by genetic means, in the form of gene constructs. Even though ribozyme-mediated gene inhibition involves a mechanism (target cleavage) that is different from the standard antisense RNAs, many of the essential steps required for gene inhibition by ribozyme and antisense RNA are identical. For example, ribozymes must exist long enough (long $t^{1/2}$) to find their target sites inside the cell, and they should locate their target through intramolecular base pairing. Furthermore, the relative concentrations of target and antisense or ribozyme affect the kinetics of target localization. Once the problem of efficient and effective targeting is solved, ribozymes will be effective RNA-inactivating agents with potentially great therapeutic applications. A polymerase chain reaction-based "in vitro evolution" technique has been recently shown to produce a population of ribozymes with 100-fold enhancement in target cleavage over the original molecule.[10]

Targets for Ribozymes in Cancer

The targets of ribozyme-mediated gene modulation have ranged from cancer cells to foreign genes that cause infectious diseases. Ribozymes have been targeted against numerous genes, including oncogenes (*ras*, c-*fos*, BCR-ABL) and drug-resistance genes (*mdr*1). Gene therapy, which involves treating a disease by altering the patient's natural genetic makeup, is fast emerging as a viable molecular technique in the treatment of cancer.

In recent years, our understanding of the features that distinguish a cancer cell from its normal tissue counterpart has increased, and a number of vital gene defects accompanying the onset of cancer have now been documented. Many genes involved in cancer exert their

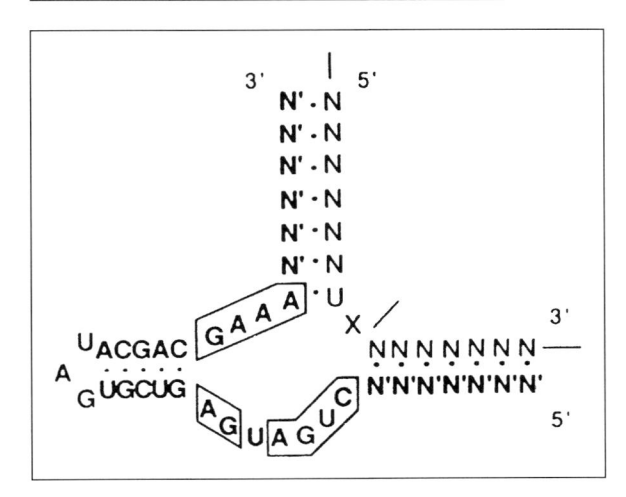

Fig. 14.1. A schematic diagram showing the structure of a typical "hammerhead" ribozyme.[15]

effect by overexpression, temporarily inappropriate expression, or in some cases, by expression of a faulty protein.

Cancer can also occur when novel sequences are generated from within the cell by mutational processes like chromosomal translocation or rearrangement. Some genes are abnormally expressed after translocation followed by fusion with other genes, for example, p210*BCR-ABL*, *bcl-2*/immunoglobulin fusion gene, and t(15;17) in promyelocytic leukemia, where the retinoic acid receptor α and zinc finger protein PML become fused. Several gene defects resulting from a single point mutation lead to activation of a proto-oncogene producing dominantly-acting transforming proteins (for instance, the *ras* oncogene). Such gene abnormalities in cancer could be potential targets for ribozyme therapy. Other genes involved in cancer exert their effect through overexpression of their normal structural proteins like c-Fos, c-Myc, N-Myc, c-erb-2, and nucleolar antigen p120. These proteins could be potential targets for antisense therapy. In addition, downregulation of MDR-1 and c-Raf1 can increase the sensitivity of the target tissue to conventional cytotoxic drugs. We have too limited a scope here to describe the ribozyme action on all different target genes tested. Here we discuss a few examples which anticipated the possibility that anti-oncogene ribozymes could be used as antineoplastic agents in gene therapy protocols.

Cellular Genes Targeted by Ribozyme Molecules

Ribozymes have been used in a number of studies to target cellular oncogenes. One study looked at the product of the c-*myc* oncogene, which is an important regulator of both cell proliferation and programmed cell death (apoptosis). Hammerhead ribozymes were shown to specifically cleave the v-*myc* but not the c-*myc* transcript in vitro. Molecular analysis revealed a reduction of v-*myc* expression in ribozyme-expressing cells, which was associated with the abrogation of hormone-induced apoptosis.[11] This confirms a direct involvement of v-*myc* in the induction of apoptosis and indicates a potential means to control apoptosis at the molecular level using a ribozyme-targeting approach.

Another study involved the activation of signal transduction pathways by mutation or overexpression of cellular oncogenes, which has been associated with neoplastic transformation. The therapeutic potential of ribozymes targeted against the activated H-*ras* oncogene as well as against the nuclear proto-oncogenes c-*fos* and c-*myc* in the FEM human melanoma cell line containing an H-*ras* mutation was evaluated. The anti-*ras* ribozyme could affect not only the proliferation but also the differentiation process of human melanoma cells in vitro. Anti-*ras* ribozyme clones showed a dendritic appearance in monolayer culture which was associated with enhanced melanin synthesis. They also reinforced the role of anti-oncogene ribozymes as suppressors of the neoplastic phenotype of melanoma cells.[12,13]

A study of EJ tumors containing the anti-*ras* ribozyme showed a reduction in tumor size and prolonged survival compared with standard EJ cells.[14] Ribozymes have been targeted against H-*ras* oncogenes, and the expression of c-H-*ras* was suppressed in cells containing ribozymes.[15] These ribozymes cleaved the target RNAs in vitro and altered the cellular pathology. In several systems, the ability of a ribozyme to specifically cleave the mRNA of the activated H-*ras* gene, and alter the malignant phenotype of an invasive human bladder cancer, was evaluated. Plasmids containing the ribozyme-encoding genes were expressed under the control of the long terminal repeats (LTR) of Rous sarcoma virus in NIH3T3 cells transfected with the activated c-H-*ras* gene. These ribozymes were found to inhibit the formation of foci (by about 50%) by cleaving the oncogene mRNA rather than by hybridizing to it. Moreover, the expression of c-H-*ras* was suppressed in cells expressing ribozymes.[16] In an EJ cell line that contained the activated H-*ras* gene, the efficacy of ribozyme action was examined in athymic (nude) mice using an orthotopic model of bladder cancer. EJ tumors containing the anti-*ras* ribozyme showed a reduction in EJ tumors expressing the H-*ras* ribozyme, characterized by a marked reduction in tumor size and invasion compared with those formed by control EJ cells.[14,17] These studies suggest that the invasive phenotype is blunted with the anti-*ras* ribozyme, delaying but not abolishing the metastatic phenotype.[14,18,19]

The tumor inhibitory activity of anti-*ras* ribozymes was also evaluated by a retroviral gene delivery system.[20] Using a tissue-specific (tyrosinase) promoter in a retroviral vector to express the anti-*ras* ribozyme in human melanoma cells was found to be superior in suppression of the human melanoma phenotype in vitro, as characterized by changes in growth, melanin synthesis, morphology, and H-*ras* gene expression. Thus, the use of tissue-specific expression of anti-oncogene ribozymes could have a potential therapeutic application in human cancers.[21] Anti-oncogene ribozymes may be useful as suppressors of tumor cell growth and inhibitors of cellular transformation.[22] A recombinant adenovirus was designed that encoded a gene cassette for the H-*ras* ribozyme. By using this virus, the phenotype in mutant H-*ras*-expressing tumor cells reverted without the need for any selection steps. The demonstration of the utility of adenoviral-mediated delivery of anti-*ras* ribozymes was very promising.[23] Currently, the therapeutic application of ribozymes to human diseases is limited by the available gene transfer systems. However, adenoviral-mediated delivery of anti-cancer ribozymes will allow the practical development of gene therapy strategies.

In a sarcoma model using a metastatic rat embryo cell line that constitutively secretes MMP-9, a hammerhead ribozyme directed against the rat MMP-9 mRNA sequence resulted in the absence of detectable MMP-9 mRNA and a loss of released 92 kDa gelatinase activity. Although these cells were no longer metastatic in a lung colonization assay, they retained their tumorigenic potential.[24] The introduction of an expression vector for a control hammerhead ribozyme had no effect. These data document the requirement of MMP-9 expression for metastasis in this system.

One study determined the ability of ribozymes to inhibit c-*fos* gene expression. The c-*fos* gene product Fos has been implicated in many cellular processes, including signal transduction, DNA synthesis, and resistance to antineoplastic agents. *fos* ribozyme (catalytic RNA) transfectants revealed decreased c-*fos* gene expression concomitant with reduced expression of thymidylate synthase, DNA polymerase beta, topoisomerase I, and metallothionein IIA mRNA. In contrast, c-*myc* expression was elevated after *fos* ribozyme action.[1] This study established a role for c-*fos* in drug resistance and in mediating DNA synthesis and repair processes by modulating the expression of these genes.

Another study used hammerhead ribozymes to the RNA of human papillomavirus type 18 (HPV-18) in an HPV-18-expressing cell line. This ribozyme affected the phenotype of HeLa cells, causing reduced growth rates, increased serum dependency, and reduced focus formation in soft agar. An increase in the intracellular concentration of the tumor suppressor protein p53 appears to indicate that this ribozyme may be effective against cancers that express HPV-18.[25,26] Moreover, p53 pre-mRNA can be modified by a specific ribozyme in vivo, suggesting a possible role for these agents in gene therapy strategies for cancer.[27]

The *p53* gene is the most commonly mutated gene yet identified in human cancers.[28] The gene product can regulate transcription and progress through the cell cycle, facilitating repair of DNA damage.[29-31] Wild type *p53* (wt*p53*) can mediate a dominant tumor suppressor effect,[32,33] but mutation of *p53* may confer a gain of function which enhances features of the malignant phenotype.[34-37]

The mutated *p53* gene product may oligomerize with wt*p53*, inactivating its tumor suppressor function, or may acquire a prolonged half life. Therefore, treatment for malignancies caused by loss of *p53* tumor suppressor gene function would ideally be achieved by introducing the wt*p53* gene into tumor cells while eliminating the endogenous mutant gene. Mutations in the *p53* gene span a wide range of the coding region; gene replacement strategies, therefore, are best targeted at the pre-mRNA level. We constructed a retroviral vector that would deliver wt*p53* into cells while expressing a ribozyme targeted to *p53* pre-mRNA, which would specifically block the endogenous mutated *p53*. We evaluated this vector as a model for *p53* gene replacement.

A ribozyme gene spanning a 52 bp sequence with *Stu*I and *Bgl*II restriction enzyme sites was designed. The catalytic domain of this *Rz5a* ribozyme recognizes a sequence at codon 187 of *p53* exon 6 close to intron 5. The flanking ribozyme sequences were antisense to the intron 5-exon 6 boundary region, determining its specificity for unspliced *p53* pre-mRNA cleavage. Two synthetic primers with little overlap (5'-CCT GAG GAG GGG CCA CTG ATG AGT CCT TTT G-3' and 5'- TGA TTG CTC TTA GGT TTC GTC CAA AAG GAC TCA-3') were used to synthesize the ribozymes by polymerase chain reaction (PCR) amplification. Ribozyme DNA thus synthesized was subcloned into a *Stu*I/*Bgl*II site of the LNSX retroviral vector, where expression of the ribozyme was under control of the SV40 promoter. A DNA fragment containing β-actin promoter and wt*p53* cDNA was subcloned into a *Bgl*II site of the same recombinant vector with the *p53* gene under control of the β-actin promoter. This vector was designed to transcribe a catalytic RNA molecule that was antisense to the intron 5-exon 6 junction sequence (thus cleaving only endogenous *p53* pre-mRNA) and to express exogenous wt *p53* cDNA. The ribozyme's catalytic activity has been shown previously to be limited to unspliced endogenous *p53* pre-mRNA, thus having no effect on *p53* mRNA. H358 *p53*-null human non-small cell lung cancer cells expressed p53 protein after transfection with *Rzp53*. After human non-small cell lung cancer cells H226Br (containing a mutated *p53* gene) were infected with the recombinant viral supernatant, they expressed both the ribozyme and exogenous wt *p53* RNA, as detected by reverse transcription-polymerase chain reaction using sequence-specific amplimers. The ribozyme component of the *Rzp53* vector mediated cleavage of *p53* pre-mRNA in vivo. *Rzp53* had a growth-inhibitory effect on transfected cells, as demonstrated by a proliferation assay.

The ribozyme has specificity for the *p53* intron 5-exon 6 boundary sequence and cleaved *p53* unspliced mRNA at codon 187 (GUC) but did not cleave mature *p53* mRNA. The ribozyme sequence was subcloned into the retroviral LNSX vector such that expression of the ribozyme was driven by the SV40 promoter. The vector also contained human *p53* cDNA, which was efficiently transcribed by the β-actin promoter. The expression of wt *p53* was evaluated by infecting the *p53*-negative H358 cell line with the *Rzp53* viral supernatant. The p53 protein expression in these infected cells was demonstrated by Western blot analysis using an α-p53 monoclonal antibody. These cells displayed a strong *p53* protein band, indicating the expression of exogenous *p53* in virus-infected cells.

The specificity of the in vitro catalytic activity of the *Rz5* ribozyme for *p53* pre-mRNA has been shown previously. We examined the effect of this ribozyme on a human NSCLC cell line, H226Br, which has a *p53* mutation at codon 254 and expresses large quantities of mutant p53 protein. H226Br cells were infected with *Rzp53* retroviral supernatant and then analyzed for the expression of ribozyme and exogenous wt *p53*. Reverse-transcriptase PCR analysis using SV40 and β-actin promoter-specific amplimers indicated that transduced H226Br cells expressed both ribozyme and exogenous wt *p53* following Southern hybridization with *p53* and ribozyme-specific probes.

To detect in vivo cleavage of the *p53* target RNA by the ribozyme, total RNA was extracted from the *Rzp53*-transduced H226Br cells 6 h or 12 h after transfection. Total RNA containing the ribozyme was used to cleave the in vitro labeled RNA substrate. The cleavage products were separated on polyacrylamide gels, which were autoradiographed. The results indicated that the total RNA contained anti-*p53* ribozymes that efficiently cleaved the *p53* pre-mRNA substrate in vitro. However, we were unable to detect cleavage products by RNase protection assay or primer extension analysis.

The concomitant expression of anti-*p53* pre-mRNA ribozyme and wild type *p53* expression in the same cell was evaluated for its effect on cell proliferation. H226Br cells were transduced with *Rzp53* viral supernatant, and their growth was monitored for 7 days. H226Br cells infected with LNSX vector only were used as a negative control. The growth rate for the *Rzp53*-transduced cells was greatly reduced compared to that of non-transduced cells or cells transduced with the empty LNSX vector. The cleavage specificity of our ribozyme relies on the unspliced *p53* RNA, and therefore it can cleave the endogenous *p53* pre-mRNA independently of the site of mutation.

With the development of a retroviral vector that induces the expression of both the wild type tumor suppressor gene and the mutant-inhibiting ribozyme, we have made an attempt to set up a model for gene replacement therapy. Treatment for malignancies caused by defects in tumor suppressor gene function would be ideally achieved through the delivery of wt *p53* at the same time that endogenous abnormal gene function is eliminated.

The precise role of *p53* mutation in the transformation process is not clear at the present time. The site of mutation appears to play a critical role in the activity of the resultant mutant. Some mutants have gain of function and are able to cooperate with activated *ras* oncogenes to increase colony formation.[34,38] However, this does not appear to be mediated by a transdominant negative effect of the protein, as cells transduced with a vector containing both wild type and mutated *p53* genes co-expressed both genes but showed no inhibition of wt *p53* growth suppression by the mutated *p53* gene.[39] Many mutations will cause loss of the transactivating activity of the protein, but others do not.[40,41] The tumor suppressor activity of wt *p53* may be retained despite the presence of a mutation in codon 248.[42,43] A vector system that mediates expression of an anti-*p53* ribozyme and restoration of wt *p53* function in the cell carrying mutated *p53* may prove useful for investigating mutant and wild type interactions and represents a novel gene replacement strategy.

Conclusion

Ribozymes are a class of RNA molecules that can perform catalytically in the absence of protein. Specifically, they can hybridize to and cleave target RNA molecules independently of cellular proteins. The cleaved target RNA cannot be translated, thereby preventing the synthesis of specific protein(s). Ribozymes targeted to the mRNA of key proteins involved in maintaining a disease state may result in its elimination. The ribozymes can be chemically synthesized and delivered directly to cells, or they can be expressed from an expression vector after either permanent or transient transfection. Future directions in ribozyme research include optimizing the design to obtain the maximal cleavage rate, increasing the specificity to prevent aberrant reactions, identifying cleavage sites within the target RNA, and delivering the ribozymes to cells of interest both in vitro and in vivo. The ribozyme-mediated inhibition of gene expression may have potential therapeutic applications in the future treatment of cancer.

References

1. Scanlon KJ, Jiao L, Funato T et al. Ribozyme-mediated cleavage of c-fos mRNA reduces gene expression of DNA synthesis enzymes and metallothionein. Proc Natl Acad Sci USA 1991; 88:10591-10595.
2. Sarver N, Cantin EM, Chang PS et al. Ribozymes as potential anti-HIV-1 therapeutic agents. Science 1990; 247:1222-1225.
3. Sioud M, Natvig JB, Forre O. Preformed ribozyme destroys tumour necrosis factor mRNA in human cells. J Mol Biol 1992; 223:831-835.
4. Kashani-Sabet M, Scanlon KJ. Application of ribozymes to cancer gene therapy (Review). Cancer Gene Ther 1995; 2:213-223.
5. Kruger K, Grabowski PJ, Zaug AJ, Sands J, Gottschling DE, Cech TR. Self-splicing RNA: Autoexcision and autocyclization of the ribosomal RNA intervening sequence of tetrahymena. Cell 1982; 31:147-157.
6. Kim SH, Cech TR. Three-dimensional model of the active site of the self-splicing rRNA precursor of tetrahymena. Proc Natl Acad Sci USA 1987; 84:8788-8792.
7. Gerlach WL, Llewellyn D, Haseloff J. Construction of a plant disease resistance gene from the satellite RNA of tobacco rinspot virus. Nature (London) 1987; 328:802-805.
8. Forster AC, Symons RH. Self-cleavage of plus and minus RNAs of a virusoid and a structural model for the active sites. Cell 1987; 49:211-220.
9. Erickson RP, Izant JG. Biology of antisense RNA and DNA. In: Erickson RP, Izant JG, eds. Gene Regulation. New York: Raven Press, 1992.
10. Beaudry AA, Joyce GF. Directed evolution of an RNA enzyme. Science 1992; 257:613.
11. Dolnikov A, King A, Luxford C, Symonds G, Sun LQ. Ribozyme-mediated suppression of v-myc expression abrogates apoptosis in transformed monocytes. Cancer Gene Ther 1996; 3:289-295.
12. Ohta Y, Kijima H, Kashani-Sabet M, Scanlon KJ. Suppression of the malignant phenotype of melanoma cells by anti-oncogene ribozymes. Journal of Investigative Dermatology 1996; 106:275-280.
13. Ohta Y, Tone T, Shitara T et al. H-*ras* ribozyme-mediated alteration of the human melanoma phenotype. Ann N Y Acad Sci 1994; 716:242-253;discussion 253-6.
14. Eastham JA, Ahlering TE. Use of an anti-*ras* ribozyme to alter the malignant phenotype of a human bladder cancer cell line. J Urol 1996; 156:1186-1188.
15. Koizumi M, Hayase Y, Iwai S, Kamiya H, Inoue H, Ohtsuka E. Design of RNA enzymes distinguishing a single base mutation in RNA. Nucleic Acids Res 1989; 17:7059-7071.
16. Koizumi M, Kamiya H, Ohtsuka E. Ribozymes designed to inhibit transformation of NIH/3T3 cells by the activated c-Ha-*ras* gene. Gene 1992; 117:179-184.
17. Kashani-Sabet M, Funato T, Tone T et al. Reversal of the malignant phenotype by an anti-*ras* ribozyme. Antisense Res Dev 1992; 2:3-15.
18. Kashani-Sabet M, Funato T, Florens VA, Fodstad O, Scanlon KJ. Suppression of the neoplastic phenotype in vivo by an anti-*ras* ribozyme. Cancer Res 1994; 54:900-902.
19. Tone T, Kashani-Sabet M, Funato T et al. Suppression of EJ cells tumorigenicity. In Vivo 1993; 7:471-476.
20. Li MX, Lonial H, Citarella R, Lindh D, Colina L, Kramer R. Tumor inhibitory activity of anti-*ras* ribozymes delivered by retroviral gene transfer. Cancer Gene Ther 1996; 3:221-229.

21. Ohta Y, Kijima H, Ohkawa T, Kashani-Sabet M, Scanlon KJ. Tissue-specific expression of an anti-*ras* ribozyme inhibits proliferation of human malignant melanoma cells. Nucleic Acids Res 1996; 24:938-942.
22. Funato T, Shitara T, Tone T, Jiao L, Kashani-Sabet M, Scanlon KJ. Suppression of H-*ras*-mediated transformation in NIH3T3 cells by a *ras* ribozyme. Biochem Pharmacol 1994; 48:1471-1475.
23. Feng M, Cabrera G, Deshane J, Scanlon KJ, Curiel DT. Neoplastic reversion accomplished by high efficiency adenoviral-mediated delivery of an anti-*ras* ribozyme. Cancer Res 1995; 55:2024-2028.
24. Hua J, Muschel RJ. Inhibition of matrix metalloproteinase 9 expression by a ribozyme blocks metastasis in a rat sarcoma model system. Cancer Res 1996; 56:5279-5284.
25. Shillitoe EJ, Kamath P, Chen Z. Papillomaviruses as targets for cancer gene therapy (Review). Cancer Gene Ther 1994; 1:193-204.
26. Chen Z, Kamath P, Zhang S, St. John L, Adler-Storthz K, Shillitoe EJ. Effects on tumor cells of ribozymes that cleave the RNA transcripts of human papillomavirus type 18. Cancer Gene Ther 1996; 3:18-23.
27. Cai DW, Mukhopadhyay T, Roth JA. Suppression of lung cancer cell growth by ribozyme-mediated modification of p53 pre-mRNA. Cancer Gene Ther 1995; 2:199-205.
28. Hollstein M, Sidransky D, Vogelstein B, Harris CC. *p53* mutations in human cancers. Science 1991; 253:49-53.
29. Diller L, Kassel J, Nelson CE et al. p53 functions as a cell cycle control protein in osteosarcomas. Mol Cell Biol 1990; 10:5772-5781.
30. Kuerbitz S, Plunkett B, Walsh W, Kastan M. Wild-type p53 is a cell cycle checkpoint determinant following radiation. Nature (London) 1992; 89:7491-7495.
31. Spandau DF. Distinct conformations of p53 are observed at different stages of keratinocyte differentiation. Oncogene 1994; 9:1861-1868.
32. Baker SJ, Markowitz S, Pearson ER, Villson JKV, Vogelstein B. Suppression of human colorectal carcinoma cell growth by wild-type p53. Science 1997; 249:912-915.
33. Cai DW, Mukhopadhyay T, Liu YJ, Fujiwara T, Roth JA. Stable expression of the wild-type *p53* gene in human lung cancer cells after retrovirus-mediated gene transfer. Hum Gene Ther 1993; 4:617-624.
34. Hinds P, Finlay C, Levine AJ. Mutation is required to activate the p53 gene for cooperation with the *ras* oncogene and transformation. J Virol 1989; 63 (2):739-746.
35. Hinds PW, Finlay CA, Quartin RS et al. Mutant *p53* DNA clones from human colon carcinomas cooperate with *ras* in transforming primary rat cells: A comparison of the "hot spot" mutant phenotypes. Cell Growth Differ 1990; 1:571-580.
36. Aaronson SA. Unique aspects of the interactions of retroviruses with vertebrate cells: CP Rhoads memorial lecture. Cancer Res 1983; 43:1-5.
37. Espevik T, Figari IS, Ranges GE, Palladino MAJ. Transforming growth factor-B1 (TGF-B1) and recombinant human tumor necrosis factor-α reciprocally regulate the generation of lymphokine-activated killer cell activity. J Immunol 1988; 140:2312-2316.
38. Robbins KC, Antonaides HN, Shshilkumar GD, Hunkapiller MW, Aaronson SA. Structural and immunological similarities between simian sarcoma virus gene product(s) and human platelet derived growth factor. Nature 1983; 305:605-608.
39. Frebourg T, Sadelain M, Ng YS, Kassel J, Friend SH. Equal transcription of wild-type and mutant p53 using bicistronic vectors results in the wild-type phenotype. Cancer Res 1994; 54:878-881.
40. Miller CW, Chumakov A, Said J, Chen DL, Aslo A, Koeffler HP. Mutant-p53 proteins have diverse intracellular abilities to oligomerize and activate transcription. Oncogene 1993; 8:1815-1824.
41. Finkel T, Der SJ, Cooper GM. Activation of *ras* genes in human tumors does not affect localization, modification, or nucleotide binding properties of p21. Cell 1984; 37:151-158.
42. Cline MJ, Slamon DJ, Lipsick JS. Oncogenes: Implications for the diagnosis and treatment of cancer. Ann Intern Med 1984; 101:223-233.
43. Duesberg PH. Retroviral transforming genes in normal cells. Nature 1983; 304:219-226.

CHAPTER 15

Inhibition of the Multidrug Resistance Phenotype by Different Delivery Systems of an Anti-*mdr* Ribozyme

Per Sonne Holm, David T. Curiel and Manfred Dietel

Introduction

In the industrial countries of the world, roughly one person in five will die of cancer; only heart diseases appear more often. Although considerable effort has been taken to improve diagnosis and treatment of cancer it becomes more and more obvious that the traditional approaches, i.e., surgery, radiation and chemotherapy, will not be able to cure all types of cancer especially after systemic distribution. A major reason for the limited success of cancer therapy was found to be the enormous functional heterogeneity of cancer cells exhibiting a variety of different characteristics, such as the potency for infiltrative growth, the possibility to metastasize, the activation of proteolytic or detoxifying enzymes and the overexpression of membrane-bound pump proteins to decrease intracytoplasmic levels of toxic drugs.

In cases where local measures, such as surgery or radiation, are no longer possible, systemic chemotherapy is the matter of choice. In many cases repeated treatments with drugs that are selectively toxic to dividing cells will kill the majority of neoplastic cells. However, therapy with cytostatic drugs often shows only limited effectiveness. Those cells that are exposed to one drug often develop a resistance not only to the specific cytostatic drug with which they have been treated and to which they were initially sensitive, but also to other drugs to which they have never been exposed.[1] In addition, the application of anticancer drugs often has the disadvantage that it unspecifically hampers normal tissue and cells, inducing severe side effects. Among the relatively great number of resistance-associated mechanisms, such as multidrug resistance-related proteins,[2,3] alteration of topoisomarase II,[4] and increased activity of glutathione-S-transferase, considerable attention in cancer research has focused on the so-called multidrug resistance phenotype (MDR).[5-7] Multidrug resistance describes the simultaneous expression of cellular resistance to a wide range of structurally and functionally unrelated lipophilic drugs. The usual pattern of cross-resistance includes a large variety of cytotoxic agents that do not have a common structure or a common intracellular target, such as anthracyclines (adriamycin), alkylating agents (melphalam), heavy metal compounds (cisplatin) and alkaloids (vinblastine). The development of this form of resistance is clinically recognized by a short period or a total lack of drug effectiveness.

Ribozymes in the Gene Therapy of Cancer, edited by Kevin J. Scanlon and Mohammed Kashani-Sabet. ©1998 R.G. Landes Company.

Generally, MDR cells appear to have a reduced ability to accumulate the different drugs, which is often accompanied by the overexpression of a membrane-bound transport protein, a P-170 kDa glycoprotein.[8,9] The elevation in the expression of this protein is mediated by elevated levels of the corresponding *mdr*1 4.5 kb mRNA.[10,11] P-170 is encoded by a small family of genes. In humans two MDR genes are described, while in hamsters and mice three genes could be identified.[12,13] The gene coding for P-glycoprotein is localized on chromosome 7.[14] By means of transfection experiments it was shown that only the *mdr*1 gene is responsible for the clinically relevant MDR.[15] P-glycoprotein consists of 1280 amino acids[16] and contains several transmembrane regions which form a pore-like structure (Fig. 15.1). P-glycoprotein has two ATP binding sites[17,18] and functions as a membrane efflux pump which reduces the intracellular concentration of cytostatic drugs.[19] In addition, it could be shown that an increased synthesis of P-glycoprotein correlates with an elevated degree of resistance.[20] Although other models for the mechanism of P-glycoprotein-mediated resistance have been proposed, the possibility that P-gp acts as a multidrug transporter has not been excluded.[21-23] At present the molecular mechanisms underlying the development of resistance are the subject of many investigations. For example, Chin et al[24] were able to show that the expression of the *mdr*1 gene is influenced by Ha-*ras* and p53.

Several types of strategies have been utilized to modulate the MDR phenotype both in vivo and in vitro. The reversing drugs are biochemically completely different from each other, including drug analogs (N-acetyl daunomycin), calcium channel blockers (verapamil), calmodulin modulators (trifluoperazine) and immunosuppressants (cyclosporine A, FK 506, PSC 833).[25-27] However, these substances are still acting in the conventional way, by limiting more or less directly the function of P-glycoprotein as an energy-dependent pump. Unfortunately, clinical studies using these compounds have been impeded by the significant toxicity and limited specificity of these chemosensitizers. The use of the anti-MDR1 monoclonal antibody MRK-16 presents another selective approach for the modulation of the multidrug resistance phenotype.[28] However, there is a considerable need to find new ways to reverse multidrug resistance.

In recent years researchers have extensively studied another alternative approach to eliminate the function of P-glycoprotein and, consequently, to reverse the resistant phenotype in tumor cells, by using antisense RNA/DNA or ribozymes.[29] Particular hammerhead ribozymes which can be applied against different target RNA sequences[30,31] provide a genuine alternative to the conventional antisense strategies[32,33] and are useful tools to inhibit unwelcome gene expressions. Compared with the RNA antisense method, hammerhead ribozymes have the advantage of cleaving the target RNA after base pairing, to subsequently emerge unchanged from the reaction and cleave several more substrate RNA molecules.[30,34] Based on these findings it seems that ribozymes are simply an advance form of antisense molecule.[35]

It is the goal of this chapter to describe the construction of a hammerhead ribozyme that is directed against the *mdr*1 mRNA which abrogates P-glycoprotein expression by tumor cells and to summarize the results obtained in vitro and in cell culture experiments. Further, this chapter will also focus on different delivery systems of the anti-*mdr* ribozyme.

Catalytic Activity of the *mdr* Ribozyme

In order to reverse the resistant phenotype in cell culture, we designed a hammerhead ribozyme recognizing the GUC triplet at position +2637 to +2639 in exon 21 of the *mdr*1 mRNA. For the in vitro analyses, it consisted of a 43 base long RNA molecule. The 5' and 3' end sequences of the ribozyme complementary to the substrate were 10 and 11 bases, respectively (Fig. 15.2). This guarantees a high specificity of the ribozyme, since a sequence of 16 nucleotides statistically is represented only once in the human genome of approximately

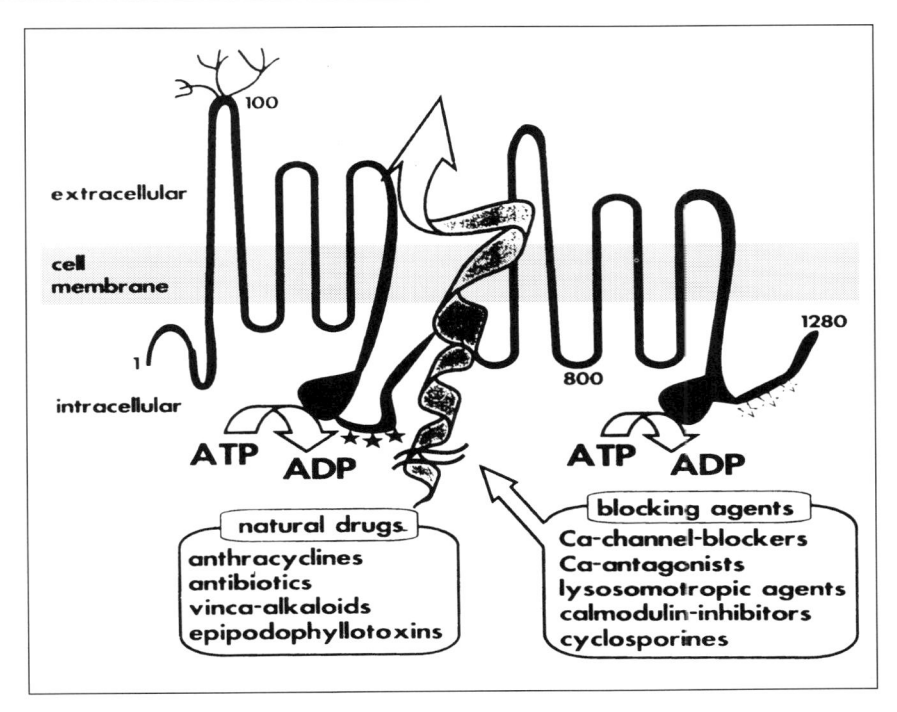

Fig. 15.1. Structural properties of the channel-forming membrane spanning P-glycoprotein. Total length is 1280 amino acids; the two halves have similar sequence and an ATP binding site each. The major classes of transported drugs and the efflux-blocking agents are indicated. The binding sites of the monoclonal antibody C-219 are marked by stars.

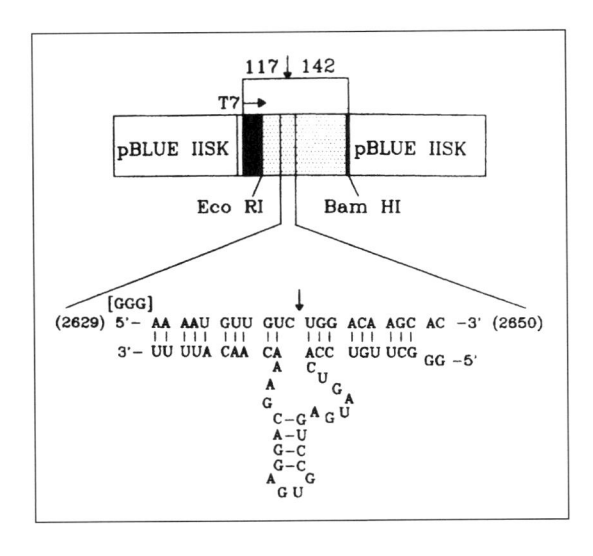

Fig. 15.2. Schematic structures of the anti-*mdr* ribozyme annealed to a part of the 259 nt of exon 21 of the *mdr*1 mRNA. The transcription plasmid derived from pBLUESCRIPT IISK was obtained as described.[47]

4×10^9 bp. The choice of the specific target site was based on the two ATP binding sites, which are suggested to be important for the function of P-glycoprotein. Before testing the ribozyme in tissue culture experiments, we investigated its ability to cleave the target sequence in a cell-free system.

Cleavage of the target RNA (259 nt transcript and a 25-mer RNA substrate) is shown in Figure 15.3A and 3B. Optimal conditions for cleavage of the 259 nt transcript by the ribozyme were approximately pH 8.0, 12 mM magnesium chloride and 52°C (data not shown). Often rather low cleavage efficiencies have been reported with large substrates (between 60 and 954 nucleotides).[36,37] For example, with a 50-fold molar excess of a hammerhead ribozyme, only about 61% of a 261 nucleotide fragment of calretinin mRNA was cleaved after incubation for 90 min at 37°C. In contrast, using only a 4-fold excess of our *mdr* ribozyme, about 70% of the 259 nucleotide fragment of *mdr*1 mRNA was cleaved after 60 min at 37°C (not shown). Further, we could observe multiple turnover. In cases when 4 nM ribozyme and 400 nM substrate were used, one ribozyme could cleave up to 12 substrate molecules within 60 min. Not only temperature, but also the sequence of hybridization (G-C content to be considered) or the length of a ribozyme influence cleavage activity. While constructing longer sequences of hybridization the K_m values remain nearly constant, whereas a clear diminution of the k_{cat} values can be observed. This is due to the fact that there is a decrease in the ribozyme's dissociation rate from the cleavage products.[38] For the time being it is difficult to evaluate whether such in vitro results are of importance in vivo.

The in vitro kinetics of cleavage reactions by hammerhead ribozymes has been studied in detail.[39] A severe limitation is the poor cleavage efficiency of large substrates, in contrast to the high activities observed with small substrates (oligoribonucleotides). In multiple turnover reactions the values of k_{cat}/K_m using short substrates are about 400-1100 mM^{-1}sec^{-1}.[30,40,41] Using a long substrate as target (985 nucleotides) Heidenreich and Eckstein[42] determined the value of k_{cat}/K_m at four orders of magnitude lower. Thus, it is assumed that large RNA molecules can form complex secondary and tertiary structures which interfere with the recognition and cleavage by hammerhead ribozymes, and might therefore contribute to the rate-limiting step.[37] In contrast, the k_{cat} values of the anti-*mdr* ribozyme for small and large RNAs were identical, whereas K_m was increased only 5-fold with the large substrate.[43] As studies of antisense oligonucleotides have already shown,[44] not all mRNA areas are equally suitable as target sequence. For reasons still unknown, the sequence here selected for the docking of the anti-*mdr* ribozyme appears to be particularly well available or recognizable to the ribozyme. Our data suggest that access of the ribozyme to the target sequence was almost as easy as with the oligonucleotide, and is in agreement with some of the computer predicted structures (not shown). However, it is not certain that in vitro results are comparable with the situation in vivo. Also, according to the latest investigations, the "targeting", i.e., the ribozyme's assignment to the same cellular compartment as the mRNA to be cut, and the RNA binding proteins play a decisive role for the ribozyme's efficacy.[45,46] At present there is no good way to predict optimal target sites, and testing of several different ribozymes with a specific mRNA may be necessary to identify suitable target sequences for biologically long substrate RNAs.

Delivery Systems of the Anti-*mdr* Ribozyme

Endogenous Delivery

The strategy for introducing antisense or catalytic RNA molecules into cells has become an important issue in cancer gene therapy. Two general mechanisms have been developed for introducing antisense or catalytic RNA molecules into target cells selectively and

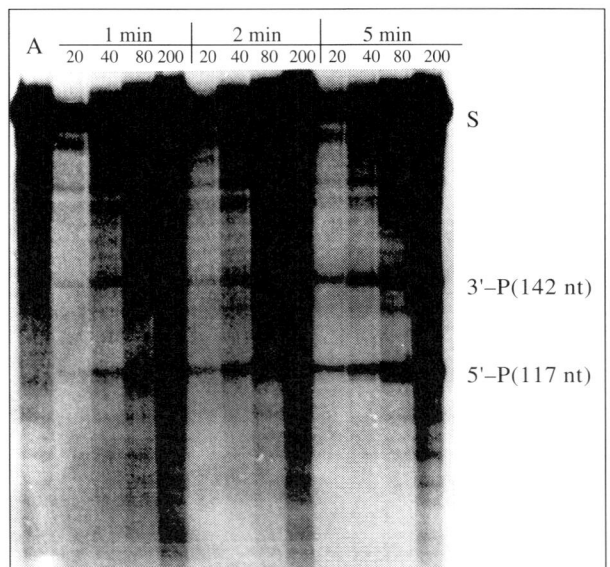

Fig. 15.3. Examples of the cleavage of the 259 nt substrate (A) and 25-mer substrate (B). 4 nM ribozyme (6 nM for 259 nt substrate) were incubated with 20, 40, 80 and 200 nM substrate for 1, 2 and 5 min. The products were analyzed on a 10% (A) or 20% (B) denaturing polyacrylamide gel. R, ribozyme; S, substrate; P, product.

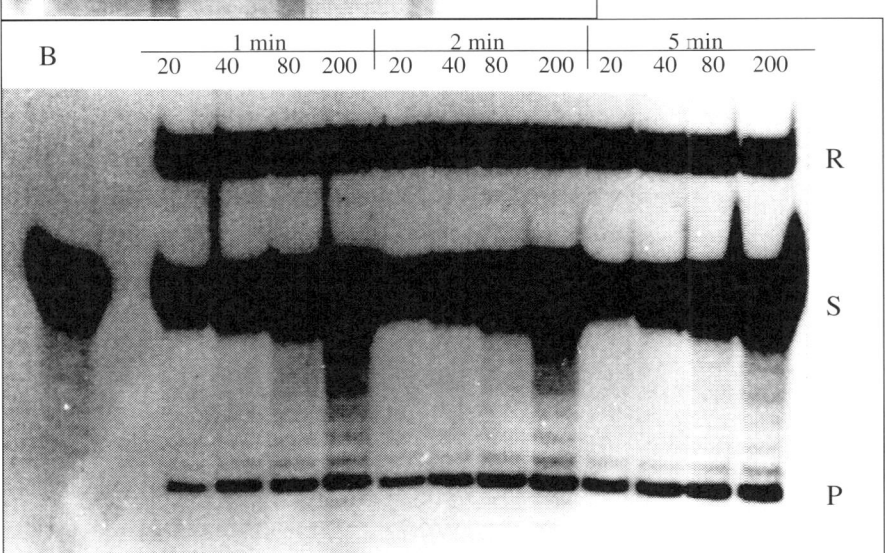

efficiently: endogenous expression of a ribozyme from a DNA template delivered by different vector systems, and exogenous delivery. Several experiments performed during the last 5 years have shown that by using different strategies the application of antisense oligonucleotides or ribozymes can induce a specific inhibition of the *mdr*1 mRNA and the P-glycoprotein, resulting in a reduced multidrug resistance.[47-51]

The use of plasmids or viral vectors is one of the most promising strategies for gene delivery and endogenous expression of ribozymes in cells. For this method, however, suitable vectors are needed, including plasmids, retroviruses, adenoviruses and adeno-associated viruses (see also Section II, Expression and Delivery of Ribozymes). The ribozyme gene is placed downstream of a strong promoter/enhancer system, so that it is highly expressed in the cells. The ribozyme can be expressed either by the polymerase II or by the polymerase III promoter-system. In spite of some advantages of the pol II promoter (poly (A) tail may prolong half life of the ribozyme), it seems that only under the control of pol III can the expression of ribozymes reach a 100- to 1000-fold excess of the ribozyme over the target RNA, which is necessary to obtain a detectable decrease in RNA levels.[52-54]

To reverse the MDR phenotype, a mammalian expression vector containing the 43 bp DNA sequence that encodes the *mdr*1 ribozyme was transfected into the human pancreatic carcinoma cell line EPP85-181RDB, which expresses the MDR phenotype. This cell line was established previously by growing the parental cells EPP85-181P in increased concentrations of daunorubicin, resulting in a 1600-fold daunorubicin resistance. After transfection and selection two cell clones that expressed the ribozyme could be isolated (EPP85-181RDB-Rb1 and EPP85-181RDB-Rb2). In these cell clones the amount of *mdr*1 mRNA expression and P-glycoprotein formation was reduced to such an extent that they were no longer detectable (Figs. 15.4 and 15.5). With reference to the IC$_{50}$ values, the resistance was reduced almost completely, whereas the clone which contained only the expression vector (EPP85-181RDB-Vec) continued to be as resistant to daunorubicin as the original resistant cell line EPP-181RDB (Fig. 15.6 and ref. 47). The almost complete reversion of the daunorubicin resistance by transfection of the *mdr*1 ribozyme excludes mechanisms of resistance other than the typical MDR, which means that the increased expression of P-glycoprotein in the EPP85-181RDB cell line is the main factor of resistance.

Adenovirus vectors are probably the most efficient tool for delivering foreign genes into mammalian cells both in vitro and in vivo. Several advantages of this vector include the infection of a wide variety of cell types, replicating and non-replicating, produced and purified in a high titer up to 5 x 10^{11} plaque forming units (PFU/ml) and the high levels of transgene expression.

To determine the feasibility of employing the adenoviral vector for anti-*mdr* ribozyme delivery, we constructed a recombinant adenovirus. The expression of the ribozyme was directed by a polymerase III promoter (Va I promoter). Forty-eight hours after infection of MCF-7Ad cells with 200 PFU AdVaIRib (>95% transduction frequency) and 200 PFU of the control virus AdCMVLacZ (recombinant adenovirus encoding the β-galactosidase reporter gene), 100-1000 ng/ml vincristine was added to the medium; cell viability was assayed after a further 72 hours (Fig. 15.7). Untransfected MCF-7Ad cells and cells infected with the control virus did not demonstrate enhanced sensitivity to vincristine, whereas the cells infected with the anti-*mdr* ribozyme induced strong sensitivity to vincristine. These results demonstrate that it is possible to downregulate *mdr* expression without any kind of selection. Together with further studies[55,56] they demonstrate the potential of an adenoviral-mediated delivery of ribozymes for cancer gene therapy. On the basis of these results, we are currently in the process of evaluating this concept in a murine model.

Despite several advantages of Ad vectors for gene therapy, there exists one drawback in using adenovirus as delivery system in vivo: its immunogenic potential.[57] To achieve the goal of using adenovirus in gene therapy, it will be necessary in the future to design Ad vectors that will prevent the induction of immune response.

Exogenous Delivery

Although much improvement in transfection has been achieved with newly developed cationic lipids,[58,59] several limitations still exist with this exogenous nonviral delivery system of ribozymes. This includes low stability, since they can easily be attacked and destroyed by the nucleases contained in the serum. Kinetic investigations, however, show that a specific insertion of 2'-modified ribonucleotides, such as 2'-fluoro, 2'-amino, 2'-*O*-methyl and

```
1  2  3  4  5  6  7
```

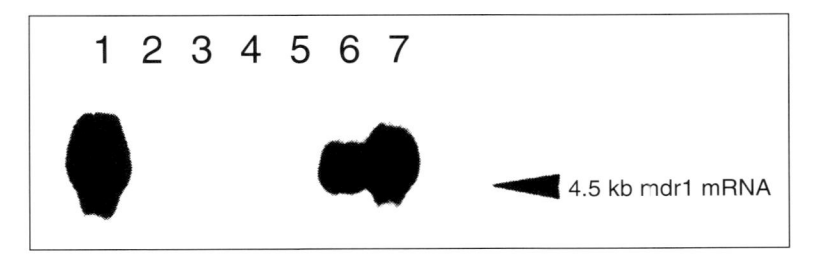

●   ●◐   ◀ 4.5 kb mdr1 mRNA

Fig. 15.4. Northern blot analysis of *mdr*1 mRNA using a 785 bp probe. The autoradiograph demonstrates no detectable signal with 10 µg of total cellular RNA of EPP85-181RDB-Rb1/2 (lanes 2 and 3) and EPP85-181P (lane 4) grown in 0.0125 µg ml^{-1} daunorubicin. The resistant cell line (EPP85-181RDB) and the cell line containing only the vector (EPP85-181RDB/Vec), when grown in 2.5 µg ml^{-1} daunorubicin, show a clear signal (lanes 1 and 7). The resistant cell line shows a weaker signal when grown in 0.025 µg ml^{-1} daunorubicin (lane 6), and almost no signal when grown in the absence of daunorubicin (lane 5).

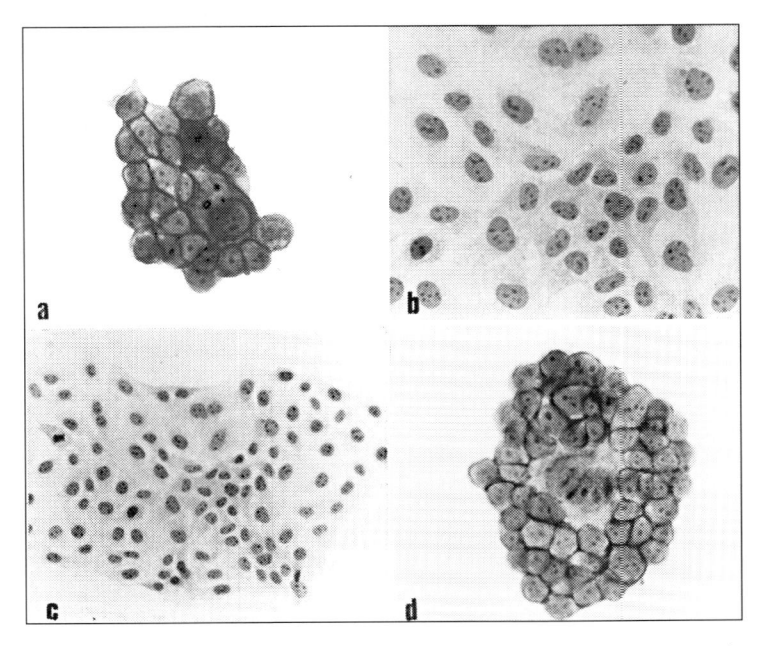

Fig. 15.5. Immunocytochemistry of P-glycoprotein in the human pancreatic cell lines EPP85-181RDB (a), EPP85-181RDB-Rb1 (b), EPP85-181P (c), EPP85-181RDB/Vec (d). The monoclonal antibody C-219 (α-P-glycoprotein) was used to label the cells; labeling of the cell membrane is seen in (a), the resistant line, and (d), the resistant line with introduced vector only; (b), with the introduced ribozyme, restores the sensitivity seen in the parental line (c). The cell clones in (a) and (d) were grown in 2.5 µg ml^{-1} daunorubicin and those in (b) and (c) in 0.0125 µg ml^{-1} daunorubicin.

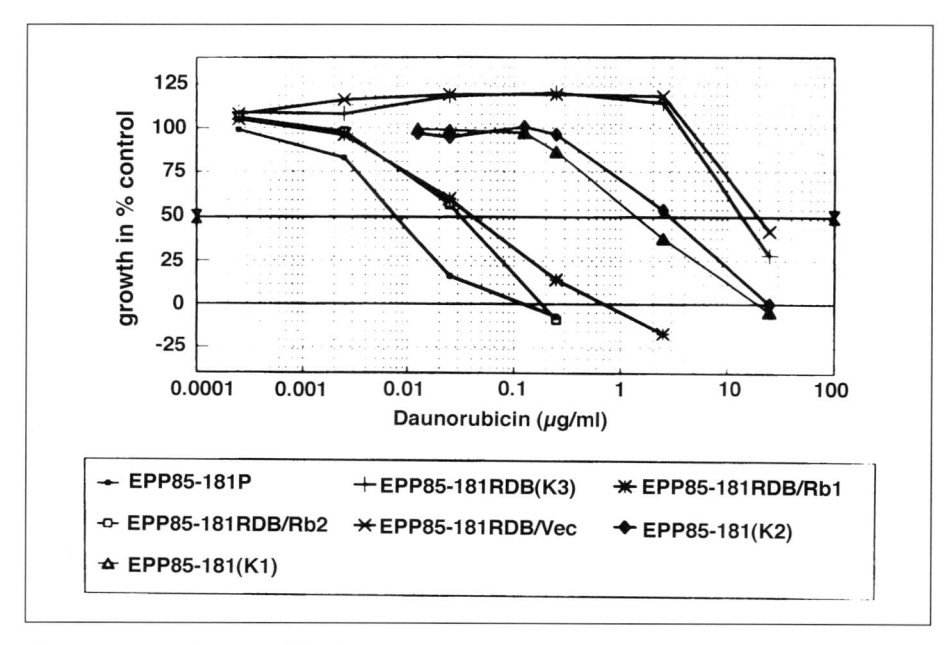

Fig. 15.6. Determination of the daunorubicin-induced IC$_{50}$ for parental and resistant cell lines (EPP85-181P, EPP85-181RDB (K1-3)), the two cell lines containing the ribozyme (EPP85-181RDB-Rb1, EPP85-181RDB-Rb2), and the cell line containing only the expression vector (EPP85-181RDB/Vec). Data points represent cell counts of cultures.

2'-deoxynucleotides within one ribozyme will increase its stability many times.[40,41,60-62] Further, the substitute must be chosen very carefully, since modifications can also decrease the cleavage activity. Another major barrier to the development of ribozymes for gene therapy is their very low permeability to cellular membranes compared to viral vector delivery. A further drawback of exogenous delivery is the fact that repeated administration is required since the delivery is transient and inefficient. Another question is how ribozymes are able to escape being trapped in the endosome. One approach to facilitate the release of DNA molecules from endosomes in order to avoid a prolonged exposure to this environment is the use of a replication-defective adenovirus.[63] Raja-Walia et al[64] reported up to 1000-fold enhanced gene transfer by using a complex of plasmid DNA/cationic lipids with a replication-deficient adenovirus. This method still remains to be performed with ribozymes.

Another strategy to increase the acceptance rate is to combine molecules at the 5' end or 3' end with cholesterol or other lipophil groups.[65] A recently proposed possibility for achieving better biological availability in the cytoplasm is the synthesis of ribozymes with hexaethylene glycol as a linker. It can be shown that hexaethylene glycol linkers can be inserted not only terminally but also in loop II of ribozymes without a significant loss of cleavage activity.[66] In what way it will influence stability and acceptance rate has still to be investigated. Based on recent findings,[67,68] several *mdr* ribozymes have been chemically synthesized which contain both hexaethylene glycol linker and 2'-modified ribonucleotides; work is in progress to determine whether an exogenous application is able to modulate the MDR phenotype.

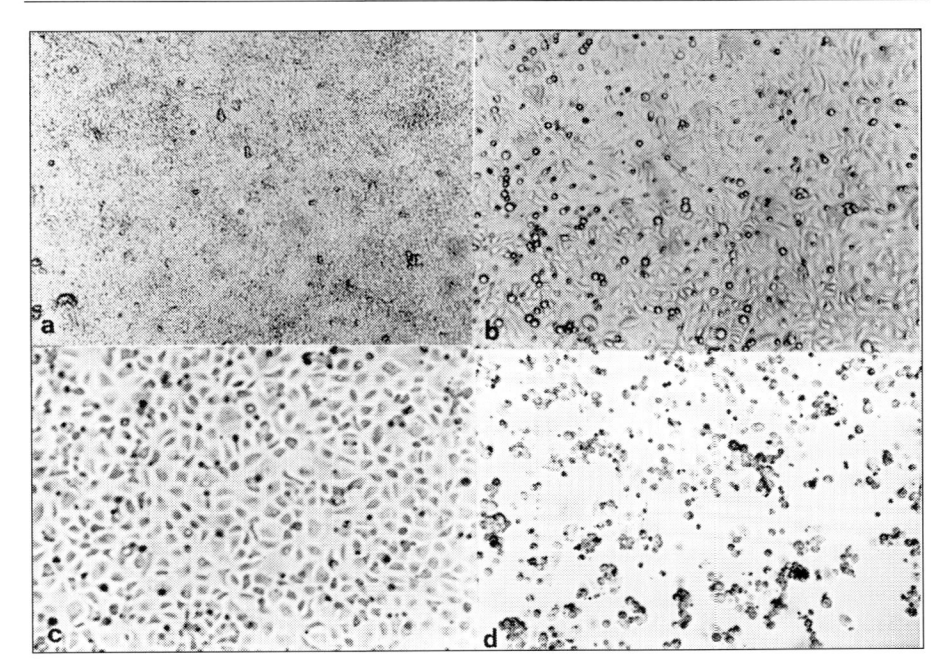

Fig. 15.7. Adenovirus-mediated delivery of an anti-*mdr* ribozyme enhances sensitivity to vincristine. MCF-7Ad cells were infected with either 200 PFU/cell of an adenovirus expressing an anti-*mdr* ribozyme (AdValrib) or 200 PFU/cell AdLacZ. Two days after infection cells were treated with vincristine. (a) Cells without any drugs or virus; (b) Cells treated with 1000 ng/ml vincristine; (c) AdlacZ +1000 ng/ml vincristine; (d) AdValrib + 100 ng/ml vincristine

Conclusion

The extremely rapid development of molecular biology and the discovery of ribozymes, combined with improvements in delivery systems, presumably opens the way to introduce ribozymes for specific antitumor therapy in vivo. The catalytic efficiency of ribozymes combined with the high efficiency of gene transfer and transgene expression in mammalian cells mediated by recombinant adenovirus may in the near future result in the development of an effective in vivo strategy for modulating the MDR phenotype in human cancer. However, there exist several basic issues which have to be solved prior to clinical trials: e.g., how can tumor cells be reached "specifically" to avoid side effects, and how is it possible to increase the rate of cellular uptake when administered by an exogenous pathway? These questions, however, reflect not only the difficulties of molecular antitumor approaches but the fundamental and general difficulties of drug-oriented treatment of malignant tumors.

Acknowledgments

We wish to thank Frau Stemmler for editorial help.

References

1. Dietel M. What's new in cytostatic drug resistance and pathology. Path Res Pract 1991; 187:892-905.
2. Cole SPC, Bhardwaj G, Gerlach JH et al. Overexpression of a transporter gene in a multidrug-resistant human lung cancer cell line. Science 1992; 258:1650-1654.

3. Grant CE, Valdimarsson G, Hipfner DR et al. Overexpression of multidrug resistance-associated protein (MRP) increases resistance to natural product drugs. Cancer Res 1994; 54:357-361.
4. Beck WT, Kim R, Chen M. Novel action of inhibitors of DNA topoisomerase II in drug resistant tumor cells. Cancer Chemoth Pramacol 1994; 34:14-18.
5. Roninson IB. The role of the mdr1 (P-Glycoprotein) gene in multidrug resistance in vitro and in vivo. Biochemical Pharmacology 1992; 43:95-102.
6. Gottesman MM, Pastan I. Biochemistry of multidrug resistance mediated by the multidrug transporter. Ann Rev Biochem 1993; 62:385-427.
7. Nielsen D, Skovsgaard T. P-Glycoprotein as multidrug transporter: A critical review of current multidrug resistant cell lines. Biochimica et Biophysica Acta 1992; 1139:169-183.
8. Ueda K, Cardarelli C, Gottesman MM, Pastan I. Expression of a full length cDNA for the human mdr1 gene confers resistance to colchicine, doxorubicin and vinblastine. Proc Natl Acad Sci USA 1987; 84:3004-3008.
9. Pastan I, Gottesman M. Multiple-drug resistance in human cancer. N Engl J Med 1987; 316:1388-1393.
10. Roninson IB, Chin JE, Choi K et al. Isolation of human mdr DNA sequences amplified in multidrug resistant KB carcinoma cells. Proc Natl Acad Sci USA 1986; 83:4538-4542.
11. Fojo AT, Ueda K, Salmon DJ et al. Expression of a multidrug resistance gene in human tumors and tissues. Proc Natl Acad Sci USA 1987; 84:265-269.
12. Riordan JR, Deuchars K, Kartner N et al. Amplification of P-glycoprotein genes in multidrug-resistant mammalian cell lines. Nature 1985; 316:817-819.
13. Gros P, Croop J, Roninson I et al. Isolation and characterization of DNA sequences amplified in multidrug resistant hamster cells. Proc Natl Acad Sci USA 1986; 83:337-341.
14. Callen DF, Baker E, Simmers RN et al. Localization of the human multiple drug resistance gene, mdr1, to 7q21.1. Hum Genet 1987; 77:142-144.
15. Pastan I, Gottesman MM, Ueda K et al. A retrovirus carrying an MDR1 cDNA confers multidrug resistance and polarized expression of P-glycoprotein in MDCK cells. Proc Natl Acad Sci USA 1989; 85:4486-4490.
16. Kartner N, Ling V. Vielfach-Resistenz von Krebszellen. Spektrum der Wissenschaft 1989; 5:64-71.
17. Gros P, Neriah YB, Croop JM et al. Isolation and expression of a complementary DNA that confers multidrug resistance. Nature 1986; 323:728-731.
18. Cornwell M, Tsudo T, Gottesman M et al. ATP-binding properties of P-glycoprotein from multidrug-resistant KB cells. FASEB J 1987; 1:51-54.
19. Fojo A, Akiyama SI, Gottesman MM et al. Reduced drug accumulation in multiply drug-resistant human KB carcinoma cell lines. Cancer Res 1985:47:3002-3007.
20. Scotto KW, Biedler JL, Melera PW. Amplification and expression of genes associated with multidrug resistance in mammalian cells. Science 1986; 232:751-755.
21. Endicott J, Ling V. The biochemistry of P-glycoprotein mediated multidrug resistance. Annu Rev Biochem 1989:58:137-171.
22. Willingham MC, Cornwell MM, Cardarelli CO et al. Single cell analysis of daunomycin uptake and efflux in multidrug-resistant and -sensitive KB cells: Effects of verapamil and other drugs. Cancer Res 1986; 46:5941-5946.
23. Hoffman MM, Wie LY, Roepe PD. Are altered pHi and membrane potential in hu MDR1 transfectants sufficient to cause MDR protein-mediated multidrug resistance. J Gen Phyiol 1996; 108:295-313.
24. Chin, K-V, Ueda K, Pastan I et al. Modulation of activity of the promoter of the human MDR1 by *Ras* and p53. Science 1992; 25:459-462.
25. Deuchars KL, Ling V. P-Glycoprotein and multidrug resistance in cancer chemotherapy. Semin Oncol 1989; 16:156-165.
26. Reymann A, Looft G, Woermann C et al. Reversal of multidrug resistance in Friend leukemia cells by dexniguldipine-HCL. Cancer Chemotherapy Pharmacology 1994; 32:25-30.

27. Dietel M, Herzig I, Reymann A et al. Secondary combined resistance to the multidrug-resistance-reversing activity of cyclosporin A in the cell line F4-6RADR-CsA. J Cancer Res Clin Oncol 1994; 120:263-271.
28. Fogler WE, Pearson JW, Volker K et al. Enhancement of recombinant human interferon alfa of the reversal of multidrug resistance by MRK-16 monoclonal antibody. J Natl Cancer Inst 1995; 87:94-103.
29. Bouffard DY, Ohkawa T, Kijima H et al. Oligonucleotide modulation of multidrug resistance. European J of Cancer 1996; 32:1010-1018.
30. Uhlenbeck OA. A small catalytic oligoribonucleotide. Nature 1987; 328:596-600.
31. Haseloff J, Gerlach WL. Simple RNA enzymes with new and highly specific endoribonuclease activities. Nature 1988; 334:585-591.
32. Stein CA, Cohen JS. Oligonucleotides as inhibitors of gene expression: A review. Cancer Res 1988; 48:2659-2668.
33. Tidd DM. Synthetic oligonucleotides as therapeutic agents. Br J Cancer 1991; 63:6-8.
34. Sarver N, Cantin EM, Chang PS et al. Ribozymes as a potential anti-Hiv-1 therapeutic agents. Science 1990; 247:1222-1225.
35. Rossi JJ, Sarver N. Catalytic Antisense RNA (Ribozymes): Their potential and use as anti-HIV therapeutic agents. In: Block T et al, ed. Innovations in Antiviral Development and the Detection of virus infection. 1992:95-109.
36. Heidenreich O, Eckstein F. Hammerhead ribozyme-mediated cleavage of the long terminal repeat RNA of human immunodeficiency virus type 1. J Biol Chem 1992; 267:1904-1909.
37. Bertrand E, Pictet R, Grange T. Can hammerhead ribozymes be efficient tools to inactivate gene function? Nucleic Acids Res 1994; 22:293-300.
38. Bertrand E, Grange T, Pictet R. Transacting Hammerhead Ribozymes In Vivo. Present Limits and Future Directions. Gene Regulation, Biology of Antisense RNA and DNA. Vol. 1. New York: Raven Press, Ltd., 1992:71-81.
39. Hertel KJ, Hershlag D, Uhlenbeck OC. A kinetic and themodynamic framework for the hammerhead ribozyme reaction. Biochemistry 1994; 33:3374-3385.
40. Paolella G, Sproat BS, Lamond AI. Nuclease resistant ribozymes with high catalytic activity. EMBO J 1992; 11:1913-1919.
41. Pieken WA, Olsen DB, Benseler F et al. Kinetic characterization of ribonuclease-resistant 2'-modified hammerhead ribozymes. Science 1991; 253:314-317.
42. Heidenreich O, Eckstein F. Hammerhead ribozyme-mediated cleavage of the long terminal repeat RNA of human immunodeficiency virus type 1. Biol Chem 1992; 267:1904-1909.
43. Holm PS, Dietel M, Krupp G. Similar cleavage effiencies of an oligoribonucleotide substrate and an mdr1 mRNA segment by hammerhead ribozyme. Gene 1995; 167:221-225.
44. Yen TJ, Machlin PS, Cleveland DW. Autoregulated instability of beta-tubulin mRNAs by recognition of the nascent amino terminus of beta-tubulin. Nature 1988; 334:580-585.
45. Sullenger BA, Cech TR. Tethering ribozymes to a retroviral packaging signal for destruction of viral RNA. Science 1993; 262:1566-1569.
46. Bertrand E, Rossi JJ. Facilitation of hammerhead ribozyme catalysis by the nucleocapsid protein of HIV-1 and the heterogeneous nuclear ribonucleoprotein A1. EMBO J 1994; 13:2904-2912.
47. Holm PS, Scanlon K, Dietel M. Reversion of the multidrug resistance in the P-glycoprotein positive human pancreatic cell line (EPP85-181RDB) by the introduction of a hammerhead ribozyme. Br J Cancer 1994; 70:239-243.
48. Scanlon KJ, Ishida H, Kashani-Sabet M. Ribozyme-mediated reversal of the multidrug-resistant phenotype. Proc Natl Acad Sci USA 1994; 91:11123-11127.
49. Cucco C, Calabretta B. In vitro and in vivo reversal of multidrug resistance in a human leukemia-resistant cell line by mdr1 antisense oligodeoxynucleotides. Cancer Res 1996; 56:4332-4337.
50. Alahari SK, Dean NM, Fischer MH et al. Inhibition of expression of the multidrug resistance associated P-glycoprotein by phosphorothioate and 5'cholesterol-conjugated phosphorothioate antisense oligonucleotides. Molecular Pharmacology 1996; 50:808-819.

51. Kobayashi H, Dorai T, Holland JF et al. Reversal of drug sensivity in multidrug-resistant tumor cells by an MDR1 (PGY1) ribozyme. Cancer Res 1994; 54:1271-1275.
52. Cotten M, Birnstiel ML. Ribozymes mediated destruction of RNA in vivo. EMBO J 1989; 8:3861-3866.
53. Lieber A, Strauss M. Selection of efficient cleavage sites in target RNAs by using a ribozymes expression library. Molecular and Cellular Biology 1995; 15:540-551.
54. Cagnon L, Cucchiarini M, Lefebre JC et al. Protection of a T-cell line from human immunodeficiency virus replication by the stable expression of short antisense RNA sequence carried by a shuttle RNA molecule. J of Acquired Immune Defiency Syndromes and Human Retrovirology 1995; 9:349-358.
55. Feng M, Cabrera G, Deshane J et al. Neoplastic reversion accomplished by high efficiency adenoviral-mediated delivery of an anti-*ras* ribozyme. Cancer Res 1995; 55:2024-2028.
56. Lieber A, Kay MA. Adenovirus-mediated exoression of ribozymes in mice. J Virology 1996; 70:3153-3158.
57. Yang Y, Nunes FA, Berensci K et al. Cellular immunity to viral antigens limits E1-deleted adenoviruses for gene expression. Proc Natl Acad Sci USA 1994; 91:4407-4411.
58. Huang L, Gao X. Cationic liposome-mediated gene transfer. Gene Therapy 1995; 2:710-722.
59. Lewis JG, Lin KY, Kothavale A et al. A serum-resistant cytofectin for cellular delivery of antisense oligodeoxynucleotides and plasmid DNA. Proc Natl Acad Sci USA 1996; 93:3176-3181.
60. Shimayama T, Nishikawa F, Nishikawa S et al. Nuclease-resistant chimeric ribozymes containing deoxyribonucleotides and phosphorothioate linkages. Nucl Acids Res 1993; 21:2605-2611.
61. Taylor NR, Kaplan BE, Swiderski P et al. Chimeric DNA-RNA hammerhead ribozymes have enhanced in vitro catalytic efficiency and increased stability in vivo. Nucl Acids Res 1992; 20:4559-4565.
62. Williams DM, Pieken WA, Eckstein F. Function of specific 2'-hydroxyl groups of guanosines in a hammerhead ribozyme probed by 2' modifications. Proc Natl Acad Sci USA 1992; 89:918-921.
63. Curiel DT, Agarwal S, Wagner E. Adenovirus enhancement of transferrin-polylysine-mediated gene delivery. Proc Natl Acad Sci USA 1991; 88:8850-8854.
64. Raja-Walia R, Webber J, Naftilan J et al. Enhancment of liposome-mediated gene transfer into vascular tissue by replication deficient adenovirus. Gene Therapy 1995; 2:521-530.
65. Mackellar C, Graham D, Will DW et al. Synthesis and physical properties of anti-HIV antisense oligonucleotides bearing terminal lipophilic groups. Nucleic Acids Res 1992; 20:3411-3417.
66. Thomson JB, Tuschl T, Eckstein F. Activity of hammerhead ribozymes containing non-nucleotidic linkers. Nucleic Acids Res 1993; 21:5600-5603.
67. Lyngstadaas SP, Risnes S, Sproat BS et al. Asynthetic, chemically modified ribozyme eliminates amelogenin, the major translation product in developing mouse enamel in vivo. EMBO J 1995; 14:5224-5229.
68. Snyder DS, Wu Y, Wang JL, Rossi JJ et al. Ribozyme-mediated inhibition of bcr-abl gene expression in a Philadelphia chromosome-positive cell line. Blood 1993; 82:600-605.

CHAPTER 16

Anti-*BCR-ABL* Ribozymes

Lance H. Leopold, Scott K. Shore and E. Premkumar Reddy

Introduction

Normal cell growth is a highly regulated process during which three important families of genes, oncogenes, growth suppressor genes, and apoptotic genes converge and cooperate to maintain homeostasis. Of these three families, oncogenes promote cell growth while growth suppressor genes and apoptotic genes provide negative growth regulation. Carcinogenesis is a multi-step process, often involving activation of oncogenes and deletion or inactivation of growth suppressor and apoptotic genes. Despite the multi-step nature of transformation, in general, restoring the function of key regulators of these cell processes can restore normal growth and differentiation in transformed cells. Among the various strategies employed to accomplish this goal, the inhibition of activated oncogenes can be accomplished by specifically targeting these sequences with complementary nucleic acid sequences that inhibit transcription and translation. The use of antisense and ribozyme molecules to inhibit transforming oncogenes has broad clinical and research applications.

Chronic myelogenous leukemia (CML) is a model disease in which to study the effects of oncogene activation, as it is characterized by the presence of the t(9,22) translocation. CML is a clonal myeloproliferative disorder which involves the hematopoietic stem cell[1] effecting the myeloid, erythroid, magakaryocytic, B lymphoid and occasionally T lymphoid blood elements.[2] In 1960, Nowell and Hungerford[3] discovered a chromosomal abnormality consistently associated with human CML, a shorter long arm of chromosome 22, and named this the Philadelphia chromosome (Ph +). More than 95% of cases of CML, as well as 15-25% of cases of ALL (acute lymphocytic leukemia), harbor the Philadelphia chromosome.[4] Molecular studies have demonstrated that during the formation of the Philadelphia chromosome, a portion of the c-*abl* gene is translocated from chromosome 9q34 to chromosome 22q11, into the *bcr* gene.[5,6] This causes the disruption of two genes and results in the generation of a new fused gene comprising portions of the *bcr* and c-*abl* genes.[7,8] The transcript of this gene either includes (b3a2) or excludes (b2a2) exon 3 of the *bcr* gene. This chimeric gene, termed *BCR-ABL*, produces an abnormal 8.5 kb RNA that encodes a 210 kDa (p210) fusion protein with increased tyrosine kinase activity compared to the normal Abl protein.[9] In addition, the p210$^{BCR-ABL}$ protein is found predominantly in the cytoplasm compared to the normal Abl protein, which is a nuclear protein. *BCR-ABL* mediated transformation is also associated with a number of alterations in cellular signal transduction pathways, which include increased binding of the Ras regulatory protein Grb-2, a block in apoptosis, and altered c-Myc regulation.[10] This new oncoprotein can transform hematopoietic cells, abrogate the growth factor dependence of myeloid cells and block the ability of these cells to differentiate.[11-14] When murine stem cells are infected with a retrovirus encoding the cDNA

Ribozymes in the Gene Therapy of Cancer, edited by Kevin J. Scanlon and Mohammed Kashani-Sabet.
©1998 R.G. Landes Company.

for the *BCR-ABL* gene and inoculated into a mouse, a disease similar to CML results.[15] Thus, BCR-ABL protein plays a crucial role in the transformation process in CML, and disruption of its synthesis is expected to result in the loss of the malignant phenotype. CML is an ideal disease for therapy targeting the *BCR-ABL* fusion gene; as the chimeric gene is the etiologic agent in CML, it is only present in leukemic cells and it occurs in over 95% of CML cases.

There are no conventional therapies that have resulted in cures in CML.[16] Up to 25% of patients receiving alpha interferon injection therapy may durably suppress the expression of the Ph-positive clones in CML.[14] Combination therapy with alpha interferon and cytarabine appears to improve the hematologic and cytogenetic responses and the survival rate in chronic phase CML.[17] However, the ability of interferon to cure CML is not proven.[18,19] Allogeneic bone marrow transplantation (BMT) using HLA identical siblings, following high dose myeloablative chemoradiotherapy is curative in up to 85% of carefully selected patients.[20,21] Notably, patients do not need to be rendered Ph-negative to have benefit or cure of CML.[22,23] Unfortunately, less than 30% of CML patients will have a normal allogeneic HLA matched donor. Current use of matched unrelated donors has resulted in high mortality due to graft-versus-host disease (GVHD) and infections.[24] Thus, the development of an autologous BMT program using Ph-negative stem cells would provide an alternative for patients without other curative options. Unpurged autologous BMTs in CML have not been successful, since Ph-positive stem cells are re-infused into the patient.[25]

Preclinical and clinical studies in humans have shown preliminary success in CML employing purged autologous marrow. Pharmacological purging with mafosphamide or 4 hydroperoxycyclophosphamide,[26] ex vivo treatment of CML marrow with gamma interferon,[27] long term culture of CML marrow,[28] removal of CD34 HLA DR positive cells from stem cells (since they appear to express the Philadelphia chromosome whereas DR negative CD34 positive cells may be largely Ph-negative),[29,30] and recent data showing that stem cells collected after chemotherapy and/or colony stimulating factor treatment have a reduction in *BCR-ABL* positive progenitor cells[31] all have resulted in transient Ph-negative hematopoeisis following high dose autografting therapy. While all of these methods have shown modest success, none of these methods are specific. The goal of antisense and ribozyme-based studies is to demonstrate the ability of these molecules to specifically suppress the *BCR-ABL* transformed phenotype while simultaneously preserving a Ph-negative stem cell pool suitable for use in autologous bone marrow transplantation.

Current Research

In the past decade, the use of antisense and ribozyme molecules to block the translation of mRNA has been developed as a strategy to inhibit viral and malignant diseases. Several groups have reported an inhibition of leukemic cell proliferation by anti-*BCR-ABL* antisense oligodeoxyribonucleotides (ODNs);[32-48] however, a specific inhibition of *BCR-ABL* gene expression has not yet been uniformly demonstrated. Of note, Vaerman et al[49] have questioned the mechanism of ODN growth inhibition in various models and suggest that the effects of ODNs are not due to an antisense effect but are sequence specific. Examination of the RNA sequence in the region of the b2a2 and b3a2 *BCR-ABL* translocations reveal several ribozyme cleavage sites in close proximity to the fusion sites (Fig. 16.1). Further, the b3a2 translocation contains a ribozyme cleavage site immediately 5' to the breakpoint region, suggesting that a ribozyme targeting this cleavage site could be specific. Recently, studies utilizing ribozymes to specifically target the *BCR-ABL* oncogene product have demonstrated in vitro, in vivo, and animal model success.[50-54] The characteristics of these first generation ribozymes are summarized in Table 16.1.

A. B2A2 BCR/ABL mRNA JUNCTION

bcr exon 2   abl exon 2

5'-CACAGCAUUCCGCUGACCAUCAAUAAGGAAG*AAGCC**CUUC**AGCGGGCC**AGUA**GCAUCUGACUU-3'

B. B3A2 BCR/ABL mRNA JUNCTION

bcr exon 3   abl exon 2

5'-GAAUGUCAUC**GUC**CACUCAGCCACUGGAUUUAAGCAGA**GUUC**AA*AA**G**CCCUUCAGCGGGCC**AGUA**GCAUCUGACU-3'

Fig. 16.1. (A) Nucleotide sequence of the b2a2 *BCR ABL* fusion gene. (B) Nucleotide sequence of the b3a2 *BCR ABL* fusion gene. The breakpoints are indicated by the asterisks. Potential ribozyme cleavage sites are NUX sequences, where N is any nucleotide and X = U, A or C. Cleavage sites targeted by ribozymes discussed are in bold. Adjacent cleavage sites result in some of the bold sequences containing four bases.

Table 16.1. Characteristics of first generation anti-BCR-ABL ribozymes

Reference	Ribozyme Target	Length of Binding Regions	Efficacy in Cell-Free Cleavage Reactions	Specificity bcr vs. abl	Transfection Method	Effects
Snyder[50]	b3a2 fusion site	5': 14 bases 3': 15 bases	25% (3hr); 69% (12 hr)	N/A ; N/A	liposomes	decrease BCR-ABL mRNA, protein, cell growth
Shore[51]	b3a2 fusion site	5': 9 bases 3': 8 bases	45% (2 hr)	N/A ; N/A	retroviral	decrease BCR-ABL kinase activity and cell number
Lange[53]	b3a2 fusion site	5': 13 bases 3': 14 bases	+ (6 hr)	0 ; N/A	liposomes	decrease BCR-ABL mRNA decrease cell proliferation over antisense controls
		5': 22 bases 3': 22 bases	0/+ (6 hr)	0 ; N/A	liposomes	decrease BCR-ABL mRNA
Wright[54]	b3a2 fusion site	5': 12 bases 3': 12 bases	77% (4 hr)	20%; N/A	N/A	N/A

Data provided is for equimolar reactions carried out at 37°C. The time points were chosen to make comparisons meaningful. When no quantification of cleavage was performed, estimates were made as follows: 0/+ = minimal, + = moderate, and ++ = extensive cleavage.

Snyder and coworkers[50] reported in 1993 on their experience with a single unit anti-*BCR-ABL* ribozyme. Their ribozyme targeted the b3a2 *BCR-ABL* mRNA sequence and overlapped the joining region. The 5' and 3' flanking arms contained 14 and 15 complementary bases respectively. In cell free experiments, this ribozyme cleaved *BCR-ABL* mRNA sequences containing the joining region. After 12 hours, they reported 69% cleavage of target RNA. It was unclear as to whether this ribozyme cleaved the normal *bcr* RNA, as no *bcr* RNA control was included. In subsequent in vivo experiments they used a DNA-RNA hybrid ribozyme which resisted nuclease cleavage. In an RNAse protection assay, their anti-*BCR-ABL* ribozyme inhibited detectable *BCR-ABL* mRNA by 49% in EM-2 cells (a human CML blast crisis cell line) treated with the anti-*BCR-ABL* ribozyme by lipofection for 48 hours. Antisense sequences targeting the same region only inhibited *BCR-ABL* mRNA by 25% in similar assays. The co-isolation of ribozyme and antisense sequences with the total RNA subsequently probed could have inhibited the probe during processing but not represented a true decrease in *BCR-ABL* mRNA. However, in an immunoprecipitation/protein kinase assay, their anti-*BCR-ABL* hybrid ribozyme eliminated the p210$^{BCR-ABL}$ signal in EM-2 cells after transfection of the ribozyme by lipofection for 72 hours. Antisense controls reduced but did not eliminate the p210$^{BCR-ABL}$ signal. In liquid culture, their hybrid ribozyme inhibited cell growth by 84% in EM-2 cells treated daily with ribozyme for 72 hours. This was marginally better than cells similarly treated with antisense control oligonucleotides. Cells plated in methylcellulose in the absence of growth factors after 72 hours of ribozyme treatment showed significant inhibition of colony formation. No antisense control data was provided for the colony studies. Additional colony studies performed with growth factors may have provided insight into the effect of ribozyme treatment on cell growth. Similarly, analysis of colonies growing after ribozyme treatment for *BCR-ABL* mRNA and protein kinase function would have been interesting. Despite the absence of certain controls which would have shed light on the specificity of their ribozyme and the omission of peripheral details as discussed, their study provided data that an anti-*BCR-ABL* ribozyme could cleave *BCR-ABL* mRNA in vitro and inhibit molecular and physiologic endpoints in cell culture conditions.

Our group had similar results with a single-unit anti-*BCR-ABL* ribozyme in cell free conditions.[51] Our ribozyme also targeted the joining regions of the b3a2 *BCR-ABL* mRNA and contained 5' and 3' complementary sequences of 9 and 8 bases respectively. In in vitro cleavage experiments, efficient cleavage of target *BCR-ABL* mRNA was demonstrated. Cleavage of *bcr* and *abl* RNA sequences was not initially reported. Subsequently, our single unit ribozyme showed evidence of cleavage activity of the *bcr* target RNA.[52]

To test the effect of constitutive expression of this ribozyme, the ribozyme cDNA sequence was inserted into several different retroviral expression vectors. Both polymerase II and III expression systems were tested. K562 cells (a human CML blast cell line) were infected with these retroviruses and subclones analyzed for *BCR-ABL* mRNA, protein kinase activity, and biological characteristics. Several subclones infected with a retrovirus expressing a tRNA/ribozyme hybrid molecule demonstrated inhibition of p210$^{BCR-ABL}$ kinase activity. RT-PCR confirmed that the ribozyme was being expressed in these cells. Furthermore, relative levels of ribozyme expressed by these subclones correlated with BCR-ABL protein inhibition (data not shown). In addition, K562 cells infected with retrovirus containing the gene for the tRNA/ribozyme construct demonstrated a 3-fold decrease in cell growth in IL-3 deficient conditions. This suggests reversal of the growth factor independence which characterizes K562 cells. The effect of this retrovirus on non-*BCR-ABL* containing cells and the growth pattern in IL-3-supplemented K562 subclones infected with the tRNA/ribozyme-containing retrovirus was not reported. While this data provided important evidence that anti-*BCR-ABL* ribozymes could be produced constitutively, it was clear that not all cells infected with a retroviral vector expressed the same levels of ribozyme. Further, high level expression of the ribozyme is necessary to obtain significant reduction in *BCR-ABL* transcripts. The lack of consistent *BCR-ABL* inhibition has led us to consider modifications to the single-unit ribozyme strategy, including a modified tRNA vector and the use of a multi-unit ribozyme (discussed below).

Lange and coworkers also published data on the effect of single-unit anti-*BCR-ABL* ribozymes targeting the b3a2 joining region as a strategy to affect CML biology.[53] They synthesized anti-*BCR-ABL* ribozymes with long and short oligonucleotide flanking arms and initially studied cleavage in a cell free system. Their short ribozyme contained 5' and 3' complementary regions of 13 and 14 bases respectively, while their long ribozyme contained complementary regions of 22 bases. While both ribozymes cleaved *BCR-ABL* mRNA, the degree of cleavage was not quantitated (although it appears to be in the range of similar single-unit ribozymes). The length of the oligonucleotide flanking arms did not appreciably affect cleavage efficiency and, despite the inclusion of numerous controls, they did not include a *bcr* substrate control. Thus, the specificity of their ribozymes can not be assessed. In vivo ribozyme transfection studies were performed in K562 cells using liposomes. Both fluorescence-labeled and [^{32}P]-labeled ribozymes could be detected in K562 cells and revealed ribozyme stability for up to 24 hours. Despite demonstrating ribozyme stability in their system, they performed six transfections in 72 hours with short or long anti-*BCR-ABL* ribozymes. K562 cell proliferation was reduced by 60% and 46% respectively, and only the short ribozyme improved the inhibition compared to antisense control oligonucleotides. In addition, the effect of their ribozymes were not assessed in other cell lines to insure the specificity of the observed effects. Quantitative PCR demonstrated a three to 5-fold reduction in intracellular *BCR-ABL* mRNA in cells similarly transfected with active ribozymes. The explanation for the increased efficiency of the ribozyme in vivo offered by the authors is that cleavage products are removed intracellularly by nucleases. Any activity of the ribozyme during the PCR reaction was not excluded (discussed further below). Further, the authors were unable to demonstrate a reduction in p210 level by Western blot or kinase assays due to very small numbers of cells used in their system, and no attempt to repeat these tests using larger quantities of cells was provided. Overall, their data confirms the potential for using ribozymes to inhibit *BCR-ABL* mRNA; however, ribozyme specificity (both in vitro and in vivo) was not explored.

Wright and coworkers published their experience with an anti-*BCR-ABL* single-unit ribozyme in cell free conditions.[54] Their ribozyme targeted the b3a2 joining region and contained 5' and 3' flanking arms of 12 bases each. At physiologic temperature, they demonstrated efficient cleavage of *BCR-ABL* from both plasmid constructs and total RNA from K562 cells. *BCR-ABL* RNA sequences from plasmid constructs were cleaved 77% and 91% by 1X and 10X ribozyme, respectively, in 4 hour cleavage reactions at 37°C. Cellular *BCR-ABL* RNA was cleaved 66% in an 8 hour cleavage reaction by ribozymes in similar concentrations. However, they also documented substantial cleavage of *bcr* RNA in similar cleavage reactions. No in vivo molecular or physiologic data is provided demonstrating the ability of their ribozyme to function in cells.

Taken together, these initial studies demonstrated the potential for ribozyme-based strategies to be useful in *BCR-ABL* transformed cells. They highlighted in vitro cleavage activity and raised appropriate concerns for ribozyme specificity. In addition, they demonstrated evidence for in vivo activity using both molecular and physiologic end points and, in specific instances, they also demonstrated improved inhibition of *BCR-ABL* transformed cells compared to antisense therapy. Despite these findings, anti-*BCR-ABL* ribozymes did not fulfill the initial enthusiasm for use in purging programs in CML. Difficulties with stability in vitro, intracellular degradation, reliable transfection techniques, and specificity needed to be overcome before clinical testing could proceed. The studies which followed these initial reports investigated these problems using several strategies. Variations in single-unit ribozyme construction,[55-58] constructing multi-unit ribozymes,[52] targeting neighboring sequences,[59] employing novel transfection techniques,[52] and improving retroviral packaging[60] have all been reported. The characteristics of these modified ribozymes are summarized in Table 16.2. Whether or not these modifications will result in a therapeutic window in which to employ a ribozyme-based purging strategy remains to be demonstrated.

Lange and coworkers synthesized four anti-*BCR-ABL* ribozymes differing in their 5' and 3' complementary regions and compared their in vitro and in vivo properties.[55] Their ribozymes targeted the b3a2 *BCR-ABL* joining region and differed from 7 to 13 bases in the 5' flanking region and from 5 to 14 3' bases in the 3' flanking region. They included a non-functional ribozyme with a mutated catalytic region as an antisense control. Maximal ribozyme efficiency was 68% in a 16 hour equimolar cleavage reaction and was demonstrated for a ribozyme with 5' and 3' flanking regions of 9 and 7 bases respectively. Ribozymes with shorter or longer flanking regions were less efficient. Despite the authors' stated concern for specificity, no data was provided on *bcr* cleavage. When their most efficient ribozyme was transfected into K562 cells by lipofection, they obtained a 77% inhibition of BCR-ABL kinase activity as measured by autophosphorylation. This was 2-fold better than their antisense control. In a follow-up study, it was shown that transfections employing liposomes inhibited K562 cell growth approximately 50% by these ribozymes.[61]

Pachuk and coworkers used two separate strategies to create ribozymes targeting non-contiguous sequences of *BCR-ABL* RNA.[56] They chose the b2a2 *BCR-ABL* mRNA in order to attempt to overcome the lack of a ribozyme cleavage site in the immediate region of the chimeric mRNA. Their ribozymes contained anchor sequences complementary to *bcr* exon 2 and a hammerhead ribozyme targeting a more distant triplet in *abl* exon 2. The only sequences that should be cleaved would contain both *bcr* and *abl* sequences. Specifically, the anchor sequences are complementary to bases in exon 2 of *bcr* just 5' to the joining region and are 31, 21, or 11 bases in length. The anchor sequences are connected to a 13 base spacer sequence, which has no complementarity to either *bcr* or *abl* RNA, and are connected to a ribozyme targeting a GUA site in *abl* exon 2. The 5' flanking region contained 9 bases and the 3' flanking region 6 bases complementary to *abl* exon 2. In cell free cleavage reactions, the ribozyme with the shortest anchor sequence was the most efficient. Of note, there was no cleavage of *abl* or *bcr* RNA by the ribozymes containing anchor sequences, and in gel shift experiments, ribozymes containing anchor sequences failed to bind to *abl* or *bcr* RNA, indicating that the specificity was due to lack of binding efficiency. These difficulties could be overcome by first denaturing the RNA and then renaturing in the presence of ribozymes, suggesting that inefficient binding was due to target RNA secondary structure. The optimal length of the anchoring sequence was not determined and may differ for each target RNA sequence, and the importance of the spacer region remains speculative.

Using a second strategy, this group constructed ribozymes which targeted the b2a2 chimeric RNA in the immediate region of the joining region by modifying the flanking arms to target a CUU sequence. The 5' and 3' flanking sequences contained 7 and 12 bases respectively, and the 3' region spanned the joining region and contained sequences complementary to both *bcr* and *abl* exons 2. In addition, a series of ribozymes with mismatches in the 3' *abl* sequences were constructed. Ribozymes with greater than 2 mismatches were unable to cleave target b2a2 *BCR-ABL* RNA. Notably, ribozymes with no or 2 mismatches were able to cleave both b3a2 and b2a2 *BCR-ABL* RNA. These ribozymes similarly showed no cleavage of *bcr* RNA sequences. Taken together, this data represents novel strategies for targeting chimeric RNA. It is noteworthy that these strategies greatly improved the specificity of these ribozymes for cleavage of the chimeric RNA. In addition, the gel shift assays and modified in vitro cleavage reactions after denaturing and renaturing the target

Table 16.2. Characteristics of modified anti-bcr-abl ribozymes

Reference	Ribozyme Target	Length of Binding Regions (Bases)	Additional Modifications	Efficacy in Cell-Free Cleavage Reactions	Specificity bcr vs. abl
Lange[55,56]	b3a2 fusion	5' : 7 ; 3' : 9	none	68% (16 hr)	N/A : N/A
	b3a2 fusion	5' : 7 ; 3' : 5	none	30% (16 hr)	N/A : N/A
	b3a2 fusion	5' : 8 ; 3' : 10	none	51% (16 hr)	N/A : N/A
	b3a2 fusion	5' : 13; 3' : 14	none	62% (16 hr)	N/A : N/A
Pachuk[56]	b2a2 abl exon 2	5' : 9 ; 3' : 31	3' arm anchors to bcr	0/+	0/+ : 0/+
	b2a2 abl exon 2	5' : 9 ; 3' : 21	3' arm anchors to bcr	+	0/+ : 0/+
	b2a2 abl exon 2	5' : 9 ; 3' : 11	3' arm anchors to bcr	++	0/+ : 0/+
Kearney[57]	b3a2 fusion	5' : 12; 3' : 12	no mismatches	77% (4 hr)	20% : N/A
	b3a2 fusion	5' : 12; 3' : 12	mismatch 1st bcr base	0% (4 hr)	0% : N/A
	b3a2 fusion	5' : 12; 3' : 12	mismatch 2nd bcr base	86% (4 hr)	4% : N/A
	b3a2 fusion	5' : 12; 3' : 12	mismatch 3rd bcr base	85% (4 hr)	13% : N/A
Kronenwett[58]	b3a2 fusion	5' : 52; 3' : 3	none	+	0/+ : 0/+
	b3a2 abl exon 2	5' : 3 ; 3' : 69	none	+	0/+ : 0/+
Leopold[52]	b3a2; three sites mismatch	63 bases total	restriction sites	95% (2 hr)	45%; 87%
James[59]	b3a2 abl exon 2	5' : 10; 3' : 20	none	11% (2 hr)	0%: 0%
	b3a2 abl exon 2	5' : 4 ; 3' : 20	none	24% (2 hr)	0%: 0%
	b3a2 fusion	5' : 10; 3' : 10	none	6% (2 hr)	0%: 0%
	b2a2 abl exon 2	5' : 10; 3' : 20	none	21% (2 hr)	0%: 7%

Data provided is for equimolar reactions carried out at 37°C. The time points were chosen to make comparisons meaningful. When no quantification of cleavage was performed, estimates were made as follows: 0/+ = minimal, + = moderate, and ++ = extensive cleavage.

RNA in the presence of ribozymes provided insight into the importance of RNA secondary structure in ribozyme binding. No data was presented regarding the in vivo efficacy of these ribozymes.

Using a similar approach, Kearney and coworkers synthesized four modified single-unit anti-*BCR-ABL* ribozymes and assessed their specificity and efficiency.[57] Their ribozymes targeted the immediate region of the b3a2 chimeric RNA and their initial ribozyme contained 5' and 3' flanking sequences of 12 bases each. Three modified ribozymes were synthesized containing single base mismatches in the 3 *bcr* bases 5' of the joining region. A fourth ribozyme targeted the b3a2 chimeric RNA, one base 3' to the joining region. The ribozyme containing a mismatch in the second base 3' to the cleavage site maintained its efficiency for cleaving *BCR-ABL* RNA but had greatly reduced catalytic activity for *bcr* target RNA. The ribozyme targeting the alternative cleavage site was also specific for *BCR-ABL* though it was less efficient. While this data demonstrates a novel approach to improve the specificity of a ribozyme targeting a chimeric RNA, no in vivo data was presented for these ribozymes.

An extensive kinetic study of antisense and ribozyme sequences targeting *BCR-ABL* sequences was recently published.[58] Ribozymes were studied which contained long (>50 bases) 5' or 3' flanking oligonucleotides, although the length of complementarity varied from 20 to 80 bases. One ribozyme, targeting a cleavage site in the immediate region of the b3a2 *BCR-ABL* junction and containing a 52 base 5' flanking arm, demonstrated efficient cleavage of *BCR-ABL* and limited cleavage of *bcr* or *abl* RNA. Notably, kinetic probing of the local folding potential of the *BCR-ABL* fusion region indicates that this region is not easily accessible for complementary DNA and RNA sequences. The authors postulate that this observation explains the lack of antisense-mediated *BCR-ABL* gene inhibition observed in human cells. This observation has been predicted by RNA secondary structure computer programs and demonstrated in other ribozyme systems.[62,63] The authors stress the importance of targeting regions of RNA that are accessible to nucleic acids.

Our group has approached the problems of efficacy, specificity, and ribozyme delivery by constructing multi-unit ribozymes and developing novel receptor-mediated transfection vehicles.[52] Because examination of the region of the b3a2 joining region reveals several GUX sequences in close proximity, we constructed single, double, and triple-unit ribozymes targeting these sequences. The intervening sequences were composed of complementary bases to the target *BCR-ABL* RNA with the exception of the restriction enzyme sites used for directional cloning. In in vitro cleavage reactions, the triple-unit ribozyme greatly improved the cleavage efficiency compared to single and double-unit ribozymes (Fig. 16.2). In fact, this ribozyme appeared to have the best cleavage efficiency of any published sequence. Because this ribozyme also targets cleavage sites in normal *abl* and *bcr* genes, it was not surprising to observe cleavage of these RNAs as well. However, the greatly improved cleavage of *BCR-ABL* may provide an opportunity to block *BCR-ABL* without significantly effecting normal gene function. Preliminary work employing liposomes to transfect ribozymes into K562 cells resulted in minimal evidence of cleavage of *BCR-ABL* transcripts, with no effect on transformed cell growth, growth-factor independence or block in differentiation.

Because of concerns about the multiple genetic abnormalities in K562 cells, we developed a simpler model of *BCR-ABL* transformation. By infecting 32D cells (a murine myeloblast cell line) with a retrovirus encoding the cDNA for *BCR-ABL*, we created a *BCR-ABL* transformed cell model containing no other genetic abnormalities. In addition, because of growing concerns about the ability of liposomes to deliver nucleic acids to the proper subcellular compartments in reasonable quantities, new transfection vehicles were investigated. By covalently linking a polylysine chain to folic acid, we created a heterobifunctional reagent capable of binding nucleic acids and cellular receptors.

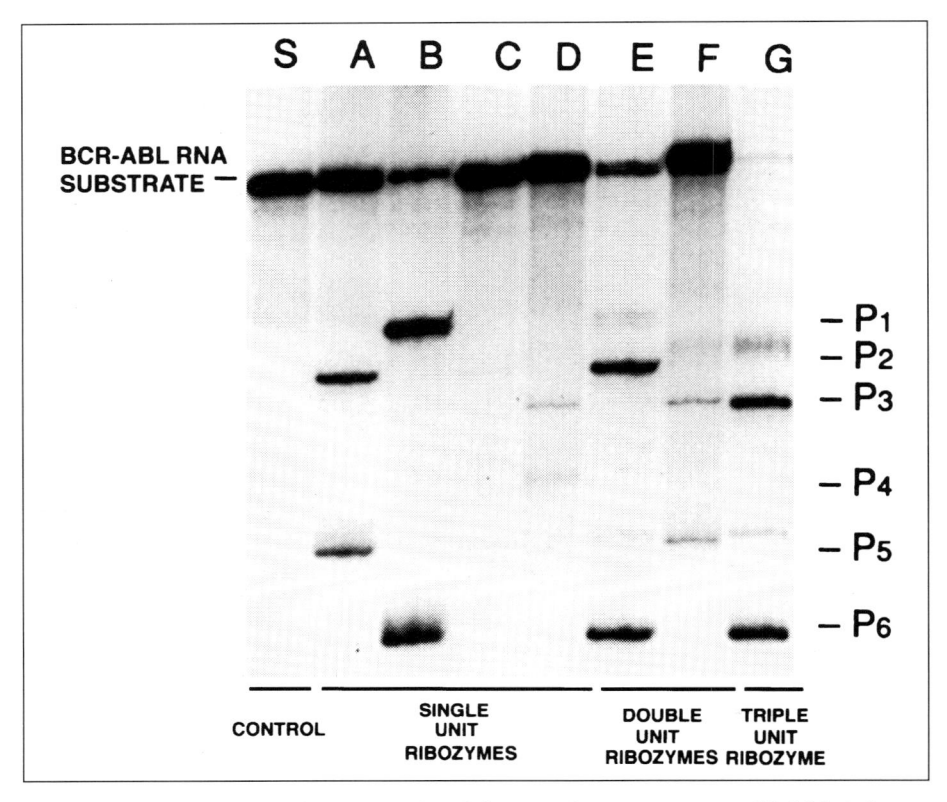

Fig. 16.2. Autoradiogram of ribozyme mediated cleavage of *BCR-ABL* mRNA. [^{32}P]-labeled *BCR-ABL* mRNA was synthesized from a plasmid vector containing a 499 bp segment of the b3a2 *BCR-ABL* chimeric gene. Substrate and ribozyme reactions were carried out in 10 µl volumes. All RNA concentrations were 100 nM. Transcribed RNAs were resuspended in 50 mM Tris-HCl, pH 7.5, containing 1 mM EDTA and heated to 95°C for 5 min, and immediately chilled on ice. Reactions were initiated by adding 1 µl of 200 mM MgCl$_2$ and stopped after 2 hours by adding 2 µl of stop solution containing 95 % formamide, 20 mM EDTA, and 2% bromophenol blue. Cleavage products were separated by electrophoresis on a 6 % denaturing gel. Lane S is a control and contains substrate without ribozymes. Lanes A, B, C, and D show cleavage products from reactions containing single-unit ribozymes targeting *bcr* exon 3, the *BCR-ABL* junction, *bcr* exon 3, and *abl* exon 2 respectively. Ribozymes A and C differ in the length of their annealing arms. Lanes E and F show cleavage products from reactions containing double-unit ribozymes targeting the *BCR-ABL* junction and either *bcr* exon 3 or *abl* exon 2, respectively. Lane G shows cleavage products from a reaction containing a triple-unit ribozyme targeting all three sites. Cleavage with double and triple-unit ribozymes releases small fragments which run at the bottom of the gel and are not shown. P1 through P6 are 314, 286, 263, 235, 212, and 184 base fragments respectively. Modified from Leopold LH et al, Blood, 1995, 85: 2162-2170.

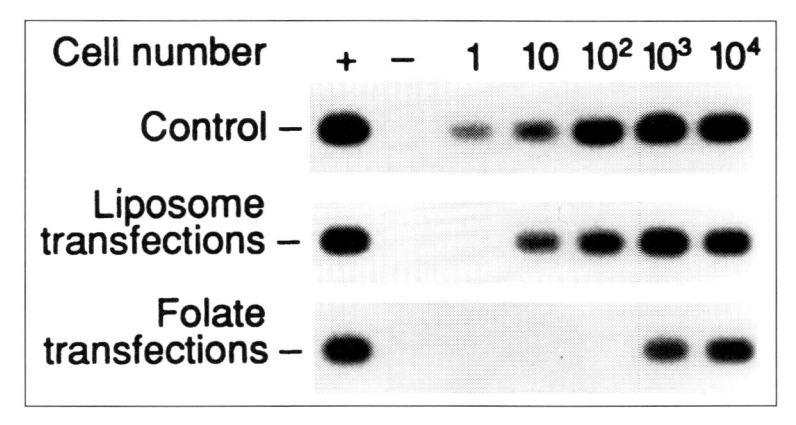

Fig. 16.3. Autoradiogram of a Southern blot of RT-PCR amplified *BCR-ABL* mRNA from transformed 32D cells transfected with ribozymes via liposomes or folic acid-polylysine vectors. From 1 to 1 x 10^4 *BCR-ABL* transformed 32D cells were added to 1 x 10^6 untransformed 32D cells. Cells were transfected with ribozymes or vectors containing no ribozymes (controls) and after 24 hours total cellular RNA was extracted. RT-PCR was performed with primers that amplified the *BCR-ABL* chimeric gene and the β-actin gene (an internal control). Southern blotting was performed with a [^{32}P]-kinased probe that detects the *BCR-ABL* breakpoint. (+) PCR control: RNA transcribed from a plasmid containing the *BCR-ABL* breakpoint region. (–) PCR control: no template addition. Modified from Leopold LH et al, Blood, 1995, 85: 2162-2170.

Transfection of the triple-unit ribozyme by folate-polylysine into *BCR-ABL* transformed 32D cells resulted in a 3 log reduction of *BCR-ABL* mRNA measured by RT-PCR and Southern blotting (Fig. 16.3). There was no evidence of ribozyme activity in the PCR amplification step when ribozymes were deliberately added to cellular RNA prior to analysis. In addition, *BCR-ABL* transformed 32D cells demonstrated growth inhibition in growth factor deficient medium when transfected daily with ribozymes by folate-polylysine uptake.[64] There was no growth inhibition seen in these cells by antisense control sequences, transfection vehicle alone, or when growth factors were provided. This model does not allow appropriate testing of the ribozyme for specificity, as murine *bcr* and *abl* sequences are not targeted by this ribozyme. Preliminary work employing clonogenic assays and normal human stem cells has failed to show any added toxicity due to the triple-unit ribozyme over that seen by transfection vehicles alone. We are continuing to investigate improved expression systems as has been recently reported.[60] These observations will be further tested using a SCID mouse model of CML.

James and coworkers have constructed ribozymes targeting the b3a2 and b2a2 *BCR-ABL* translocations with modified complementary flanking oligonucleotides.[59] They observed, in in vitro cleavage reactions, that ribozymes targeting 9 bases 3' and 3 bases 5' to the joining region of the b3a2 *BCR-ABL* sequence were specific at physiologic temperature. The ribozyme targeting 9 bases 3' of the junction had a 3' flanking sequence containing 20 bases and a 5' sequence with 10 bases. The ribozyme targeting the immediate joining region had 5' and 3' flanking arms of 10 bases each. By reducing the length of the 5' flanking region of the ribozyme targeting 9 bases 3' of the joining region to 4 bases, efficacy improved from 11% to 24% cleavage without cleavage of normal *abl* sequences. They also observed that similar ribozymes with short noncomplementary bases on the ends of otherwise identical ribozymes (resulting from the cloning strategy used) slightly improved efficacy of cleavage. In subsequent reports,[65,66] they have shown that transfection of this modified ribozyme into *BCR-ABL* transformed 32D cells failed to affect *BCR-ABL* mRNA levels by RT-PCR or RNAse protection assay. Despite these observations, cell growth was inhibited in a dose-related manner and survival of SCID mice transplanted with ribozyme-treated 32D *BCR-ABL* cells had prolonged survival compared to control treated mice.

Other recent data demonstrates the potential effectiveness of constitutive expression of ribozymes targeting *BCR-ABL* mRNA. Liu and coworkers recently reported the results of transfection studies employing retroviral expression systems for anti-*BCR-ABL* ribozymes in K562 cells.[67] They developed ribozymes which target the immediate joining region and the *bcr* translation initiation site, and expressed these ribozymes in pLXSN vector containing the SV promoter connected to a rabbit hemoglobin intron. They report high infection efficiency of K562 cells and inhibition of K562 cell growth in culture, soft agar, and a SCID mouse model by both ribozyme-expressing retroviruses.

Snyder and coworkers have reported on the effectiveness of an anti-*BCR-ABL* hairpin ribozyme which targets the p190 mRNA found in acute lymphoblastic leukemia patients (ALL).[68] Despite lack of ribozyme specificity data, transfection studies employing liposomes in p190-expressing cells demonstrated decreased levels of p190 protein and growth inhibition.

Our group has also recently reported preliminary results with tRNA/ribozyme hybrid molecules expressed from the retroviral vector DCt5T' (Fig. 16.4).[69] When the triple-unit anti-*BCR-ABL* ribozyme is cloned into the 3' tRNA tail and expressed in in vitro systems fully functional ribozymes are produced. Electroporation of this vector into K562 cells resulted in the isolation of several subclones expressing ribozymes and containing reductions in *BCR-ABL* transcripts. Experiments are currently in progress to study the effects of these vectors on p210*Bcr abl* protein levels and growth factor independent growth of transfected cells.

In summary, these initial experiences with anti-*BCR-ABL* ribozymes have demonstrated the challenges that are faced by researchers applying antisense and ribozyme strategies to inhibit oncogenes. Despite initial success in in vitro cleavage reactions, the issues of efficacy and specificity remain key problem areas in ribozyme development. Delivering ribozymes to cells and subcellular locations are critical issues being explored to improve the efficacy of ribozyme-based therapies. Delivery methods employing ribozymes as drugs and first generation models employing constitutive expression strategies have not demonstrated reliable inhibition of *BCR-ABL* transformed cells, whether assayed by molecular or biologic end points. Whether or not modifications to these approaches will improve on current results will determine the role that antisense and ribozyme strategies play in treating malignant diseases. These issues are discussed further below.

Future Directions

As our knowledge of RNA trafficking improves, additional strategies for ribozyme design and delivery will be developed. The problem of improving ribozyme efficacy, specificity, cellular delivery, co-localization with target RNA, and efficient expression are critical areas of ongoing research. Strategies for improving these properties of anti-*BCR-ABL* ribozymes are discussed.

Modifications in ribozyme design continue to be relevant issues to improve efficacy and specificity. Although targeting the joining region has been the most common strategy for ribozyme design, this has not guaranteed specificity. Considering the relative inaccessibility of this site due to RNA secondary structure,[70] targeting other cleavage sites remains an attractive option for improving efficacy. The use of RNA-folding programs can assist in the

Fig. 16.4. RT-PCR analysis from K562 cells infected with retroviral constructs encoding triple-unit ribozymes. K562 cells were electroporated with retroviruses encoding tRNA/ribozyme hybrid molecules from the DCt5T' vector. Cells were plated and grown in the presence of neomycin to select for clones containing DNA coding for ribozymes. hrIL-3 (5 pmol/μl) was provided in the media to prevent negative selection, as cells with low levels of BCR-ABL tyrosine kinase may become growth factor dependent. Single cells were isolated, expanded and screened for the production of ribozymes by RT-PCR employing primers antisense to the multi-unit ribozyme. Southern blots were performed with [^{32}P]-labeled oligonucleotides specific for ribozymes, *BCR-ABL*, and actin DNA. Panel A shows the results of PCR analysis for the presence of the triple-unit ribozyme in cells electroporated with the DCt5T' retroviral construct. Lanes 1, 2, 3, and 8 demonstrate the presence of ribozymes in these clones. K562 parental cells contain no ribozymes. The positive plasmid control contains ribozyme bands with prolonged exposure. In Panel B, *BCR-ABL* PCR analysis is shown. Clones 1 and 8 inhibited *BCR-ABL* mRNA production. K562 cells and plasmid controls also demonstrated the presence of *BCR-ABL* mRNA sequences. Panel C shows the results of β-actin gene amplification and is presented to show that similar quantities of mRNA were used in RT and PCR reactions.

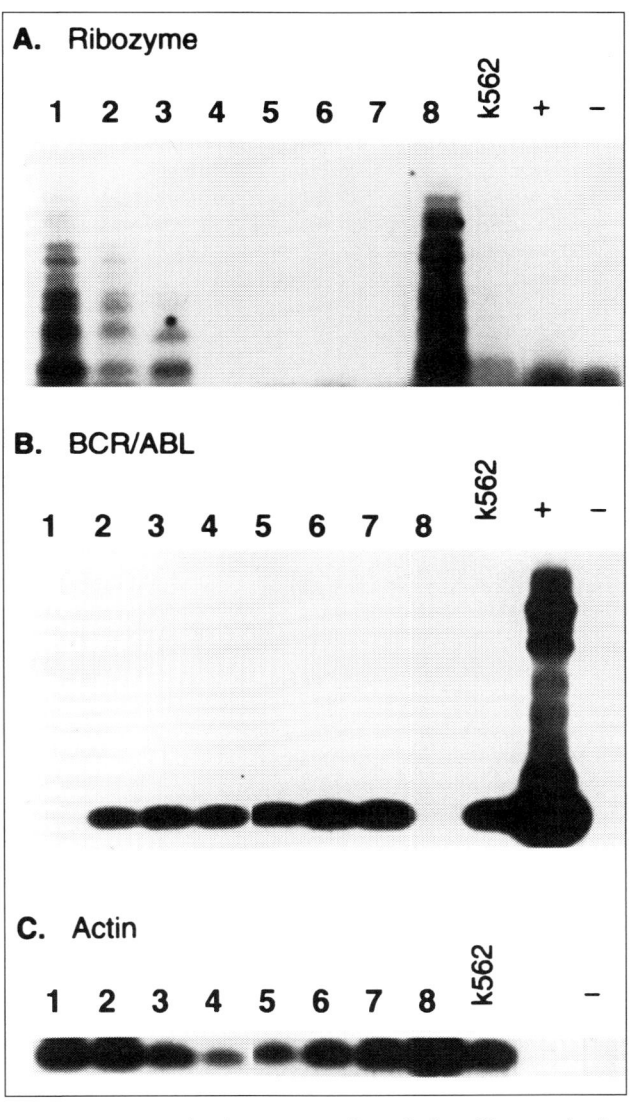

identification of accessible cleavage sites. Further, employing anchoring sequences, varying the length of the oligonucleotide flanking arms, targeting multiple cleavage sites, and including extra or mismatched sequences have had unpredictable effects on ribozyme efficacy and specificity.[71] These modifications have largely been a process of trial and error, and combinations of these strategies may optimize efficacy and maintain specificity.

Other aspects of ribozyme design impact on ribozyme efficacy and specificity. Mutations in the target RNA may be a strategy which malignant cells employ to develop resistance to ribozyme-based therapy. Analogous to the application of combination therapies for various malignant and viral diseases, targeting several sites for ribozyme cleavage may be necessary to prevent the emergence of resistant clones. Further, the role of intracellular RNA binding proteins is beginning to be explored. The heterogeneous nuclear-ribonuclear protein hnRNP A1 is associated with RNAs in the nucleus and cytoplasm, and in in vitro cleavage reactions facilitate ribozyme cleavage by enhancing product release from ribozyme flanking oligonucleotides.[72,73] This enhancement may be limited by the degree of complementarity between ribozyme and target RNA and may be unavailable for ribozymes employing mismatching or anchoring strategies. Empirical testing is required to answer these questions.

Ribozymes can be delivered to cells as therapeutic agents or as genes encoding these sequences. Further, gene therapy can be accomplished through both viral and non-viral methods. There are various physico-chemical methods to facilitate RNA uptake into large amounts of cells including liposomes and cationic lipids, and heterobifunctional reagents binding to cell surface molecules and nucleic acids. Liposomal strategies are limited by being nonspecific, only transiently affecting target RNA levels, and delivering the majority of their contents to endosomes where RNA degradation may occur.[74] As there appears to be a requirement for a large excess of ribozymes in vivo applications, liposomal strategies may be limited.[75] Receptor-mediated uptake and employing heterobifunctional reagents can improve the intracellular effectiveness of ribozymes by improving intracellular trafficking and half life.[52] The specificity of such reagents can be improved by employing antibody-mediated uptake. Such a vector would contain an antibody (which binds to cells) attached to liposomes or polylysine (which binds to RNA).[76] The CD34 antigen would be an ideal target for such a vector since the transformed stem cell in CML is CD34 positive. In addition, an antibody targeting the HLA-DR antigen could be upregulated by interferon and may allow increased ribozyme uptake. These strategies may target the malignant clone which is HLA-DR positive, while sparing the normal stem cell compartment which is HLA-DR negative. Further, targeting multiple receptors may optimize ribozyme delivery.

Ribozyme gene therapy can employ both viral and non-viral methods. Gene therapy has the potential to improve ribozyme co-localization with target RNA as the ribozyme is produced by the same cellular transcription machinery. However, concerns about releasing competent viruses, transcription silencing, low infection/transduction rates, disrupting normal cellular genes during viral integration, and the need for the target cell to divide to allow viral integration are some of the concerns facing the development of retroviral gene-based therapies. Retroviral vectors employ RNA polymerase II or III based systems with constitutive, tissue-specific, and inducible promoters. Packaging strategies must consider sequences for termination, capping, RNA processing, and RNA transport to subcellular compartments. Including bacterial operator-repressor systems or tissue-specific promoters may add expression control. In addition, variations in the viral expression system may reduce competition between inserted promoters and viral long terminal repeats (LTRs).

Alternative viral vectors and non-viral techniques have also been developed to overcome several of the problems associated with retroviral systems. Adeno-associated virus has a higher transduction efficiency than traditional retroviral vectors, and its integration can be directed. Adenovirus systems can deliver genes to cells for transient expression, as integration is not necessary for gene activation. In addition, gene guns, liposomes, and heterobifunctional reagents can all deliver genes of various sizes to cells. While these nonviral methods generally have higher transduction efficiency and avoid the issue of release of competent retroviruses, random insertion, transcription repression, and toxicity remain ongoing concerns.

Despite improvements in viral and non-viral expression systems, comparatively little is known about intracellular RNA transport. mRNA has a heterogeneous distribution in cells and trafficking may be accomplished by sequences in the 3' untranslated region of mRNAs. Including these localization signals in ribozyme expression systems may improve the co-localization of ribozymes with target RNA. In addition, mRNA processing involves small nuclear RNA in the cell nucleus. These sequences could be included in ribozyme transcription units to improve nuclear ribozyme and target interactions.

CML remains a model disease in which to consider using ribozyme-based therapy to inhibit the disease-causing oncogene. Despite advances, only allogeneic BMT is curative in CML. As the properties that affect ribozyme efficacy and specificity become better defined and the intracellular signals that govern RNA trafficking become understood, the improvements in gene therapy and RNA delivery strategies can be applied to helping patients overcome this otherwise fatal disease.

References

1. Golde DW, Chaplin RE. Chronic myelogenous leukemia: Recent advances. Blood 1985; 65:1039.
2. Fialkow PJ, Jacobson RJ, Papayannopoulou T. Chronic myelocytic leukemia. Clonal origin in a stem cell common to the granulocyte, erythrocyte, platelet and monocyte/macrophage. Am J Med 1977; 63:125.
3. Nowell PC, Hungerford DA. A minute chromosome in human chronic granulocytic leukemia. Science 1960; 132:1497-1499.
4. Kurzrock R, Gutterman JU, Talpaz M. The molecular genetics of Philadelphia chromosome-positive leukemias. New Engl J Med 1988; 319:990-998.
5. Rowley JD. A new consistent chromosomal abnormality in chronic myelogenous leukemia identified by quinacrine flourescence and Giemsa staining. Nature 1973; 243:290-293.
6. deKlein A, Geurts van Kessel A, Grosveld G et al. A cellular oncogene is translocated to the Philadelphia chromosome in chronic myelogenous leukemia. Nature 1982; 300:765-767.
7. Heisterkamp N, Stephenson JR, Geoffen J et al. Localization of the c-abl oncogene adjacent to a translocation breakpoint in chronic myeocytic leukemia. Nature 1983; 306:239-42.
8. Schtivelman E, Lifshitz B, Gale RP et al. Fused transcript of abl and bcr genes in chronic myelogenous leukemia. Nature 1985; 315:550-553.
9. Konopka JB, Watanabe SM, Witte ON. An alteration of the human c-abl protein in K562 cells unmasks associated tyrosine kinase activity. Cell 1984; 37:1035-1042.
10. Kantarjian HM, Deisseroth A, Kurzrock R et al. Chronic myelogenous leukemia: A concise update. Blood 1993; 82,3:691-703.
11. McLaughlin J, Chianese E, Witte ON. In vitro transformation of immature hematopoietic cells by the P210 BCR-ABL oncogene product of the Philadelphia chromosome. Proc Natl Acad Sci USA 1987; 84:6358.
12. Daley GQ and Baltimore D. Transformation of an interleukin 3-dependent hematopoietic cell line by the chronic myelogenous leukemia-specific p210bcr abl protein. Proc. Natl. Acad. Sci. USA 1988; 85:9312-9316.
13. Cannistra S. Chronic myelogenous leukemia as a model for genetic basis for cancer. Hematol Oncol Clin North Am 1990; 4:337.
14. Kantarjian HM, Deisseroth A, Kurzrock R, Estrov Z, and Talpaz M. Chronic myelogenous leukemia: A concise update. Blood 1993; 82:691-703.

15. Daley GQ, Van Etten RA, Baltimore D. Induction of chronic myelogenous leukemia in mice by the p210*bcr abl* gene of the Philadelphia chromosome. Science 1990; 247:824-830.
16. Lichtman MA. Chronic myelogenous leukemia and related disorders. In: Williams WJ et al, eds. Hematology. 4th ed. New York: McGraw-Hill, 1990:205-212.
17. Guilhot F, Chastang C, Michallet M et al. Interferon alpha-2b combined with cytarabine versus interferon alone in chronic myelogenous leukemia. N Engl J Med 1997; 337:223-9.
18. Talpaz M, Kantarjian H, McCredie K et al. Hematologic remission and cytogenetic improvement induced by recombinant human interferon alpha in chronic myelogenous leukemia. N Eng J Med 1986; 314:1065-1069.
19. The Italian Cooperative Study Group on Chronic Myeloid Leukemia. Interferon alfa-2a as compared with conventional chemotherapy for the treatment of chronic myeloid leukemia. N Eng J Med 1994; 330:820-25.
20. Butturini A, Keating A, Goldman J et al. Autotransplants in chronic myelogenous leukemia: Strategies and results. The Lancet 1990; 335:1255-1258.
21. Gale RP, Butturini A. How do transplants cure chronic myelogenous leukemia? Bone Marrow Transplantation 1992; 9:83-85.
22. Pichert G, Alyea EP, Soiffer RJ et al. Persistence of myeliod progenitor cells expressing BCR-ABL mRNA after allogeneic bone marrow transplantation for chronic myelogenous leukemia. Blood 1994; 84,7:2109-2114.
23. Miyamura K, Tahara T et al. Long persistent *bcr-abl* positive transcript detected by polymerase chain reaction after marrow transplant for chronic myelogenous leukemia without clinical relapse: A study of 64 patients. Blood 1993; 81,4:1089-1093.
24. Marks DI, Cullis JO, Ward KN et al. Allogeneic bone marrow transplantation for chronic myeloid leukemia using sibling and volunteer unrelated donors. Ann Int Med 1993; 119:207-214.
25. Reiffers J, Trouette R, Marit G et al. Autologous blood stem cell transplantation for chronic granulocytic leukemia transformation: A report of 47 cases. Brit J Haematology 1991; 77:339-345.
26. Marcus RE, Goldman JM. Autografting in chronic granulocytic leukemia. Clinics in Haematology 1986; 15:235-247.
27. McGlave PB, Arthur D, Miller WJ et al. Autologous transplantation for CML using marrow treated ex vivo with recombinant human interferon gamma. Bone Marrow Transplantation 1990; 6:115-120.
28. Barnett MJ, Eaves CJ, Phillips GL et al. Successful autografting in chronic myeloid leukemia after maitenance of marrow in culture. Bone Marrow Transplantation 1989; 4:345-351.
29. Berenson R. Transplantation of stem cells enriched by immunoadsorption. Third International Symposium on Bone Marrow Purging and Processing, San Diego, Oct 4, 1991 (Abstract).
30. Verfaillie CM, Miller WJ, Boylan K et al. Selection of benign primitive hematopoietic progenitors in chronic myelogenous leukemia on the basis of HLA-DR antigen expression. Blood 1992; 79:1003-1010.
31. O'Brien SG, Goldman JM. Current approaches to hematopoietic stem-cell purging in chronic myeloid leukemia. Journal of Clinical Oncology 1995; 13,3:541-546.
32. Taj AS, Martiat P, Dhut S et al. Inhibition of $P210^{BCR-ABL}$ expression in K562 cells by electroporation with an antisense oligonucleotide. Leuk Lymphoma 1990; 3:201.
33. Skorski T, Szczylik C, Malaguarnera L et al. Gene-targeted specific inhibition of chronic myeloid leukemia cell growth by BCR-ABL antisense oligodeoxynucleotides. Folia Histochem Cytobiol 1991; 29:85.
34. Mahon FX, Belloc F, Reiffers J. Antisense oligomers in chronic myeloid leukaemia. Lancet 1993; 341:566.
35. Kirkland MA, O'Brien SG, McDonald C et al. BCR-ABL antisense purging in chronic myeloid leukaemia. Lancet 1993; 342:614.
36. Maekawa T, Murakami A, Kimura S et al. Clonal suppression of human leukemia cell growth by antisense oligodeoxynucleotide phosphorothioates. J Cell Biochem 1993; 197 (suppl 17E).

37. Skorski T, Nieborowska-Skorska M, Barletta C et al. Highly efficient elimination of Philadelphia leukemic cells by exposure to *bcr-abl* antisense oligodeoxynucleotides combined with mafosfamide. J Clin Invest 1993; 92:194.
38. Vaerman JL, Lewalle P, Martiat P. Antisense inhibition of p210 *bcr-abl* in chronic myeloid leukemia. Stem Cells 1993; 11:89 (suppl 2).
39. DeFabritiis P, Amadori S, Calabretta B et al. Elimination of clonogenic Philadelphia-positive cells using BCR-ABL antisense olgodeoxynucleotides. Bone Marrow Transplant 1993; 12:261.
40. Smetser TFCM, Skorski T, Van de Locht LTF et al. Antisense BCR-ABL oligonucleotides induce apoptosis in the Philadelphia chromosome positive cell line BV173. Leukemia 1994; 1:129.
41. Skorski T, Nieborowska-Skorska M, Nicolaides NC et al. Suppression of Philadelphia leukemia cell growth in mice by *bcr-abl* antisense oligodeoxynucleotides. Proc Natl Acad Sci USA 1994; 91:4504.
42. Okabe M, Kunieda Y, Miyagishima T et al. BCR-ABL oncoprotein-targeted antitumor activity of antisense oligonucleotides complementary to BCR-ABL mRNA and herbimycin A, an antagonist of protein tyrosine kinase: Inhibitory effects on in vitro growth of Phl-positive leukemia cells and BCR-ABL oncoprotein-associated transformative cells. Leuk Lymphoma 1993; 10:307.
43. Bedi A, Zehnbauer BA, Barber JP et al. Inhibition of apoptosis by BCR-ABL in chronic myeloid leukemia. Blood 1994; 83:2038.
44. Thomas M, Kosciolek B, Wang N et al. Capping of *bcr-abl* antisense oligonucleotides enhances antiproliferative activity against chronic myeloid leukemia cell lines. Leuk Res 1994; 18:401.
45. McGahon A, Bissonnette R, Schmitt M et al. BCR-ABL maintains resistance of chronic myelogenous leukemia cells to apoptotic cell death. Blood 1994; 83:1179.
46. Tari AM, Tucker SD, Deisseroth A et al. Liposomal delivery of methylphosphonate antisense oligonucleotides in chronic myelogenous leukemia. Blood 1995; 84:601.
47. O'Brien SG, Kirkland MA, Melo JV et al. Antisense BCR-ABL oligomers cause non-specific inhibition of chronic myeloid leukemia cell lines. Leukemia 1994; 8:2156.
48. Smetsers TFCM, Van de Locht LTF, Pennings AHM et al. Phosphorothioate BCR-ABL antisense oligonucleotides induce cell death, but fail to reduce cellular *bcr-abl* protein levels. Leukemia 1995; 9:118.
49. Vaerman JL, Lammineur C, Moureau P et al. BCR-ABL antisense oligodeoxyribonucleotides suppress the growth of leukemic and normal hematopoietic cells by a sequence-specific but nonantisense mechanism. Blood 1995; 86:3891-3896.
50. Snyder DS, Wu Y, Wang JL et al. Ribozyme-mediated inhibition of *bcr-abl* gene expression in a Philadelphia chromosome-positive cell line. Blood 1993; 82:600-605.
51. Shore SK, Nabissa PM, Reddy EP. Ribozyme-mediated cleavage of the BCRABL oncogene transcript: in vitro cleavage and in vivo loss of P210 protein-kinase activity. Oncogene 1993; 8:3183-3188.
52. Leopold LH, Shore SK, Newkirk TA et al. Multi-unit ribozyme-mediated cleavage of *bcr-abl* mRNA in myeloid leukemias. Blood 1995; 85:2162-2170.
53. Lange W, Cantlin EM, Finke J et al. In vitro and in vivo effects of synthetic ribozymes targeted against BCR-ABL mRNA. Leukemia 1993; 7:1786-1794.
54. Wright L, Wilson SB, Milliken S et al. Ribozyme-mediated cleavage of the *bcr-abl* transcript exprressed in chronic myelogenous leukemia. Exp Hematology 1993; 21:1714-8.
55. Lange W, Daskalakis M, Finke J et al. Comparison of different ribozymes for efficient and specific cleavage of BCR-ABL related mRNAs. FEBS Letters 1994; 338:175-178.
56. Pachuk CJ, Yoon K, Moellling K et al. Selective cleavage of *bcr-abl* chimeric RNAs by a ribozyme targeted to non-contiguous sequences. Nucleic Acids Research 1994; 22:301-307.
57. Kearney P, Wright LA, Milliken S et al. Improved specificity of ribozyme-mediated cleavage of *bcr-abl* mRNA. Experimental Hematology 1995; 23:986-989.
58. Kronenwett R, Haas R, Sckakiel G. Kinetic selectivity of complementary nucleic acids: *bcr-abl*-directed antisense RNA and ribozymes. J Mol Biol 1996; 259:632-644.

59. James H, Mills K, Gibson I. Investigating and improving the specificity of ribozymes directed against the bcr-abl translocation. Leukemia 1996; 10:1054-1064.
60. Thompson JD, Ayers DF, Malmstrom TA et al. Improved accumulation and activity of ribozymes expressed from a tRNA-based RNA polymerase III promotor. Nucleic Acids Research 1995; 23:2259-2268.
61. Lange W. Cleavage of BCR-ABL mRNA by synthetic ribozymes—effects on the proliferation rate of K562 cells. Klin Padiatr 1995; 207:222-224.
62. Perriman R, Delves A, Gerlach WL. Extended target-site specificity for a hammerhead ribozyme. Gene 1992; 113:157.
63. Fedor JJ, Uhlenbeck OC. Substrate sequence affects "hammerhead" RNA catalytic efficiency. Proc Natl Acad Sci USA 1990; 87:1668.
64. Leopold LH, Shore SK, Reddy EP. Multi-unit anti-BCR-ABL ribozyme therapy in chronic myelogenous leukemia. Leukemia and Lymphoma 1995; 18:179-184.
65. James HA, Twomey CM, Mills KI et al. Specificity of ribozymes against the bcr-abl mRNAs in vitro. Biochemical Society Transactions 1996; 24:409S.
66. Mills KI, Walsh V, Gilkes AF et al. In vitro ribozyme treatment of 32D cells expressing a bcr-abl construct prolongs the survival of SCID mice. Proceedings of Amer Soc Hematolgy 1996; 2296, Abstract.
67. Liu JH, Cheng SC, Chu CJ et al. Retrovirally transduced ribozymes suppress the growth of chronic myelogenous leukemic cell line. Proceedings of Amer. Society of Hematology 1996; 816, Abstract.
68. Snyder DS, Wu Y, McMahon R et al. Ribozyme-mediated inhibition of a Philadelphia-chromosome positive acute lymphoblastic leukemia cell line expressing the p1'90 bcr-abl oncogene. Proceedings of the American Society of Hematology 1996; 821, Abstract.
69. Leopold LH, Shore SK, Krishnaraju J et al. Retroviral expression of a triple-unit anti-bcr-abl ribozyme inhibits bcr-abl RNA expression in K562 cells. Proceedings American Society of Oncology 1997; 1956, Abstract.
70. Mahone FX, Ripoche J, Pigeonnier et al. Inhibition of chronic myelogenous leukemia cells harboring a bcr-abl b3a2 junction by antisense oligonucleotides targeted at the b2a2 junction. Exp Hematol 1995; 23:1608-1611.
71. Zoumadakis M, Neubert WJ, Tabler M. The influence of imperfectly paired helices I and III on the catalytic activity of hammerhead ribozymes. Nucleic Acids Res 1994; 22:5271-5278.
72. Herschlag D, Khosla M, Tsuchihashi Z et al. An RNA chaperone activity of non-specific RNA binding proteins in hammerhead ribozyme catalysis. EMBO J. 1994; 13:2913-2924.
73. Bertrand E, Rossi JJ. Facilitation of hammerhead ribozyme catalysis by the nucleocapsid protein of HIV-1 and heterogeneous nuclear ribonuclear protein A1. EMBO J. 1994; 13:2904-2912.
74. Cameron F, Jennings P. Specific gene suppression by engineered ribozymes in monkey cells. Proc Natl Acad Sci USA 1989; 86:9139-9143.
75. Cotten M, Birnstiel ML. Ribozyme mediated destruction of RNA in vivo. EMBO J 1989; 8:3861-3866.
76. Renneisen K, Leserman L, Matthes E et al. Inhibition of human immunodeficiency virus-1 in vitro by antibody-targeted liposomes containing antisense RNA to the env region. J Biol Chem 1990; 265:163337-42.

CHAPTER 17

Potential Design and Facilitation of Hammerhead Ribozyme Turnover by Cellular Proteins

Mouldy Sioud

Introduction

Phenotypic inhibition of gene expression is an important experimental method to determine the function of genes and could have a great impact upon the treatment of diseases in which an undesirable overproduction of a protein is implicated in the pathogenesis. Some of the major problems of the currently used drugs include both their specificity and cytotoxicity. In the case of cancer chemotherapy, for example, the ratio of the toxic dose to the therapeutic dose is relatively low, indicating that a large number of cellular targets may be affected by any chemotherapeutic drug. Therefore, there is a need for increasing the specificity of any medication, since it would be desirable to affect only proteins causing diseases without harming normal cells.

Because of the specificity of Watson-Crick base pairing, in principle strategies based upon nucleic acids targeted at a gene involved in diseases such as cancer should interfere only with the function of this gene. In this area three major approaches have been used to downregulate the expression of genes. The first is the use of antisense DNA or RNA,[1] the second approach involves the formation of a triple helix[2] and the third is ribozyme-mediated RNA cleavage.[3-5] For therapeutic application, cleavage of mRNA by ribozymes is likely to be more promising than the two other strategies mentioned above. Ribozymes not only complex with target sequences via complementary antisense arms, but also hydrolyze the target RNA. Thus, ribozymes have the potential to work like molecular scissors to snip a messenger RNA that contains the genetic code for synthesizing a disease-causing protein.

Ribozyme application has revealed a number of important results in vitro, in tissue culture and in vivo.[6-11] However, despite this significant progress, there is still a lot to learn in order to optimize ribozyme function in the complex intracellular environment. The intracellular ribozyme activity can be affected by a number of potential intracellular factors such as the ability of the ribozyme to co-localize with target RNA,[12] the accessibility of the target sites[13] and the effect of endogenous proteins upon ribozyme catalysis.[14-17] Studies that address these current obstacles are likely to lead to successful applications of ribozymes. This chapter addresses some of these problems and summarizes our experimental approaches towards designing active ribozymes against mRNAs coding for proteins involved in the pathogenesis and/or perpetuation of autoimmunity and cancer.

Ribozymes in the Gene Therapy of Cancer, edited by Kevin J. Scanlon and Mohammed Kashani-Sabet.
©1998 R.G. Landes Company.

General Aspects for Ribozyme Design

In principle, ribozymes can be designed to cleave any RNA sequence as long as the target molecule contains the nucleotide triplet NUX, where N and X can be any nucleotide, except G for X. Cleavage occurs most efficiently after the GUC triplet in vitro. However, considerable disparity appears to exist between in vitro and in vivo results.[18] This could be due, in part, to differential intracellular structural properties of ribozymes and/or their substrates.

An important feature of synthetic ribozymes is the length and base composition of their antisense arms. For turnover reasons, this length is usually chosen to be 6 to 8 nucleotides (nt) on either side of the cleavage site, so dissociation and a complete catalytic cycle can occur. In general, the free energy for RNA duplex formation between a ribozyme and its target RNA should be less than -16 kcal/mol for efficient catalytic cycling to occur. Thus, it would appear that an AU-rich ribozyme target complex is more desirable than, for example, a GC-rich complex, since the latter will have a high binding energy with only few base-pairs. Despite these assumptions, there are cases where hammerhead ribozymes with long antisense arms were found to be more active in the cell as compared to shorter derivatives.[19] In accordance with this observation, an IL-2 ribozyme with 16 nt as antisense arms was found to be less active when compared with ribozymes having 21 or 27 nt antisense arms.[16] Since all ribozymes had the same catalytic core and were targeted to the same site, the differences in the cell activity most likely reflect the rate of the ribozyme/substrate association. Further analysis of the target site suggested that an important part of the chosen IL-2 site (11 nt) is present within a double-stranded RNA region, which limited the binding of the short ribozymes.[20] Interestingly, extension of the hammerhead ribozyme antisense arms with nucleotides which base pair with the single-stranded regions facilitated its binding to longer RNA substrates. In another example, a ribozyme directed to the protein kinase A (PKA) RI-α subunit with antisense arms covering 18 nucleotides of the target RNA cleaved the in vitro transcribed PKA mRNA less efficiently when compared to a similar ribozyme with antisense arms covering 21 nucleotides (unpublished results). In our opinion it seems that ribozymes with long arms are more effective in binding longer target mRNAs than shorter ones.

Another problem for ribozymes having short antisense arms is reduced intracellular specificity. Therefore, for each site it is essential to define the minimal length of ribozyme antisense arms. Such length should be tested for binding to in vitro transcribed mRNA in a cell-free system representative of those that would be generated in vivo, since in vivo activity of ribozymes seems to differ from predictions derived from in vitro experiments. In this connection, it was recently shown that a minimum length of 51 nt in the antisense arm was required for both antisense and ribozyme-mediated inhibition of HIV-1 replication.[21]

A current difficulty with in vivo use of ribozymes arises in part from insufficient knowledge about intracellular ribozyme structures and stability. In many cases ribozymes were transcribed with additional long sequences which would dramatically increase the number of potentially inactive ribozyme conformations. Ribozymes flanked by a minimal length such as short stable hairpins have been expressed in the cell.[8] Such 3' stem-loop structures were found to increase the lifetime of the ribozyme in the cell by protecting the transcripts from 3' exonucleases.[22]

Our initial idea of adding hairpin structures to ribozymes (e.g., T7 terminator) was recently adapted by Gavin and Gupta,[23] where ribozymes with 3' hairpins targeted to the polycistronic Sendai virus P/C mRNA were found to be both more active and more resistant to intracellular nucleases. The major advantage of incorporating nucleotides which form stable secondary structures at the 3' end of ribozymes is that they can be synthesized as part of any ribozyme using conventional DNA/RNA synthesis chemistry.

In general ribozymes can be delivered to the cells either endogenously as genes coding ribozymes or exogenously[8,16] by transfection. In the latter case both in vitro transcribed ribozymes and chemically synthesized ribozymes have been used. In order to reduce the cost of chemically synthesized ribozymes, a smaller version of the hammerhead ribozyme, in which stem-loop II has been replaced by a short linker, has been developed and shown to be active both in vitro and in cells.[24,25] Due to their reduced size, these ribozymes may be useful as pharmaceutical agents.

Effect of Proteins on Ribozyme Cleavage

The simplified catalytic cycle of a hammerhead ribozyme as shown in Figure 17.1 consists mainly of:
1. sequence-specific binding to the target RNA via complementary antisense sequence;
2. site-specific hydrolysis of the cleavable motif of the target strand; and
3. release of the cleavage products, which gives rise to another catalytic cycle (turnover).

In contrast to in vitro experiments, the turnover of the ribozyme in the cell seems to be weak, since the ratio of ribozyme vs. target RNA was found to be relatively high (>100) for activity to occur in the cell.[8,11] Thus, there is a need to search for trans-acting factors that could assist the ribozyme catalysis intracellulary.

We have been interested in developing ribozymes against cytokines such as the tumor necrosis factors (TNF-α), as well as searching for cellular proteins with potential facilitation of RNA catalysis and/or stability. The pleiotropic activity of TNF-α is mediated by its ability to activate some transcription factors, in particular NF-κB, which controls the transcription of many inflammatory cytokines and growth factors[26] such as the granulocyte macrophage colony stimulating factor (GM-CSF).

During our studies with ribozymes, we have observed that a hammerhead ribozyme directed against human TNF-α specifically binds to a cellular protein as compared to other ribozymes and RNA molecules tested.[15] The ribozyme maintained its in vitro cleavage activity despite its strong binding to the protein. Thus, neither the binding of the ribozyme to its substrate nor the cleavage step seems to be hampered by the protein. Further analysis identified this major protein as the glyceraldehyde-3-phosphate dehydrogenase (GAPDH).[16] This protein strongly enhances ribozyme catalysis by increasing the ribozyme annealing to their target RNAs (association) as well as by increasing the product dissociation as summarized in Figure 17.2. The effect of GAPDH on RNA was attributed to its RNA chaperone activity.[16] Furthermore, our results indicated that GAPDH also binds to RNAs in a nonspecific and a specific manner. Interestingly, the nonspecific binding of GAPDH to ribozymes in general was found to be adequate for the cleavage enhancement to occur in vitro. However, tissue culture and in vivo experiments suggest that a high affinity RNA binding site for GAPDH is required for its effect upon ribozyme catalysis. This is not a major problem, since the facilitation by GAPDH upon ribozyme catalysis could be achieved by including a cis-appended GAPDH high-affinity binding RNA site to any ribozyme.[9] Since ribozymes act by recognizing and annealing to one RNA target sequence, it is conceivable that proteins able to affect RNA conformations can enhance their activity and specificity in vivo. This observation is further supported by the finding that the heterogeneous nuclear ribonucleoprotein (hnRNP) A1 can enhance the rate of the hammerhead ribozyme catalysis in vitro.[17]

As mentioned above, the binding of IL-2 ribozymes with short arms to in vitro transcribed full length IL-2 mRNA or longer targets (e.g., 500 nt) was found to be weaker when compared to ribozymes with long antisense arms and directed to the same site.[20] These results have suggested that IL-2 mRNA may adopt a conformation that prevents the binding

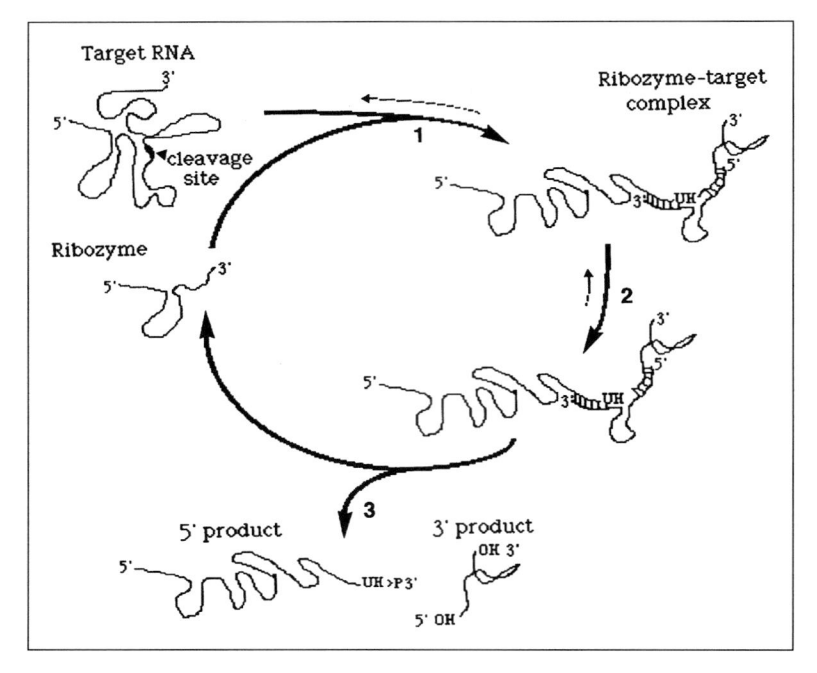

Fig. 17.1. Schematic representation of the catalytic cycle of a hammerhead ribozyme. The ribozyme binds the substrate (1) and cleaves it at a specific site determined by its antisense arms (2). Following cleavage the products can dissociate from the ribozyme (3). Thus the ribozyme can perform another catalytic cycle.

of the ribozyme with short arms (e.g., 14 nt), but not ribozymes with longer arms (e.g., 18 nt). Interestingly, the binding problem arising from the IL-2 mRNA secondary and/or tertiary structure was overcome in vitro by the addition of GAPDH (Fig. 17.3). The question remains as to why GAPDH did not assist the IL-2 ribozymes with short antisense arms in the cell.[20] The answer is not surprising, since our data have suggested that a high affinity binding RNA site for GAPDH is required for its activity in the cell and in vivo.[9,16] Such a high affinity RNA binding site for GAPDH would localize the protein near the ribozyme and ensure its interaction with the ribozyme and/or targeted RNA.

Ribozymes as Gene Therapy in Cancer Treatment

The use of ribozymes in cancer therapy has focused mainly on the inhibition of tumor-specific oncogenes and multi-drug resistance genes (see ref. 27 for review). These early studies have suggested that there are many appropriate targets for ribozyme strategies in cancer therapy. As mentioned above, TNF-α seems to regulate the expression of GM-CSF, which is expressed by a wide range of cells following activation.[28] However, in some pathological conditions such as certain myeloid leukemias and inflammations, GM-CSF is constitutively expressed and may play a pathological role.[29,30] Ribozymes targeted to human TNF-α mRNA were found to inhibit both the expression of GM-CSF in primary leukemic cells from patients with juvenile myelomonocytic leukemia and GM-CSF dependent colony formation by JMML cells (Iversen and Sioud, submitted for publication).

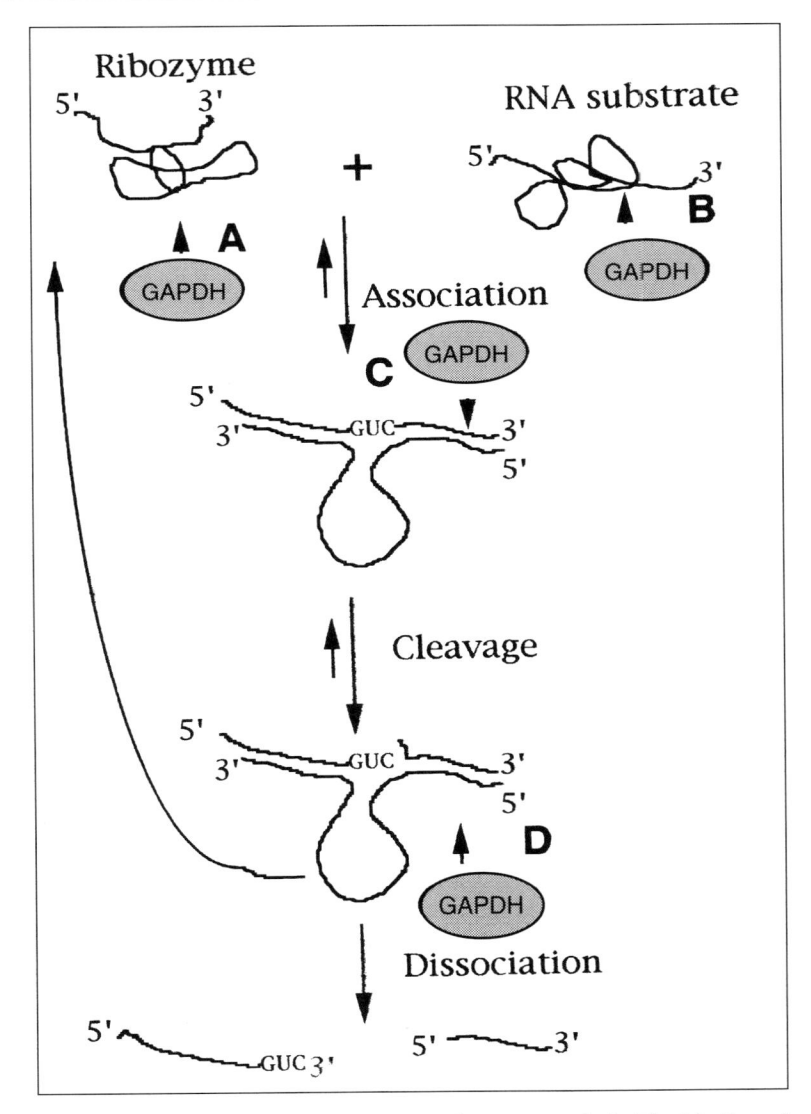

Fig. 17.2. Potential effect of GAPDH on ribozyme catalysis. The binding of GAPDH to the ribozyme (A) and/or the substrate (B) may modulate their secondary structures and direct the annealing process (C). Following cleavage, GAPDH would also facilitate the dissociation step (D). These two activities seem to depend on the length of the RNA duplexes. For details see ref. 16.

Fig. 17.3. In vitro facilitation of RNA catalysis by GAPDH. PhosphorImager printout of 6% polyacrylamide denaturing gel showing the in vitro cleavage activity of the 500 nt target IL-2 mRNA by an IL-2 ribozyme (+) with 14 nt as antisense arms in the absence (lane 2) or in the presence of various concentrations of GAPDH (lanes 3 to 8) for 60 min at 37°C. Lane 1 contains only the 500 nt substrate. Maximum effect of GAPDH was seen at concentrations of 70 to 150 ng/μl (lanes 6 and 7, respectively). For more details see refs. 16 and 20.

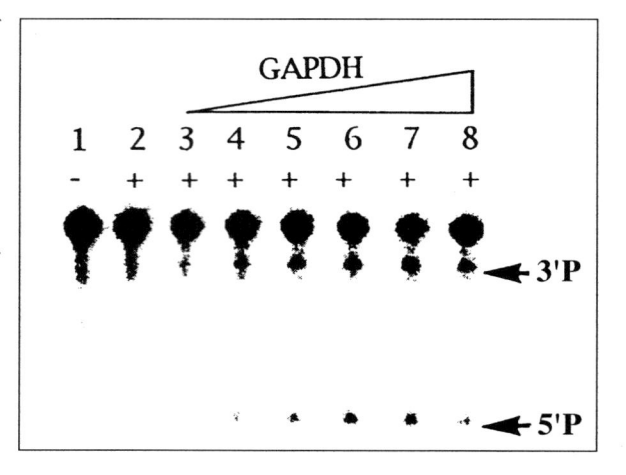

Since 1986, we have been interested in investigating the molecular mechanism by which anti-tumor drugs and newly discovered prokaryotic antibiotics kill cells.[31] The molecular target of, for example, the epipodophyllotoxins (e.g., VP16, VM26) was identified as DNA topoisomerase II, an enzyme involved in DNA replication repair and transcription. Interestingly, the cleavage activity of VP16 was found to be similar to ciprofloxacin, an inhibitor of bacterial DNA gyrase.[32] More recently, epipodophyllotoxins and other drugs known to interact specifically with actin, tubulin, DNA or DNA topoisomerase II were found to also activate the apoptosis machinery of eukaryotic cells.[33] However, despite their promising activity in cell death, their toxicity remains the major problem in cancer chemotherapy. Thus, there is a need for developing novel tools that specifically induce apoptosis in cancer cells.

The susceptibility of cells to apoptosis seems to be determined by the relative levels and interactions between the Bcl-2 related proteins, such as Bax, Bcl-x_L, Bad, Bag, Bak, and Bik, some of which protect from cell death (Bcl-x_L) while other members of the family, such as Bax, promote apoptosis.[34] The interactions and the expression of these proteins can be affected by different activation pathways, for example those involving the protein kinase C (PKC).

In order to determine which PKC isoform is involved in apoptosis we have used as a model a rat glioma cell line called BTCn.[35] This cell line has the properties that seem relevant for a model of aggressive human gliomas. The BTCn cell line gives both subcutaneous and brain tumors in syngeneic BD IX rats. As shown in Figure 17.4C, a hammerhead ribozyme targeted to the PKC-α isoform induced apoptosis in all BTCn cells as detected by the TUNEL-method.[36] This method is based on the fact that apoptotic cells contain free 3' ends of double-stranded DNA due to the endonuclease digestion of genomic DNA at the nucleosomal intervals. Such 3' ends can be used as substrate by the terminal deoxynucleotidyl transferase. In this assay apoptotic cells would show nuclear staining as shown in Figure 17.4. By introducing 2'-amino pyrimidine residues into a catalytically active protein kinase Cα ribozyme, we have designed a ribozyme that is over 14,000-fold more stable than its unsubstituted version yet retains most of its biological activity. A single injection of the modified ribozyme into a glioma solid tumor almost completely inhibited tumor growth.[37]

The growth of new blood vessels from an existing vascular supply in the tissue is a process called angiogenesis. This process is an essential component of tumor growth.[38] The newly formed blood vessels, in addition to their nutritional role, also provide an exit route

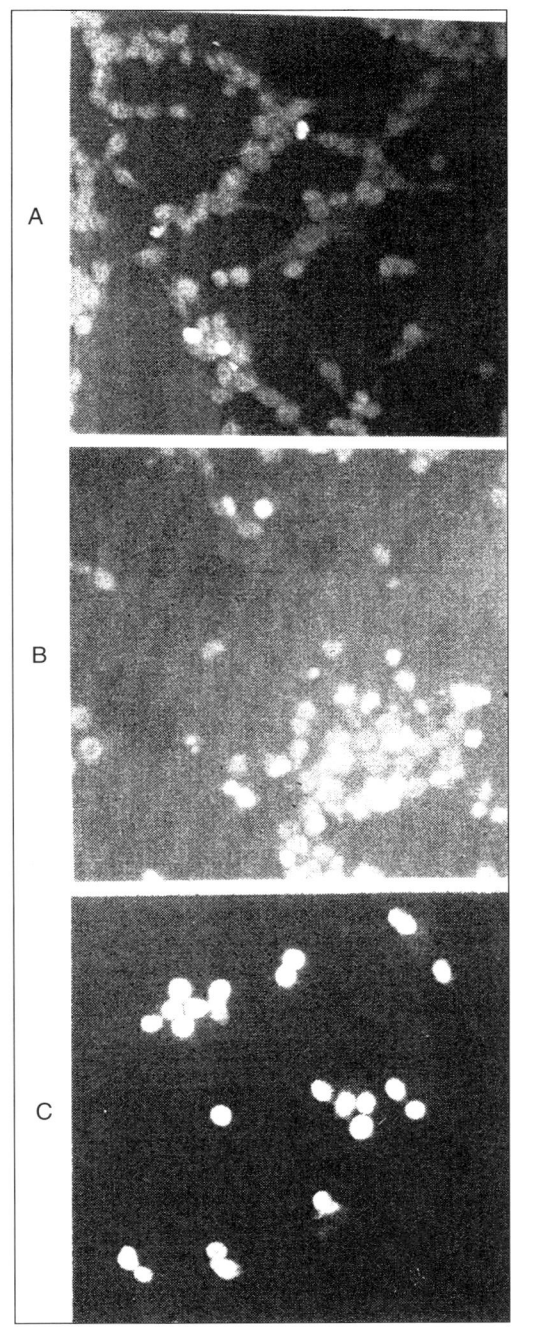

Fig. 17.4. Induction of apoptosis by a PKC-α specific ribozyme directed to the CUC at codons 10 and 11. BTCn cells were transfected with only DOTAP (liposomal transfection reagent Chemical name N-[1-(2,3-Dioleoloxy)propyl]-N, N, N-trimethylammonium methylsulfate) (A), the mutant ribozyme (B) or the ribozyme (C) for 48 hours in slide flasks. Following transfection, cells were fixed with ETOH for 5 min and then permeabilized with 0.1% saponin in PBS containing 1% BSA fraction V for 10 min. Following washing with PBS, the apoptotic cells were detected using a commercially available in situ cell death fluorescein detection kit (Boehringer, Mannheim, Germany) based on terminal deoxynucleotidyl transferase (TdT)-mediated dUTP-FITC nick end labeling (TUNEL). Briefly, permeabilized cells were incubated in the TUNEL reaction for 30 min. Following washing with PBS, samples were covered with antifade and mounting medium for fluorescence microscopy analysis.

for metastasizing tumor cells into the systemic circulation. Given the importance of such a process in tumor progression, inhibition of the factor promoting angiogenesis may lead to the development of new anti-cancer therapy. Many factors, such as the vascular endothelial growth factor (VEGF), basic fibroblast factor (BFF) and TNF-α, were found to stimulate the angiogenesis process.[39] We are currently studying the effect of synthetic ribozymes against VEGF on tumor growth and vascularization. Our ongoing experiments indicate that tumor vascularization can be inhibited by ribozymes. Using a similar strategy, it was suggested recently that pleiotropin (PTN) is a factor that could be responsible for melanoma angiogenesis and metastasis.[40] This study supports a direct link between these two processes; however it remains to be demonstrated that such a link exists in other tumors.

In conclusion, the described set of experiments indicate: firstly, that both synthetic ribozymes and genes encoding ribozymes can be delivered to cells in an active form; secondly, that endogenous cellular proteins can provide protection and catalysis enhancement for hammerhead ribozymes; and thirdly, that both the machinery of apoptosis and angiogenesis in cancer cells can be targeted specifically by ribozymes. Furthermore, our data emphasize the importance of detailed structural investigations of ribozyme target RNAs. Thus, we need to learn more about the traffic of RNA inside the cell, as well as the target secondary structures and the cellular factors that can facilitate ribozyme catalysis and stability. In addition, we should address the problem of delivery of preformed ribozymes. Presently, cationic lipids seem to be the most versatile method.

Acknowledgments

This work was supported in part by grants from Gene Shears Pty. Inc, The Norwegian Research Council, The Norwegian Womens Public Health Organization, The European Union (Biotech program) and currently by the Norwegian Radium Hospital.

References

1. Wagner RW. Gene inhibition using antisense oligonucleotides. Nature 1994; 372:333-335.
2. Helene C, Thuong NT, Harel-Bellan A. Control of gene expression by triple helix-forming oligonucleotides: The antigen strategy. Ann New York Acad Sci 1992; 660:27-36.
3. Cech T. The chemistry of self-splicing RNA and RNA enzymes. Science 1987; 236:1532-1539.
4. Uhlenbeck OC. A small catalytic oligonucleotide. Nature 1987; 328:596-619.
5. Haseloff J, and Gerlach WL. Simple RNA enzymes with new and highly specific endoribonuclease activities. Nature 1988; 334:585-591.
6. Cameron FH, Jennings PA. Specific gene suppression by engineered ribozymes in monkey cells. Proc Natl Acad Sci USA 1989; 83:8859-8862.
7. Sarver N, Cantin EM, Chang PS et al. Ribozymes as potential anti HIV-1 therapeutic agents. Science 1990; 247:1222-1225.
8. Sioud M, Drlica K. Prevention of HIV-1 integrase expression in *E.coli* by a ribozyme. Proc Natl Acad Sci USA 1991; 88:7303-7307.
9. Sioud M. Ribozyme modulation of lipopolysaccharide-induced tumor necrosis factor-α production by peritoneal cells in vitro and in vivo. Eur J Immunol 1996; 26:1026-1031.
10. Scanlon KJ, Ishida H, Kashani-Sabet M. Ribozyme-mediated reversal of the multidrug-resistant phenotype. Proc Natl Acad Sci USA 1994; 91:11123-11127.
11. Cotten M, Birnstiel ML. Ribozyme mediated destruction of RNA in vivo. EMBO J 1989; 8:3861-3866.
12. Sullenger BA, Cech TR. Tethering ribozymes to a retroviral packaging signal for destruction of viral RNA. Science 1993; 262:1566-1569.
13. Taylor NR, Rossi JJ. Ribozyme mediated cleavage of an HIV-1 gag RNA: The effects of non-targeted sequences and secondary structure on ribozyme cleavage activity. Anti Res Dev 1991; 1:173-186.

14. Tsuchihashi Z, Khosla M, Herschlag D. Protein enhancement of hammerhead ribozyme catalysis. Science 1993; 262:99-102.
15. Sioud M. Interaction between tumor necrosis factor α ribozyme and cellular proteins. J Mol Biol 1994; 242:619-629.
16. Sioud M, Jespersen L. Enhancement of hammerhead ribozyme catalysis by glyceraldehyde-3-phosphate dehydrogenase. J Mol Biol 1996; 257:775-789.
17. Bertrand EL, and Rossi JJ. Facilitation of hammerhead ribozyme catalysis by the nucleocapsid protein of HIV-1 and the heterogeneous nuclear ribonucleoprotein. EMBO J 1994; 13:2904-2912.
18. Kawasaki H, Ohkawa J, Tanishige N et al. Selection of the best target site for ribozyme-mediated cleavage within a fusion gene for adenovirus E1A-associated 300 kDa protein (p300) and luciferase. Nucleic Acids Res 1996; 24:3010-3016.
19. Crisell P, Thompson S, James W. Interaction of HIV-1 replication by ribozymes that show poor activity in vitro. Nucleic Acids Res 1993; 21:5251-5255.
20. Sioud M. Effects of variations in length of hammerhead ribozyme antisense arms upon the cleavage of longer RNA substrates. Nucleic Acids Res 1997; 25:333-338.
21. Hormes R, Homann M, Oelze I et al. The subcellular localization and length of hammerhead ribozymes determine efficacy in human cells. Nucleic Acids Res 1997; 25:769-775
22. Sioud M, Opstad A, Zhao JQ et al. In vivo decay kinetic parameters of hammerhead ribozymes. Nucleic Acids Res 1994; 22: 5571-5575.
23. Gavin DK, Gupta KC. Efficient hammerhead ribozymes targeted to the polycistronic Sendai virus P/C mRNA. J Biol Chem 1997; 272:1461-1472.
24. McCall MJ, Hendry P, Jennings PA. Minimal sequence requirements for ribozyme activity. Proc Natl Acad Sci USA 1992; 89:5710-5714.
25. Sioud M, Opstad A, Hendry P et al. A minimised hammerhead ribozyme with activity against interleukin-2 in human cells. Biochem Biophys Res Com 1997; 231: 397-402.
26. Baeuerle PA, Henkel T. Function and activation of NF-κB in the immune system. Annu Rev Immunol 1994; 12:141-179.
27. Poeschla E, Wong-Staal F. Antiviral and anticancer ribozymes. Curr Opin Oncology 1994; 6:601-606.
28. Gasson JC. Molecular physiology of granulocyte-macrophage colony stimulating factor. Blood 1991; 77:1131-1145.
29. Young DC, Wagner K, Griffin JD. Constitutive expression of the granulocyte-macrophage colony stimulating factor gene in acute myeloblastic leukemia. J Clin Invest 1987; 79:100-106.
30. Xu W, Firestein GS, Taetle R et al. Cytokines in chronic inflammatory arthritis. II. GM-CSF in rheumatoid synovial effusions. J Clin Invest 1989; 83:876-882.
31. Sioud M, Baldacci G, Forterre P et al. Antitumor drugs inhibit the growth of halophilic archaebacteria. Eur J Biochem 1987; 69:231-236.
32. Sioud M, Forterre P. Ciprofloxacin and etoposide (VP16) produce a similar pattern of DNA cleavage in a plasmid of an Archaebacterium. Biochemistry 1989; 28:3638-3641.
33. Hannun YA. Apoptosis and the dilemma of cancer chemo-therapy. Blood 1997; 89:1845-1853.
34. Kroemer G. the proto-oncogene Bcl-2 and its role in regulating apoptosis. Nature Med 1997; 3:614-620.
35. Mella O, Bjerkvig R, Schem BC et al. A cerebral glioma model for experimental therapy and in vivo invasion studies in syngeneic BD IX rats. J Neuro-Oncology 1990; 9:93-104.
36. Gavrieli Y, Shermen Y, Ben-Sasson SA. Identification of programmed cell death in situ via a specific labelling of nuclear DNA fragmentation. J Cell Biol 1989; 119:493-498.
37. Sioud M, Børensen R. A nuclease-resistant protein kinase Cα ribozyme blocks glioma cell growth. Nature Biotech 1998; 16:556-561.
38. Folkman J. Fighting cancer by attacking its blood supply. Scient American 1996; 275:116-119.

39. Levis CE, Leek R, Harris A et al. Cytokine regulation of angiogenesis in breast cancer: The role of tumour-associated macrophages. J Leuk Biol 1995; 57:747-751.
40. Czubayko F, Schulte AM, Berchem GM et al. Melanoma angiogenesis and metastasis modulated by ribozyme targeting of the secreted growth factor pleiotrophin. Proc Natl Acad Sci USA 1996; 93:14753-14758.

CHAPTER 18

Human Papillomaviruses

E.J. Shillitoe

Introduction

Several viruses are susceptible to the effects of ribozymes. These include HIV,[1,2] bovine leukemia virus,[3] tobacco mosaic virus,[4] and lymphocytic choriomeningitis virus.[5] However, all of these are RNA viruses. Thus both the viral genome and its RNA transcripts could serve as targets. For DNA viruses the susceptibility to ribozymes could be very different, and indeed very little work has been done in that area. However there is one example of a DNA virus in which several investigators have explored a role for ribozymes, and that is the papillomavirus group.

Papillomaviruses

Human papillomaviruses (HPVs) are one of the largest groups of viruses. Over 70 types are now recognized. They are the focus of a very large research effort, and new information is continually summarized and made available through the Los Alamos online database (http://hpv-web.lanl.gov/). The HPVs can be classified in several ways, but it is useful to consider some of them as being "low risk" and some as being "high risk" viruses. The low risk HPVs are responsible for warts and similar superficial lesions, while the high risk HPVs are found in dysplastic and malignant lesions. They include HPV-16, HPV-18 and HPV-33, and are found in cervical cancers and some oral cancers. Other HPVs, such as types -6 and -11 seem to be of an intermediate risk and occur in conditions, such as laryngeal papillomatosis, which are generally benign but can occasionally become malignant.

An important question is whether the high risk HPVs are the cause of the malignancy in which they are found, or whether they are simply present in a latent or passenger state. The question is made difficult by the fact that HPVs are sometimes found in normal tissues. However it does seem clear that in cervical cancer the HPVs are largely responsible for the malignancy. The viruses are present in over 90% of cervical cancers.[6] Several large case-control epidemiological studies have confirmed the association of high risk HPV types and cervical cancer.[7,8] The malignant tissues continually express high levels of the viral RNA.[9] It is of course likely that other factors are also involved in the development of the cancer, but since the virus is at least partly responsible, then any anti-HPV techniques could protect patients against cervical cancer, or might be helpful as part of its treatment.

In the case of oral cancer the role of the virus is not quite so clear. Many studies have shown the presence of HPV DNA in the tumors.[10] For example, one study found HPV DNA in 49% of patients and 8% of control subjects.[11] Another study found HPV in 29% of oral cancers and no control tissues.[12] Only one epidemiological study has used a carefully matched

---

Ribozymes in the Gene Therapy of Cancer, edited by Kevin J. Scanlon and Mohammed Kashani-Sabet. ©1998 R.G. Landes Company.

control group and, although it found a low incidence of HPV generally, it did find a significantly higher prevalence of HPV in the cancer as compared to the control subjects.[13] No studies have reported that the viral genes are actually being expressed in oral cancer, and this is a significant defect in the virological studies of that disease.

Studies in vitro have confirmed the clinical suspicion that the high risk HPVs are oncogenic. These viruses can transform normal human keratinocytes in vitro to a malignant phenotype, in a step-wise fashion. Initial infection of the cells leads to a cell line which expresses viral genes and has an immortal phenotype in which the cells can not make tumors in nude mice.[14] They do, however, have an increased frequency of mutations, which makes them more susceptible to the effects of chemical carcinogens.[15] If these cells are then exposed to carcinogens they undergo changes that do make them tumorigenic. Theses changes include amplification of the HPV sequences.[16] This sequential development of the malignant phenotype may be an in vitro equivalent of the changes that happen in vivo as HPV-associated cancers develop.

The progression of HPV-immortalized cells to cancer may involve genetic factors that are not well understood. Two studies have failed to find changes in the expression level of HPV genes or the E7 protein during the progression of cells from immortal to malignant.[17,18] Thus other genetic changes could have been occurring. Indeed, one study found that expression of the *myc* oncogene was increased in one HPV-immortalized cell line[14] and possibly other genes were activated at the same time.

The Viral Genome

The genome of all HPVs is very similar, and is illustrated in Figure 18.1. It is composed of about 8 kb of double stranded DNA, and all genes are on the same strand. Some genes are designated 'E' since they have similarities to the early genes of other small DNA viruses, and some are designated 'L', and are similar to the late, structural genes of other viruses. The remainder of the genome is designated as the 'long control region' (LCR) or 'upstream regulatory region' (URR). This region is the major enhancer and promoter region for the viral genes, although minor promoters do exist elsewhere.

Mechanism of Oncogenesis

The molecular mechanism by which HPVs produce cancer has been elucidated in some detail. The most important genes are the E6 and E7 genes. These encode small proteins which together are necessary and sufficient for oncogenesis.[19] When cells are transformed by HPVs the viral RNA must be expressed continuously for them to stay transformed.[20] The E6 and E7 genes are expressed as a single transcript, which is spliced (Fig. 18.2). The effect of the splice is to produce two different E6 proteins, one of which is shorter and has a frame shift beyond the splice acceptor site. The significance of the splice is not certain, although it may allow more efficient initiation of translation of the E7 protein.[21,22]

The E6 gene product binds to the p53 tumor-suppressor protein,[23] and the E7 gene product binds to the Rb tumor-suppressor protein.[24] The effect of the binding of E6 to p53 is to activate an enzyme pathway, the ubiquitin system, which then digests the p53 protein. Thus the half life of p53, which is normally 3 h or more, is reduced to around 15 min in tumor cells which express HPVs.[25,26] The effect of binding E7 is to inactivate the Rb protein by preventing its normal interactions with other cell proteins.[19,24] These effects of E6 and E7 are not unique to HPVs, but are in fact the mechanisms that are used by several of the small DNA tumor viruses.[27]

Although the high risk HPVs are found in many persons, the cancers that are associated with them are relatively rare. Thus there must be other factors that determine the development of HPV-associated cancers. One critical factor appears to be the level of expres-

Human Papillomaviruses 225

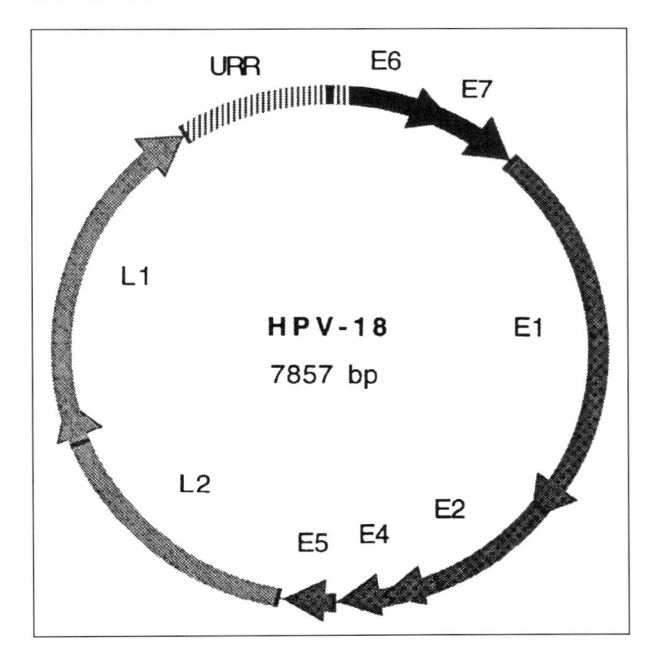

Fig. 18.1. Gene map of HPV-18, which is one of the high risk papillomaviruses. This map shows the features that are common to HPV-16, HPV-18 and other HPVs that are associated with some human carcinomas. The genome is around 8 kbp. The upstream regulatory region (URR) controls expression of the small E6 and E7 proteins, whose continual expression is necessary for malignancy. The other genes are probably involved in viral replication and viral structure, but are not associated with human cancers. They are often lost when the viral genome becomes integrated into the chromosome of human cancer cells.

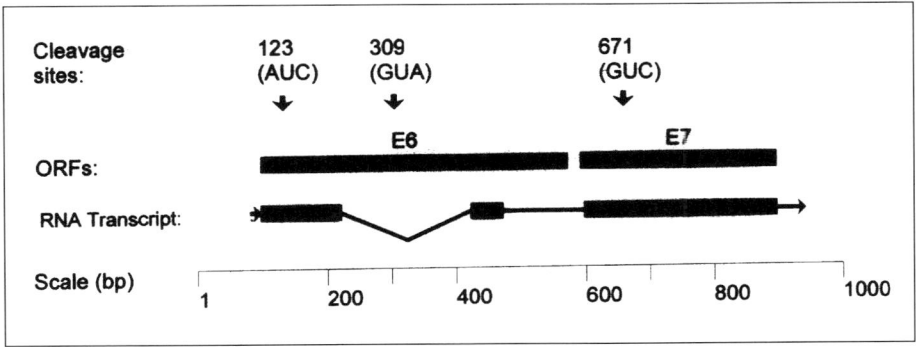

Fig. 18.2. Partial map of the HPV-18 genome, showing the open reading frames (ORFs) for the E6 and E7 genes, together with the RNA transcript with a splice in the E6 region.[70] The vertical arrows indicate the three target sites at nucleotides 123, 309 and 671 at which ribozymes can be effective in inhibiting the growth of HPV-18-expressing cancer cells.

sion of the transforming genes.[28] Expression levels may be increased in cervical cancers by mutation or other modifications to the viral genome.[29] In many cervical cancer cell lines, the viral DNA is integrated into the cellular chromosome and the integration routinely truncates the E2 gene of the virus. The E2 gene product is a repressor of high risk HPV gene expression,[30] although regions of the protein have the potential to act as transcriptional activators.[31] Thus, in cancers it is possible that the function of the integration at the E2 gene site is to produce a truncated E2 gene product which has a stimulating effect on the expression of the E6 and E7 genes.[29,32] Another mechanism of overexpression can happen in laryngeal papillomas which have become malignant. The HPV that is present in those lesions has been reported to show duplications in the URR which thereby increase its strength as a gene expression enhancer.[33] In some cervical cancers other changes in the URR can lead to increased expression of viral genes. The binding sites for the transcriptional repressor YY-1 are mutated in some cases, and this leads to over-expression of viral genes.[34] In oral cancer cell lines that contain DNA of HPVs there is frequent deletion of sequences from suppressor regions of the URR, which leads to greater activity.[35] Thus HPV-associated cancers often show over-expression of the transforming genes because of mutations or other changes in the viral genome.

Anti-Papillomavirus Gene Therapy

Since the molecular mechanism by which HPVs stimulate the growth of tumor cells are known, several targets for new types of therapy have been revealed. These could include use of mutated URRs for expression of suicide genes, or development of proteins that could interrupt the effects of the E6 and E7 proteins.[36] In the present context, however, the important targets are the RNA transcripts that encode the E6 and E7 proteins.

Antisense Inhibition of Expression of HPV-Genes

One of the earliest ways of blocking gene expression specifically was by the use of antisense RNA. These molecules, transcribed from the opposing strand of DNA from the one used in gene expression, can hybridize to the sense strand and inhibit translation. Several workers have shown that antisense RNA can inhibit the expression of the transforming genes of papillomaviruses.

The first study of this type used cDNA sequences of HPV-16, which were cloned into expression vector plasmids and then transferred to the HPV-16-expressing cervical cancer cell line, C4-1.[37] Expression of antisense RNA was then induced by dexamethasone. Expression of sense RNA was shown to be reduced, as was expression of the HPV-proteins, and growth of the cells was reduced. The interpretation of the experiments was complicated by the fact that the dexamethasone by itself had effects on the C4-1 cells, but nevertheless the work showed that HPV RNA was a reasonable molecule to target for future research into HPV-associated cancers.

In a follow-up study it was reported that the tumorigenicity of the cells was reduced by the effects of the antisense sequences.[38] Antisense-transduced cell lines were implanted into nude mice so as to form tumors, and some mice were given dexamethasone in the drinking water so as to induce expression of the antisense sequences. Those mice developed tumor nodules which were significantly smaller. Surviving tumor cells were shown to be expressing the antisense RNA, which therefore was not completely inhibitory to the tumors.

Another group showed that synthetic antisense oligonucleotides could also inhibit expression of HPV in cancer cells.[39] They made phosphorothioate oligonucleotides that represented the start codon regions of the E6 and E7 genes of HPV-18. These were shown to inhibit the growth of cervical and oral cancer cells that carry DNA of HPV-18 but without effects on other cells. Either the blocking of E6 or E7 had some effect, but blocking both together was the most effective. As might be expected, the synthetic oligonucleotides were rapidly degraded, despite the protection of the phosphorothioate modification, and repeated application was necessary. Once the oligonucleotides were degraded the cells recovered and grew as rapidly as before.

As with HPV-16, it is possible to express antisense RNA to HPV-18 from expression vector plasmids, and another study introduced such plasmids into the HeLa cell line, which expresses HPV-18.[40] Cell lines were developed that expressed antisense sequences to either the E7 gene, or to both E6 and E7. The antisense-expressing cells showed slower growth, reduced formation of colonies in soft agar and increased serum requirements, which all indicate a loss of the transformed phenotype. These effects were not seen in tumor cells that lacked HPV sequences.[40]

These early results have been confirmed by other workers. It has been shown that synthetic antisense sequences to HPV-16 E6 and E7 could inhibit the transformed phenotype of the cervical cancer cell lines CaSki and SiHa. Both in vitro parameters of transformation and tumorigenicity in nude mice were reduced.[41] Others have investigated the effects of synthetic oligonucleotides directed against the start codon of the E7 gene of HPV-16.[42] In a rabbit reticulocyte assay system the antisense oligonucleotide did reduce the translation of the E7 protein. When the gene that encoded the antisense sequence was introduced into CaSki cells by lipofection, the HPV RNA transcript was lost from the cells and was replaced by two shorter transcripts. This was interpreted as meaning that RNase H degradation had been activated. This interesting observation seems to be unique in antisense studies and deserves further attention. Curiously, no change was found in the protein levels of E7 in the cells and it was not reported whether any changes occurred in the phenotype of the cells. The level of the receptor for epidermal growth factor has been found to fall in HeLa cells that are transfected with antisense genes for E6 and E7, although the exact pathway has not been investigated.[43]

Although confirmatory studies on the effects of antisense to E6 and E7 have been reported,[44,45] not all workers have been able to detect anti-HPV effects from the use of antisense RNA. One group found significant nonspecific effects from the use of synthetic antisense oligonucleotides,[46] and in fact nonspecificity of phosphorothioate-modified antisense molecules is a critical problem with numerous targets.[47]

Inhibition of HPV by Ribozymes

Since antisense RNA shows some effects in the inhibition of papillomaviruses, it seems very likely that ribozymes would also show an effect, and possibly be more potent. The first demonstration that this could be possible came from a study of the cottontail rabbit papillomavirus.[48] It was found that a ribozyme directed at the E6/E7-containing RNA transcript of that virus could cleave the transcript in vitro. This early work on rabbit papillomaviruses has not been continued, and more recent interest has centered on the human high-risk papillomaviruses. Their DNA sequence shows a very large number of potential target sites, as might be expected.[36]

HPV-16 RNA transcripts were first shown to be cleavable by in vitro studies, using very short synthetic targets. One study examined the use of a self-trimming construct that could cut itself out of a longer transcript.[49] This anti-HPV ribozyme could then cut various length HPV-16 transcripts in vitro, but the efficiency depended on the length of the target. A very short target of 171 nucleotides (nt) was cut efficiently, with 64% reduction of the target under the conditions of the assay. However, a target of 360 nt fragment was reduced by only 25%, and a target of 686 nt was not cut at all. The natural HPV RNA transcripts in cancer cells are much longer than any of these, being, for example, 3.4 and 1.6 kb in HeLa cells,[40] which appears to raise doubts about the use of ribozymes in cancer cells. Another study showed that ribozymes directed to the region of the start codons of the E6 and E7 genes of HPV-16 did cleave the target RNA in vitro when it was in the form of a partial-length 202 base transcript.[50] Simultaneous cleavage by both ribozymes was also demonstrated. Ribozymes in this case were expressed from a plasmid which contained adeno-associated virus sequences and which could presumably be used to produce a virus vector.

Ribozymes that can cleave the RNA transcript of HPV-18 have been examined in some depth.[51,52] Two ribozymes were designed so as to be directed at the first possible target sites in the E6 and E7 coding regions respectively, while a third target site was selected as being in a region of minimal secondary structure, according to computer predictions. The full-length

RNA transcript of HPV-18 was then expressed in *E. coli* cells, and a ribozyme was expressed simultaneously from a different plasmid. The results showed that the most effective ribozyme was the one directed against the region of minimal secondary structure, named Rz309.[51] As well as being most effective in the *E. coli* assay, Rz309 was also the most effective when used to cut HPV RNA in vitro that had been extracted from HeLa cells. The ability to cut the full-length transcript was considered to be significant and implied a potential use for inhibiting the tumorigenicity of the cells. The fact that the most effective ribozyme was the one selected from a computer prediction is of course interesting, but is not a conclusive demonstration that secondary structure issues can be avoided in this simple way. It is also noteworthy that Rz309 is directed to a region of the transcript that is removed by splicing (Fig. 18.2). This implies that either the cleavage by the ribozyme happens early after transcription, before splicing has occurred, or else that the unspliced E6 product is essential for tumor cell growth.

The same three ribozymes were then cloned into an eukaryotic shuttle vector and transferred to HeLa cells. Each of the ribozymes showed inhibitory effects on the cells, but again it was Rz309 which was most effective. It caused a decrease in the intracellular concentration of the HPV-18 RNA transcript and a corresponding increase in the intracellular concentration of the p53 gene product. The cells showed reduced growth rates, increased serum dependency, and reduced focus formation in soft agar.[52] All of these changes suggest a reduced potential to be malignant. Thus Rz309, and other ribozymes, were judged to have potential as anti-tumor agents for treatment of HPV-associated tumors.

Another group has cloned an anti-HPV-16 ribozyme into a plasmid vector, under control of the RSV-LTR promoter.[53] The construct was transfected into C4-1 cervical cancer cells. By the use of an RNase protection assay it was found that the level of HPV-16 E7 RNA was reduced by around 90%. In contrast, an antisense-expressing plasmid reduced expression only around 20%. Although no measurements were taken of the effects of this on cellular phenotype, these results also seem to be promising.

Delivery Methods for Anti-HPV Ribozymes

Any method for delivery of anti-HPV ribozymes will have to take account of the type of tissue and tumor in which HPV is found. In the early stages of cervical or oral cancer, the virus is found in epithelium which is relatively thin and accessible, and thus it might seem to be a simple matter to transduce the affected cells. In practice, no effective method has emerged. The most straightforward technique is the use of particle bombardment, in which a helium-powered 'gene gun' is used to fire DNA-coated gold beads into the epithelium. Although this is simple and fast, the penetration of the beads does not reach the basal layers of the epithelium, which is where cell division takes place.[54] Thus the transduced cells are lost within a few days. Improvements to the gene gun technology might allow more effective transfer of DNA, in which case it could become a very useful technique.

An alternative method for transduction of tissues is the use of virus vectors. Retroviruses can be used to transduce oral and cervical cells in culture and, by careful selection, transduced cell lines can be developed. Many workers have shown that retrovirus vectors can introduce functional ribozymes into cells so as to inhibit the effects of HIV,[55-58] SIV,[59] the *ras* oncogene[60] or the *BCR/ABL* fusion gene.[61] However there have been no in vivo experiments to suggest that retroviruses will be used in treatment of HPV-associated human carcinomas.

Adenovirus vectors provide an alternative to retroviruses. Adenovirus vectors have been used to introduce ribozymes to cells so as to inhibit growth hormone,[62] transferase genes,[63] the hepatitis C virus[64] or the *ras* oncogene.[65] Adenoviruses readily transduce oral or cervical cancer cells in vitro, and will diffuse through solid tumors to some extent.[66,67] However, in vivo their efficiency is rather limited, since they do not replicate in the tumor and are limited to the area where they were deposited. They have not been able to transduce the basal cell layer of epithelia in an effective way.[66] Our recent experience suggests that expression of anti-HPV ribozymes from adenovirus vectors can be obtained readily, yet they are not always functional for cleavage of the target transcript. This is probably associated with sub-compartmental distribution within the cancer cell, secondary structure of the ribozyme, or stability of the ribozyme, and this problem must be solved before further progress is possible (Shillitoe et al, in preparation).

In addition to a suitable delivery method, suitable gene promoters and enhancers will be needed for proper expression of ribozymes in cancers that express HPV. The desirable properties of such promoters are known in some detail. Presumably powerful expression will be necessary, so as to obtain a suitable excess of ribozyme sequences relative to target sequences, but the level of expression has not been determined accurately. Presumably specificity of expression will be less important. Since ribozymes show specific actions rather than nonspecific, they would not be expected to produce untoward effects if they become expressed in other cells apart from the tumor cells. Thus strength of a promoter will be more important than cell type specificity.

Tissue specific promoters for expression of anti-*ras* ribozymes in melanomas has been attempted using the tyrosinase promoter.[68] Tissue-specific promoters for cervical or oral cancer have not been identified—however one candidate is the secretory leukoprotease inhibitor gene promoter which is active in many carcinomas.[69] Alternatively, papillomavirus promoters might be expected to serve as tumor-specific promoters in cells that express papillomavirus genes. Indeed one group has demonstrated that in oral cancer cells that contain HPV DNA, the promoter regions of the virus have generally undergone mutations that make them more active in HPV-containing carcinomas.[35] These promoters can now be examined for their ability to direct tumor-specific expression of ribozymes.

Future Directions for Research

Although encouraging progress has been made in the development of ribozymes that will target expression of HPVs in human cancer cells, there are still many issues to be resolved before human therapy will be possible. In the case of oral cancer it is not entirely clear that the presence of HPV DNA is a cause, or partial cause, of the tumor. It has not been shown that the DNA is expressed as RNA, and of course unless this occurs then there will be no role for ribozymes. In the case of cervical cancer, a critical issue is the mode of delivery of ribozyme genes. Injection of adenovirus vectors into solid tumors seems to be the best available method so far, but it has not been shown to produce regression of HPV-associated tumors that are grown in nude mice. The long pre-malignant phase that is seen in many cervical cancers does provide an opportunity for the use of ribozyme therapy, but so far there are no reports of how the dysplastic tissues could be transduced. Another important question is the way that expression of ribozymes can be optimized within a tumor cell. The sub-cellular localization, the length of flanking arms, the expression level that is needed and the role of post-transcriptional processing will all need to be addressed. Although the use of ribozymes in management of HPV-containing cancers is under investigation, there are several questions that must be answered before their future role will be clear.

Acknowledgment

Original work referred to in this review was supported by PHS grant R01 DE10842.

References

1. Homann M, Tzortzakaki S, Rittner K, Sczakiel G, Tabler M. Incorporation of the catalytic domain of a hammerhead ribozyme into antisense RNA enhances its inhibitory effect on the replication of human immunodeficiency virus type 1. Nucl Acids Res 1993; 21:2809-2814.
2. Ventura M, Wang P, Ragot T, Perricaudet M, Saragosti S. Activation of HIV-specific ribozyme activity by self-cleavage. Nucl Acids Res 1993; 21:3249-3255.
3. Cantor GH, McElwain TF, Birkebak TA, Palmer GH. Ribozyme cleaves *rex/tax* mRNA and inhibits bovine leukemia virus expression. Proc Natl Acad Sci USA 1993; 90:10932-10936.
4. de Feyter R, Young M, Schroeder K, Dennis ES, Gerlach W. A ribozyme gene and an antisense gene are equally effective in conferring resistance to tobacco mosaic virus on transgenic tobacco. Mol General Genet 1996; 250:329-338.
5. Xing Z, Whitton JL. Ribozymes which cleave arenavirus RNAs: Identification of susceptible target sites and inhibition by target site secondary structure. J Virol 1992; 66:1361-1369.
6. zur Hausen H. Papillomaviruses in anogenital cancer as a model to understand the role of viruses in human cancers. Cancer Res 1989; 49:4677-4681.
7. Lorincz AT, Reid R, Jenson AB, Greenberg MD, Lancaster W, Kurman RJ. Human papillomavirus infection of the cervix: Relative risk associations of 15 common anogenital types. Obstet Gynecol 1992; 79:328-337.
8. Munoz N, Bosch FX, DeSanjose S et al. The causal link between human papillomavirus and invasive cervical cancer: A population-based case-control study in Colombia and Spain. Int J Cancer 1992; 52:743-749.
9. Stoler MH, Rhodes CR, Whitbeck A, Wolinsky SM, Chow LT, Broker TR. Human papillomavirus type 16 and 18 gene expression in cervical neoplasias. Human Pathol 1992; 23:117-128.
10. Miller CS, White DK. Human papillomavirus expression in oral mucosa, premalignant conditions, and squamous cell carcinoma: A retrospective review of the literature. Oral Surg Oral Med Oral Pathol Oral Radiol and Endo 1996; 82:57-68.
11. Yeudall WA, Campo MS. Human papillomavirus DNA in biopsies of oral tissues. J Gen Virol 1991; 72:173-176.
12. Brandsma JL, Abramson AL. Association of papillomavirus with cancers of the head and neck. Arch Otolaryngol- Head Neck Surg 1989; 115:621-625.
13. Maden C, Beckmann AM, Thomas DB et al. Human papillomaviruses, herpes simplex viruses, and the risk of oral cancer in men. Am J Epidemiol 1992; 135:1093-1102.
14. Park NH, Min BS, Li SL, Huang MZ, Cherick HM, Doniger J. Immortalization of normal human oral keratinocytes with type 16 human papillomavirus. Carcinogenesis 1991; 12:1627-1631.
15. Shin KH, Tannyhill RJ, Liu X, Park NH. Oncogenic transformation of HPV-immortalized human oral keratinocytes is associated with the genetic instability of cells. Oncogene 1996; 12:1089-1096.
16. Park NH, Gujuluva CN, Baek JH, Shin KH. Combined oral carcinogenicity of HPV-16 and benzo(a) pyrene: An in vitro multistep carcinogenesis model. Oncogene 1995; 10:1061-1067.
17. Inoue H, Kondoch G, Kamakura CR, Yutsudo M, Hakura A. Progression of rat embryo fibroblast cells immortalized with transforming genes of human papillomavirus type 16. Virology 1991; 180:191-198.
18. Hurlin PJ, Kaur P, Smith PP, Perez-Reyes N, Blanton RA, Mc Dougall JK. Progression of human papillomavirus type 18-immortalized human keratinocytes to a malignant phenotype. Proc Natl Acad Sci USA 1991; 88:570-574.
19. Munger K, Phelps WC, Bubb V, Howley PM, Schlegel R. The E6 and E7 genes of the human papillomavirus type 16 together are necessary and sufficient for transformation of primary human keratinocytes. J Virol 1989; 63:4417-4421.
20. Crook T, Storey A, Almond N, Osborn K, Crawford L. Human papillomavirus type 16 cooperates with activated *ras* and *fos* oncogenes in the hormonally dependent transformation of primary mouse cells. PNAS 1988; 85:8820-8824.

21. Sedman SA, Barbosa MS, Vass WC et al. The full-length E6 protein of human papillomavirus type 16 has transforming and trans-activating activities and cooperates with E7 to immortalize keratinocytes in culture. J Virol 1991; 65:4860-4866.
22. Myers F, Androphy E. The E6 protein. In: Myers G, Bernard HU, Delius H, Baker C, Icenogel J, Halpern A, eds. Human Papillomaviruses. Los Alamos NM:Los Alamos National Laboratories, 1995:III-47—III-57.
23. Scheffner M, Werness BA, Huibregtse JM, Levine AJ, Howley PM. The E6 oncoprotein encoded by human papillomavirus types 16 and 18 promotes the degradation of p53. Cell 1990; 63:1129-1136.
24. Dyson N, Howley PM, Munger K, Harlow E. Human papillomavirus-16 E7 oncoprotein is able to bind to the retinoblastoma gene product. Science 1989; 243:934-936.
25. Hubbert NL, Sedman SA, Shiller JT. Human papillomavirus type 16 E6 increases the degradation rate of p53 in human keratinocytes. J Virol 1992; 66:6237-6241.
26. Band V, Dalal S, Delmolino L, Androphy EJ. Enhanced degredation of p53 protein in HPV-6 and BPV-1 E6-immortalized human mammary epithelial cells. EMBO J 1993; 12:1847-1852.
27. Nevins JR, Vogt PK. Cell transformation by viruses. In: Fields BN, Knipe DM, Howley PM, eds. Fundamental Virology. Philadelphia PA: Lippincott-Raven, 1996:267-310.
28. Liu TJ, El-Naggar AK, McDonnell TJ et al. Apoptosis induction mediated by wild-type p53 adenoviral gene transfer in squamous cell carcinoma of the head and neck. Cancer Res 1995; 55:3117-3122.
29. Johnson MA, Blomfield PI, Bevan IS, Woodman CBJ, Young LS. Analysis of human papillomavirus type 16 E6-E7 transcription in cervical carcinomas and normal cervical epithelium using the polymerase chain reaction. J Gen Virol 1990; 71:1473-1479.
30. Bernard BA, Bailly C, Lenoir MC, Darmon M, Thierry F, Yaniv M. The human papillomavirus type 18 (HPV18) E2 gene product is a repressor of the HPV18 regulatory region in human keratinocytes. J Virol 1989; 63:4217-4324.
31. Bouvard V, Storey A, Pim D, Banks L. Characterization of the human papillomavirus E2 protein: evidence of trans-activation and trans-repression in cervical keratinocytes. EMBO J 1995; 13:5451-5459.
32. Schneider-Maunoury S, Croissant O, Orth G. Integration of human papillomavirus type 16 DNA sequences: A possible early event in the progression of genital tumors. J Virol 1987; 61:3295-3298.
33. DiLorenzo TP, Tamsen A, Abramson AL, Steinberg BM. Human papillomavirus type 6a DNA in the lung carcinoma of a patient with recurrent laryngeal papillomatosis is characterized by a partial duplication. J Gen Virol 1992; 73:423-428.
34. May M, Dong X, Beyer-Finkler E, Stubenrauch F, Fuchs PG, Pfister H. The E6/E7 promoter of extrachromosomal HPV16 DNA in cervical cancers escapes from cellular repression by mutation of target sequences for YY1. EMBO J 1994; 13:1460-1466.
35. Chen Z, Storthz KA, Shillitoe EJ. Mutations in the long control region of human papillomavirus DNA in oral cancer cells, and their functional consequences. Cancer Res 1997; 57:1614-1619.
36. Shillitoe EJ, Lapeyre JN, Adler-Storthz K. Gene therapy—its potential in the management of oral cancer. Oral Oncol-Eur J Cancer B 1994; 30B:143-154.
37. Von Knebel Doeberitz M, Oltersdorf T, Schwarz E, Gissman L. Correlation of modified human papilloma virus early gene expression with altered growth properties in C4-1 cervical carcinoma cells. Cancer Res 1988; 48:3780-3786.
38. Von Knebel Doeberitz M, Rittmuller C, zur Hausen H, Durst M. Inhibition of tumorigenicity of cervical cancer cells in nude mice by HPV E6-E7 anti-sense RNA. Int J Cancer 1992; 51:831-834.
39. Steele C, Cowsert LM, Shillitoe EJ. The effects of human papillomavirus type-18-specific antisense oligonucleotides on the transformed phenotype of human carcinoma cell lines. Cancer Res 1993; 53:2330-2337.
40. Steele C, Sacks PG, Adler-Storthz K, Shillitoe EJ. Effect on cancer cells of plasmids that express antisense RNA of human papillomavirus type 18. Cancer Res 1992; 52:4706-4711.

41. Tan TMC, Ting RCY. In vitro and in vivo inhibition of human papillomavirus type 16 E6 and E7 genes. Cancer Res 1995; 55:4599-4605.
42. Lappalainen K, Pirila L, Jaaskelainen I, Syrjanen K, Syrjanen S. Effects of liposomal antisense oligonucleotides on mRNA and protein levels of the HPV 16 E7 oncogene. Anticancer Res 1996; 16:2485-2492.
43. Hu G, Liu W, Mendelsohn J et al. Expression of epidermal growth factor receptor and human papillomavirus E6/E7 proteins in cervical carcinoma cells. J Natl Cancer Inst 1997; 89:1271-1276.
44. Hu G, Liu W, Hanania EG, Fu S, Wang T, Deisseroth AB. Suppression of tumorigenesis by transcription units expressing the antisense E6 and E7 messenger RNA (mRNA) for the transforming proteins of the human papillomavirus and the sense mRNA for the retinoblastoma gene in cervical carcinoma cells. Cancer Gene Ther 1995; 2:19-32.
45. Madrigal M, Janicek MF, Sevin BU et al. In vitro antigene therapy targeting HPV-16 E6 and E7 in cervical carcinoma. Gynecol Oncol 1997; 64:18-25.
46. Storey A, Oates D, Banks L, Crawford L, Crook T. Anti-sense phosphorothioate oligonucleotides have both specific and non-specific effects on cells containing human papillomavirus type 16. Nucl Acids Res 1991; 19:4109-4114.
47. Stein CA. Phosphorothioate antisense oligodeoxynucleotides: questions of specificity. Trends Biotechnol 1996; 14:147-149.
48. Wisotzkey JD, Krizenoskas A, DiAngelo S, Kreider JW. Cleavage of cottontail rabbit papillomavirus E7 RNA with an anti-E7 ribozyme. Biochem Biophys Res Commun 1993; 192:833-839.
49. He YK, Lu CD, Qi GR. In vitro cleavage of HPV16 E6 and E7 RNA fragments by synthetic ribozymes and transcribed ribozymes from RNA-trimming plasmids. Fed Eur Biochem Soc 1993; 322:21-24.
50. Lu D, Chatterjee S, Brar D, Wong KK. Ribozyme-mediated in vitro cleavage of transcripts arising from the major transforming genes of human papillomavirus type 16. Cancer Gen Ther 1994; 1:267-277.
51. Chen Z, Kamath P, Zhang S, Weil MM, Shillitoe EJ. Effectiveness of three ribozymes for cleavage of an RNA transcript from human papillomavirus type-18. Cancer Gen Ther 1995; 2:263-271.
52. Chen Z, Kamath P, Zhang S, St John L, Adler Storthz K, Shillitoe EJ. Effects on tumor cells of ribozymes that cleave the RNA transcripts of human papillomavirus type 18. Cancer Gene Ther 1996; 3:18-23.
53. Huang Y, Kong Y, Wang Y, Qi G, Lu C. Stable expression of anti-HPV 16 E7-ribozyme in CV-1 cell lines. Chinese J Biotechnol 1996; 12:215-220.
54. Shillitoe EJ, Hinckle CC, Noonan S, Marini F, Kellman R. Use of particle bombardment for transduction of normal and malignant oral epithelium. Cance Gene Ther 1997; 5:176-182.
55. Zhou SZ, Li Q, Stamatoyannopoulos G, Srivastava A. Adeno-associated virus 2-mediated transduction and erythroid cell-specific expression of a human beta-globin gene. Gene Ther 1996; 3:223-229.
56. Thompson JD, Ayers DF, Malmstrom TA et al. Improved accumulation and activity of ribozymes expressed from a tRNA-based RNA polymerase III promoter. Nucl Acids Res 1995; 23:2259-2268.
57. Yu M, Leavitt MC, Maruyama M et al. Intracellular immunization of human fetal cord blood stem/progenitor cells with a ribozyme against human immunodeficiency virus type 1. Proc Natl Acad Sci USA 1995; 92:699-703.
58. Dropulic B, Lin NH, Martin MA, Jeang KT. Functional characterization of a U5 ribozyme: Intracellular suppression of human immunodeficiency virus type 1 expression. J Virol 1992; 66:1432-1441.
59. Heusch M, Kraus G, Johnson P, Wong-Staal F. Intracellular immunization against SIV_{mac} utilizing a hairpin ribozyme. Virology 1996; 216:241-244.
60. Li M, Lonial H, Citarella R, Lindh D, Colina L, Kramer R. Tumor inhibitory activity of anti-*ras* ribozymes delivered by retroviral gene transfer. Cancer Gene Ther 1996; 3:221-229.

61. Shore SK, Nabissa PM, Reddy EP. Ribozyme-mediated cleavage of the BCRABL oncogene transcript: In vitro cleavage of RNA and in vivo loss of P210 protein-kinase activity. Oncogene 1993; 8:3183-3188.
62. Lieber A, Kay MA. Adenovirus-mediated expression of ribozymes in mice. J Virol 1996; 70:3153-3158.
63. Hayashi S, Nagasaka T, Katayama A et al. Adenovirus-mediated gene transfer of antisense ribozyme for alpha (1,3)galactosyltransferase gene and alpha (1,2)fucosyltransferase gene in xenotransplantation. Transplant Proc 1997; 29:2213-.
64. Lieber A, He CY, Polyak SJ, Gretch DR, Barr D, Kay MA. Elimination of hepatitis C virus RNA in infected human hepatocytes by adenovirus-mediated expression of ribozymes. J Virol 1996; 70:8782-8791.
65. Feng M, Cabrera G, Deshane J, Scanlon KJ, Curiel DT. Neoplastic reversion accomplished by high efficiency adenoviral-mediated delivery of an anti-*ras* ribozyme. Cancer Res. 1995; 55:2024-2028.
66. Clayman GL, Trapnell BC, Mittereder N et al. Transduction of normal and malignant oral epithelium by an adenovirus vector: The effect of dose and treatment time on transduction efficiency and tissue penetration. Cancer Gen Ther 1995; 2:105-111.
67. Mitchell MF, Hamada K, Sastry KJ et al. Transgene expression in the rhesus cervix mediated by an adenovirus expressing beta-galactosidase. Am J Obstet Gynecol 1996; 174:1094-1101.
68. Ohta Y, Kijima H, Ohkawa T, Kashani-Sabet M, Scanlon KJ. Tissue-specific expression of an anti-*ras* ribozyme inhibits proliferation of human malignant melanoma cells. Nucl Acids Res 1996; 24:938-942.
69. Garver RJ, Goldsmith KT, Rodu B, Hu PC, Sorscher EJ, Curiel DT. Strategy for achieving selective killing of carcinomas. Gene Ther 1994; 1:46-50.
70. Schneider-Gadicke A, Schwarz E. Different human cervical carcinoma cell lines show similar transcription patterns of human papillomavirus type 18 early genes. EMBO J 1986; 5:2285-2292.

Index

A

Adeno-associated virus (AAV) 95, 101-118, 156, 162, 193, 212, 231
Adenoviral vector 101, 102, 129-131, 137, 144, 148, 151, 155, 158-160, 191
Adenovirus 43, 95, 101-114, 129-131, 137, 138, 143-147, 156-158, 160, 178, 199-201, 208, 215, 225
Antisense 4, 10, 24, 27, 34, 41, 42, 44, 45, 47, 51, 52, 62, 67, 69, 70, 81, 83, 85-87, 91, 92, 98, 99, 107, 129, 140, 141, 143, 145, 148, 149, 156, 158, 159, 160, 162, 169, 172, 173, 177, 179, 180, 183, 192, 193, 200, 201, 203, 206, 208, 209-211, 215, 216, 220, 221, 223, 227, 229, 230, 232
Apoptosis 126, 138, 155, 160, 166, 168, 177, 195, 218, 219, 220
Asymmetric hammerhead ribozyme 8-10

B

β-actin promoter 129, 137, 179, 180
BCR-ABL 61, 62, 65-71, 73, 74, 177, 195, 199
Bioconjugates 51
Bioerodible polymer 54
Bladder cancer 125-131, 135, 178
Breast cancer 55, 135-139
BT-474 cell 137, 138

C

C-erbB-2 135-139, 151, 152, 153
Catalytic activity 4, 8, 9, 17, 24, 26-28, 30, 32, 34, 62, 144, 146, 153, 158, 159, 179, 180, 184, 203
Catalytic RNA 3, 11, 15, 30, 32, 34, 79, 101, 135, 144, 152, 153, 165, 175, 176, 178, 179, 186
Cationic lipid 41-45, 52, 54, 156, 188, 190, 208, 220
CD34 97, 102, 113, 116
Cell culture 30, 34, 41, 43, 44, 47, 94, 97, 157, 161, 184, 199
Cervical cancer 223, 225-229
Chronic myelogenous leukemia (CML) 61, 62, 69, 74, 195, 196, 199, 200, 205, 208, 209
Cis-acting ribozyme 166
Clinical trial 95-98, 113, 129, 130, 136, 144, 165, 166, 191

D

Dimeric minizyme 62-74

E

Electroporation 45, 136, 156, 157, 206
Endonuclease 8, 9, 176, 218
Exonucleases 214

F

Folate-polylysine 43, 205
Folding 3, 5, 17, 19, 25, 26, 203, 208

G

G418 90, 105, 156, 157
Glioma 9, 114, 116, 218
Glyceraldehyde-3-phosphate dehydrogenase (GAPDH) 9, 215-218

H

Hairpin ribozyme 3, 15-21, 93, 135, 206
Helper virus 23, 90, 102, 103, 109
HIV 88, 91-97, 105, 108, 110, 116, 165, 214, 223, 228
Host range 95, 102, 112

I

Interleukin-2 (IL-2) 96, 97, 165, 166, 214-216, 218
Intraarticular 45-48, 50
Intraocular 47
Intravenous 9, 49-52, 55, 112
Iontophoresis 49

K

Kinetic analysis 74

L

L6 61, 62, 65-67, 69, 74, 87, 90, 94, 114
Liposome 8, 44, 52-55, 74, 156, 158, 170, 198, 200, 201, 203, 205, 206, 208, 209
Lung cancer 151-153, 155-158, 179

M

Metal ion requirement 5
Minizyme 8, 62-74, 159, 160
Multidrug resistance (MDR) 177, 183, 184, 187, 188, 190, 191

N

Nanoparticle 42, 47, 49

O

Oncogene. *See* BCR-ABL; C-erbB-2; Ras
Oral cancer 223, 224, 226, 228, 229

P

P-glycoprotein 184-189
p53 89, 126, 127, 138, 151-153, 155, 160, 166, 179, 180, 184, 224, 228
Packaging 87-92, 94, 95, 104, 105, 107-109, 116, 144, 158, 159, 201, 208
Papillomavirus 180, 223-227, 229
PHb Apr-1-neo 129, 151, 156
Polycations 42, 43
Probasin 169, 170
Promoter 69, 71, 73, 74, 80, 84, 87-91, 93, 101-112, 114, 116, 129, 137, 145, 147, 157, 158, 160, 168, 169, 178-180, 188, 206, 208, 224, 228, 229
Prostate cancer 165, 166, 168-170
Protein kinase C (PKC) 218, 219

R

Ras (ras) 126-131, 135, 136, 143-147, 151-153, 155-160, 175-178, 180, 184, 195, 228, 229
  H-Ras 151
  K-Ras 151, 152
Required bases 15
Retroviral vector 87, 89-93, 95-97, 101, 116, 155, 178-180, 199, 206, 208, 209
Ribozyme transfection 200
RNA polymerase I 87, 166-170
RNA polymerase II 23, 24, 104, 105, 188, 208
RNA polymerase III 69, 71, 74, 87, 104, 105, 166, 188
RT-PCR 81, 82, 156, 199, 205-207

S

Southern blot 205, 207

Structure 5, 6, 10, 11, 15-21, 23-32, 46, 62-65, 67, 72-74, 91, 92, 94, 105, 116, 153, 158, 159, 167, 175-177, 183-186, 201, 203, 206, 214, 216, 217, 220, 225, 227-229
Sustained release 47, 55

T

Tat 91, 93-95, 116
Tissue-specific expression 178
Titer 87, 90, 92, 104, 107-111, 114, 137, 156, 159, 188
TNF-α 215, 216, 220
Transduction 90, 95-97, 102, 104, 109, 112-114, 116, 126, 129, 131, 137, 138, 144, 155, 165, 177, 178, 188, 195, 208, 209, 228
Transitional cell carcinoma 125
Triple ribozyme 166, 168-170
tRNA 3, 69, 71-74, 92, 105, 108, 110-112, 116, 166, 199, 200, 206, 207
tRNAVal promoter 71-74, 93
Tumor suppressor gene 89, 126, 128, 131, 138, 151-153, 160, 166, 176, 179, 180

V

Vascular endothelial growth factor (VEGF) 41, 45-47, 126, 128, 220